PRESCRIBING HIV PREVENTION

T0173091

Critical Cultural Studies in Global Health Communication

Global changes in migratory patterns, the increasing health inequalities faced by the poor, the health risks faced by communities at the margins of global societies, and the communicative nature of health problems have drawn additional attention to the relevance of studying health communication processes across global cultures. This series will challenge West-centric ideals of health and human behavior by publishing theoretically provocative, pedagogically critical volumes addressing the intersection of communication principles and practices with health concepts and structures. The intent of the series is foregrounding knowledge that creates openings for transforming structures of injustice and exploitation underlying global health inequalities. Manuscript proposals should be addressed to Series Co-editor Mohan J. Dutta at cnmhead@nus.edu.sg

General Editors

Mohan J. Dutta, *National University of Singapore*
Ambar Basu, *University of South Florida*

Series Titles

Volume 1 *Prescribing HIV Prevention: Bringing Culture into Global Health Communication*, Nicola Bulled

Volume 2 *Neoliberal Health Organizing: Communication, Meaning, and Politics*, Mohan J. Dutta

Information on these titles and other volumes in the Critical Cultural Studies in Global Health Communication Series can be obtained from the Left Coast Press, Inc. (www.LCoastPress.com).

Prescribing HIV Prevention

Bringing Culture into Global Health Communication

Nicola Bulled

Left Coast
Press Inc.

Walnut Creek, California

LEFT COAST PRESS, INC.
1630 North Main Street, #400
Walnut Creek, CA 94596
www.LCoastPress.com

Left Coast
Press Inc.

Copyright © 2015 by Left Coast Press, Inc.
All rights reserved. No part of this publication may be reproduced,
stored in a retrieval system, or transmitted in any form or by any
means, electronic, mechanical, photocopying, recording, or otherwise,
without the prior permission of the publisher.

ISBN 978-1-61132-362-7 hardback
ISBN 978-1-61132-363-4 paperback
ISBN 978-1-61132-364-1 institutional eBook
ISBN 978-1-61132-732-8 consumer eBook

Library of Congress Cataloging-in-Publication Data:
Bulled, Nicola, 1981- author.
   Prescribing HIV prevention : bringing culture into global health communication /
Nicola Bulled.
       pages cm. -- (Critical cultural studies in global health communication ; vol. 1)
   ISBN 978-1-61132-362-7 (hardback : alk. paper) -- ISBN 978-1-61132-363-4 (pbk.
: alk. paper) -- ISBN 978-1-61132-364-1 (institutional ebook) -- ISBN 978-1-61132-
732-8 (consumer ebook)
   1. HIV infections--Lesotho--Prevention. 2. HIV infections--Social aspects--Lesotho.
3. AIDS (Disease)--Lesotho--Prevention. 4. AIDS (Disease)--Social aspects--Lesotho.
5. Communication in medicine--Lesotho. I. Title. II. Series: Critical cultural studies in
global health communication ; vol. 1.
   RA643.86.L5B85 2014
   362.19697'920096885--dc23
                          2014024213

Printed in the United States of America

⊖™ The paper used in this publication meets the minimum requirements of American
National Standard for Information Sciences—Permanence of Paper for Printed Library
Materials, ANSI/NISO Z39.48–1992.

CONTENTS

FIGURES

TABLES

The gate lock clicked and the car drove away. They were gone. This was the first time our parents had left us alone for an evening—no baby sitters, no staying at a friend's house—just three girls, alone. The moment signified our maturation into responsible teenagers, except I was twelve, and my sister and her friend were just turning fourteen. We had been planning the events of this Saturday night all week. We made pizza and rented a movie—*Sarafina!* We understood that *Sarafina!* was the story of youth in Soweto, the mega-township on the other side of Johannesburg from where we lived in Benoni. We had picked *Sarafina!* mostly because of Whoopi Goldberg, the American comedian/singer. We loved Whoopi as Dolores Van Cartier, a showgirl turned nun in the film *Sister Act*. *Sarafina!* promised to be a similarly uplifting Hollywood-style musical, just with a more local and recognizable feel.

We were horribly mistaken.

The 1992 film *Sarafina!*, based on the original Broadway production, centers around the riots in Soweto in the late 1970s. Inspired by their teacher, Mary Masombuka (the role played by Whoopi Goldberg[1]), the youth of Soweto rise up in opposition to the implementation of Afrikaans as the language of instruction in public schools.[2] On June 16, 1976, an estimated 20,000 students took part in the demonstrations. The event is most well recognized by the iconic image of 12-year-old Hector Pieterson being carried by Mbuyisa Makhubo after he was shot by South African police.

Sarafina! was filmed on location in Soweto and Johannesburg, revealing that not far beyond the bolted doors, barred windows, seven-foot high walls, and electric fence of my modest Benoni home, a war was raging. Soweto was not so much a place to us, more an idea. We had never been there, but knew it to be a place where we should not go. It featured prominently on the nightly news. When the violence was really out of control, the giant, yellow, military-style 'hippo' police vehicles slowly made their way into the danger zones of the townships, tear gas canisters dispersed toyi-toyi-ing crowds, and police (both black and white) brutally beat people with their rubber batons.[3]

The story of *Sarafina!* offered justification for the uprisings and ongoing violence occurring on a daily basis throughout South Africa during my childhood. The images and the story provided a different lens through which

I could see my own world. I grew up in middle class neighborhoods, insulated from apartheid realities. Like many of my childhood friends, I knew nothing about the pass system, did not know who Steve Biko was, thought Nelson Mandela was a terrorist who failed to blow up the Koeberg nuclear power station, and could not identify with the iconic image of him burning his pass in protest against apartheid policies restricting the movements of non-whites. I had come to believe that the systems in place in South Africa were appropriate and necessary. The protests and violence of black youth, as portrayed in *Sarafina!*, threatened to destabilize the system. I had come to believe that the black youth were the perpetrators of violence and I was the victim. The *Sarafina!* narrative suggested otherwise. It was not until this moment, watching a collection of singing youth on the screen inspired by their teacher, someone I too admired, that I began to realize that the situation in South Africa was not 'normal.'

This childhood experience reflects the complexity of 'communication' that I attempt to unravel, or at least pull at the strings of, in this book. The structural realities that are present in our everyday—the apartheid-state, poverty, joblessness, the position of women, the threat of HIV infection—influence our individual awareness, understandings, and behaviors. Communication is not just about the message or the individual receiver, but rather a far more complex interaction involving the construct of the message and the situational context of the receiver. The ability of *Sarafina!* to communicate to me the realities of the apartheid state was likely related to a combination of my age at the time; the lack of parental presence; the medium of film; a U.S. film star providing an 'outsider' commentary on my local world; the recognizable locations, geography, and languages; and the defied expectations for an uplifting musical.

This book offers an ethnographic examination of communication related to the most pressing threat in southern Africa from the last four decades— HIV/AIDS. Here I focus on the small southern African Kingdom of Lesotho, which is situated within the borders of South Africa. In this work, I explore how the knowledge of HIV prevention is transmitted from global health institutions (where much knowledge is coalesced) to local youth. I offer a perspective on the power dynamics generated by varied access to health knowledge and the distinct roles participating in health communication. The research is largely the product of a personal journey. During my initial engagement in Lesotho, as a novice public health practitioner, I assumed a position of authority over HIV prevention knowledge given my science-based Western education. However, in working closely with individuals locally, I came to realize the limitations of current message-based health education strategies. One of these limitations is the static construction of expertise as exclusively in the hands of the message producers and disseminators. I argue that social, political, economic, educational and even current communication structures have defined for us our roles in knowledge circulation including what 'expert' knowledge is and who can hold claim to 'expertise.' Given the unequal access to health knowledge, including avenues to be producers and disseminators of knowledge, health education messages can themselves establish and perpetuate the social stratifications that contribute to disease.

HIV serves as my focus as, being born the same year that AIDS was first discovered in 1981, I have not known of a time when HIV was not part of the world's health landscape. I spent my early childhood years in South Africa, the country with largest number of people living with HIV and AIDS, at 5.6 million (UNAIDS 2012). South Africa's legacy of apartheid (economic, political, gender, and racial/ethnic inequality, migratory labor practices, and high rates of sexual violence) has significantly contributed to the country's current disease burden (Poku and Whiteside 2004). Chris Hani, a prominent anti-apartheid activist, recognized as early as 1990 that, following the demise of white supremacy, HIV would be South Africa's new peril and the limiting factor in South Africa's successful transition to democracy. Indeed, HIV is perhaps the most apparent indictor of the dramatic and enduring effect that apartheid policies had on the South African society. It is a personal identification with South Africa, an intellectual curiosity about the social dynamics of disease, and a professional frustration with the continued failures of HIV containment efforts that inspire my eagerness to understand the limitations of current approaches in an effort to inform future strategies.

Lesotho, and not South Africa, is the geographic setting of this exploration for a number of reasons. Practicalities brought me to Lesotho. I left South Africa with my family in 1994, just a few months after the first democratic elections. I returned for the first time in 2004, joining a group of faculty and students from Boston University's School of Public Health to work on HIV prevention initiatives in Lesotho. Returning to the same location in 2010, to conduct an ethnographic study of HIV prevention initiatives, allowed me to reflect on the presumptions I had made in my role as a health educator and the limitations of current models of health communication. Politics kept me out of South Africa. To have left South Africa during the tenuous transitional phase to democracy and then to return with a Western education is perceived by some as a further expression of the unfair advantage of my race.[4] The people of Lesotho experienced the oppression of the apartheid state, being reliant on South Africa for migratory labor and the import and export of goods. However, they endured less of the everyday violence. Consequently, with my American accent, I could operate in the Lesotho context less burdened by historical racial prejudices.

In my role as a global public health practitioner in Lesotho, I believed that by transferring knowledge about HIV to local youth I could contribute to curbing the local epidemic. I was certain that if people understood the risks related to HIV infection they could make rational choices—the classic 'hypodermic model' (Patton 1996) and 'empty vessel' fallacy (Paul 1955, Polgar 1963). My enthusiasm was well received, but it was clear that I could offer little to address effectively the issues that contribute to sustaining the local HIV epidemic—unemployment, poverty, and economic and gender inequality. In addition, while my students lacked a full comprehension of the biology of the virus, they were exposed on a daily basis to the effect of the virus on individual and social bodies that I could not fully comprehend.

In returning to Lesotho six years later to conduct the ethnographic research that forms the foundation of this book, I became increasingly aware of how I functioned as an actor in the process of health communication. My personal subjectivities—my upbringing, education, ethnicity, and gender— affected my relationships and even transformed my research (Delamont 1992). Linda Tuhiwai Smith (1999, 176), author of *Decolonizing Methodologies: Research and Indigenous Peoples*, noted that in cross-cultural context power differentials between researcher and the researched are inherent and special care should be taken to ameliorate their effects, stating:

> Researchers are in receipt of privileged information…they have the power to distort, to make invisible, to overlook, to exaggerate and to draw conclusion based not on factual data, but on assumptions, hidden value judgments, and often downright misunderstandings. They have the potential to extend knowledge or to perpetuate ignorance.

She described features that ought to characterize a researcher working in a cross-cultural context including respecting people, being present among people, being slow to speak and eager to learn, not flaunting knowledge, being cautious, not trampling on people's dignity, and being generous.

Colonial legacies from a British protectorate, and more recent histories as a safe haven for South African anti-apartheid activists, have formed the foundations of racial power divides in the country. Ninety-nine point nine-nine percent of Basotho are black. Europeans and Americans comprise a large proportion of development workers, and Asian immigrants own a large portion of Lesotho's textile industry. Both of these groups are highly visible given their phenotypes and ethnicity, their white four-wheel drive vehicles (in the case of development workers), and their propensity to congregate in certain coffee shops and restaurants in Maseru, the country's capital city. Their status as business owners or managers and their generous international salaries offer the perception that all non-black people are wealthy. This is further confirmed by the situation in South Africa where Basotho have historically found employment as mine workers with white managers or domestic laborers in white homes. In South Africa, whites hold the majority of the country's wealth. In 2008, per capita personal income for a white South African averaged 75,300 South African Rand (ZAR), as compared to 9,800 ZAR for a black South African (Holborn 2010).

In rural areas of Lesotho, returning migrant laborers provide accounts of these economic divisions and their corresponding social divisions along racial lines. Similar racial distinctions in rural areas are seen in the form of tourists or Peace Corp volunteers. Predominantly white South African tourists, or European and American development workers looking for some adventure on the weekends, venture into Lesotho's mountainous terrain to hit the ski slopes, trek on ponies, or ride dirt bikes, all-terrain vehicles, and motorbikes. Since 1967, 2,000 Peace Corps volunteers, certainly not all white, have been scattered throughout Lesotho's ten districts. Peace Corps volunteers live in modest accommodations; however, they still possess items such as radios, iPods, laptops, and sleeping bags that display their material status.

Differences in skin color similarly define researcher/participant positioning in Lesotho. My white skin, English parents, and South African upbringing connected me with multiple former oppressors. My American education and citizenship added yet another association with a present-day global power. For many students I engaged with for this research, I was the first white person with whom they had ever directly interacted. The youth felt that, as an American, I was connected to what is locally considered the epicenter of modernity, the home of many music, film, and television celebrities. I always disappointed people with my lack of US popular culture knowledge. I was also perceived as someone who had money, or items of value, which I could withhold or dispense to whomever I chose. Thus, careful considerations of power differentials resulting from my skin color, extensive Western education, relative economic status, and current country of origin, projected into my daily interactions. The Lesotho Ministry of Health Ethics Board does not allow researchers to pay participants, so this eased the conversations regarding economic inequities between myself and my informants. However, I was careful to ensure that youth were clear on what I was allowed to give them for their participation so they would not have expectations regarding activities or rewards.

The majority of the conversations that inform the research for this book took place in English. Using English as the language of communication may have generated or further perpetuated the divisions between myself and my informants. However, I purposefully selected a study population—students at the Lesotho College of Education (LCE)[5]—proficient in English. English is the primary language of education in Lesotho. As a result, all LCE students are required to achieve a certain standard in their qualifying high school English examinations prior to entrance into the teaching college. My informants were randomly selected, thus students were not selected or self-selecting based on their abilities to communicate in English. I preferred not to use a translator, despite the difficulty of some conversations resulting from the range of abilities to communicate in English as well as exposure to a different English accent. It was more important for me to interact directly with my student informants rather than use an intermediary, as this contact allowed me to acknowledge openly my inadequacies with respect to language (many of the students were proficient in English and Sesotho, and could also communicate in isiZulu and isiXhosa), and ultimately provided a means of equalizing power.

By revisiting the population of youth in Lesotho as an anthropologist conducting research, rather than as a public health practitioner with an agenda to improve health conditions using specific indicators of success, I could take more time to be cautious and devote greater effort to listening and learning. Spending a significant time in the geographic region (as a child, a public health practitioner, and anthropological researcher) means that I have a greater appreciation for the multiple complex facets of the local context and can reflect upon the dynamics central to the impact of health education. As an anthropologist, my training and perspectives uniquely position me to uncover the nuances involved in studying the social, economic, and political aspects of HIV. The discipline examines the historical frame, larger social contexts, and how these multiple dimensions interact in the creation of meanings, logics, and behavioral norms within communities.

In my research, I adopt a mixed-method approach to data collection, combining qualitative ethnographic techniques (i.e., interviews, self-generated questions, and pile sorts) and quantitative techniques (survey). Collecting data in different ways serves multiple purposes (see Bryman 2006; Greene, Caracelli, and Graham 1989; Mertens 2005; Pearce 2002; Tashakkori and Teddlie 2003). Ethnography brings to light the features of the culture, telling us what parameters merit investigation. Systematic collection of data, for example through surveys, is necessary to test hypotheses about how those features work. In combination, ethnography tells us what parameters to study, surveys quantify those parameters, and ethnography helps to interpret and flesh out the survey results.

Data gathered between 2010 and 2012, which are cited periodically in this book, take advantage of a unique, 'natural' experimental situation in which LCE students were arbitrarily assigned to the rural (Thaba-Tseka) or urban (Maseru) campuses for three years, irrespective of whether they are from rural or urban environments. The assignment process generated four distinct groups of youth: students from either urban or rural backgrounds who either remained in or left the environment in which they were socialized as children. Only students between the ages of 18 and 26 years were included in any component of the study. The random assignment process allowed me to assess how varying access to disparate spheres of communication, as well as distinct social and material capital, impacts disease risk. By comparing groups I could assess the effects of HIV knowledge on disease risk, while considering confounding factors associated with distinct social environments that have been shown to impact HIV risk, including elements of social control such as curfews, privacy, and access to sexual partners (Amuyunzu-Nyamongo and Magadi 2006; Browning 2005; Burgard and Lee-Rife 2009; Modo 2001; Upchurch et al. 1999).

In keeping with the traditions and conventions of anthropology, I have masked the identity of some of my sources both for their protection and to emphasize the human collective. I name only those individuals who have already entered the public record, identifying others using pseudonyms or their social roles. My deepest gratitude goes out to all those who agreed to talk with me, and were so generous with their time as well as tolerant and patient with my tedious questioning of their realities. Though I do not claim to speak *for* the youth in Lesotho, and they may not agree with everything I write, I present their words and situations as I perceive them with the intent to present their voice and thereby "give life to frozen words" (Das 2007, 8-9). This book, with its faults and omissions, aims to shine a much-needed spotlight on the plight of youth in Lesotho and those in similar communities and situations throughout the world and to challenge global public health practitioners to reconsider the assumptions inherent in our approaches.

Acknowledgments

None of what lies in the subsequent pages of this book would have been possible without the generosity of those who agreed to give me their time, supplied me with documents, communicated their knowledge, and responded to the hypotheses I submitted to them, although sometimes with the discouraging statement—"Go back and do more research." I thank not only government workers and college officials with overburdened schedules, but also the administrative staff who thoughtfully offered me a seat, a place to have tea, and a moment in time to recognize that humanity and life exist much the same everywhere. To all the students that were brave enough to trust a stranger to guard their secrets, fears, and future dreams, I hope I have proved a worthy confidante.

I am indebted to my mentor, Merrill Singer. His thoughtful comments, careful guidance, and constant support have challenged me and moved my work in fruitful directions. His dedication to my development has proven time and again that nothing is gained by not trying. This book certainly would not have been possible without his encouragement and his often repeated phrase— "What do you have to lose?" I am grateful as well for the efforts of my advisors,

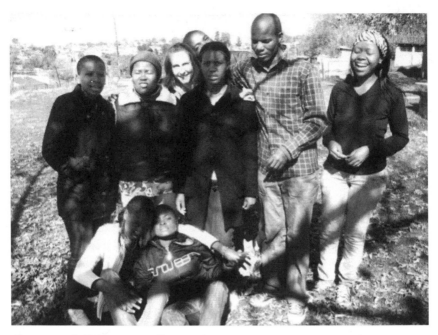

Figure 0.1. LCE-Maseru students and me.

Pamela Erickson and Stephen Schensul, whose perceptive observations in prior versions of this manuscript forced me to reconsider my assumptions.

A special thanks to Fiona Vernal, who tenderly brought me to a deeper understanding of southern African history and politics. Her care in showing me the perspective of the 'other' during a painful time in my own country's history, without judgment or prejudice for my ignorance of, part in, or benefit from the persecution of others, allowed for a conscious self-reflection on my own subjectivities and their impact on my relationships with people in Lesotho. With her guidance I have been able to consider how my own history influences my perceptions of the people whose stories I retell in this text. She has also shown me that I should never get too lost in academia, being cautious not to forget that life continues regardless of how much we deconstruct and analyze it from a distance.

I have also benefited from the insights of many friends, colleagues and students with whom I have either discussed this work or shared portions of it along the way, including Jill Chidley, Nora Kenworthy, Alexandra Collins, Leah Krohn, Antonie Du Toit, Philreen Du Toit, Marie Brault, Ann Cheney, Ruthanne Marcus, Cindy Frank, Pascalina Mabitle, Mamathe Jobo, Keneoe 'Mota, Motena Putsoa, 'Mme Hlalefang, Toni Mokhele, Peter Böxkes, the members of my Medical Anthropology Writing Group, the audiences at many conferences and talks where I have presented my work, and the anonymous reviewers of the works (including this one) that I have submitted for publication.

I am grateful to the faculty, staff, and students in the Anthropology Department at the University of Connecticut (UCONN), especially Francoise Dussart, Rich Sosis, W. Penn Handwerker, Richard Wilson, and Sarah Willen, who have been instrumental in furthering my education and challenging my insights. Special thanks to Sally McBrearty, the UCONN department chair, for being willing to take a chance by admitting to her program a doctoral student with limited prior experience in the discipline; to the faculty at Boston University School of Public Health who first entrusted me to serve as one of the founding students of their now well establish Lesotho-Boston-Health-Alliance; and to my editors Mohan Dutta and Ambar Basu who have encouraged me to look beyond my own discipline to see overlapping theoretical perspectives and principles in others.

Some of the chapters that make up this book are revised and rewritten versions of previously published articles. In revising these texts and contextualizing them within a larger argument and somewhat different frame, that of health education, I have sought to offer more depth and bring forth different perspectives and analyses. In particular, this text draws on the following published pieces:

Bulled, Nicola. (2013) (Re)distribution of blame: Examining the politics of biomedical HIV knowledge in Lesotho. *Critical Arts* 27(3): 267-287.

Bulled, Nicola. (2013) New lives for old: Modernity, biomedicine, traditional culture and HIV prevention in Lesotho. *Global Discourse* 1-16.

This research was made possible by the Fulbright Institute for International Education, the Dean Ross McKinnon Endowment from the College of Liberal Arts and Sciences at UCONN, and additional departmental and school funding from the UCONN. My capacity to bring this project to closure was greatly enhanced by a D43 TW009359 NIH/Fogarty International Center Fellowship with the University of Virginia's Center for Global Health.

The Prescription for HIV Prevention

While biomedicine and epidemiology have made possible an understanding of HIV pathology, these specialized fields of knowledge have been unable to prevent the persistent spread of HIV throughout the world.[1] Since it was recognized over 40 years ago, 75 million people have become infected with HIV, more than 36 million people have died of AIDS, and 16 million children are considered AIDS orphans. At the end of 2012, 35.3 million people were estimated to be living with HIV/AIDS, and approximately 2.3 million new infections had occurred (UNAIDS 2012). It is by far the most dramatic epidemic since the Black Plague devastated Europe 500 years ago. Author and journalist Adam Hochschild describes the epidemic by saying, "If a war had killed 20 million soldiers, and left 28 million more dying of wounds, we'd call it the worst such tragedy since World War II. This is the scale of AIDS...the greatest health crisis of our time" (comment on Stephanie Nolen's *28: Stories of AIDS in Africa*, 2008).

Genetic tracing and social history place the beginnings of the human form of the immunodeficiency virus—HIV—in Central Africa in the 1920s (Pepin 2011). However, June 5, 1981 is generally referred to as the beginning of the HIV/AIDS pandemic. On this date, the U.S. Centers for Disease Control and Prevention (CDC) reported the first cases of rare pneumonia among a small group of young men in Los Angeles (Gottlieb et al. 1981). Since that moment, the extensive dedication devoted to understanding HIV has resulted in the building of knowledge and global awareness of the disease at a pace never before experienced.

Just one month after the *Morbidity and Mortality Weekly Report* (Gottlieb et al. 1981) publication of the observed disease cluster, the CDC reported a highly unusual occurrence of rare skin cancer, Kaposi's sarcoma (CDC 1981). Both conditions were later determined to be AIDS-related. By 1982, the CDC formally established the term Acquired Immune Deficiency Syndrome (AIDS) and identified four primary disease 'risk factors': anal sex among

Nicola Bulled, "The Prescription for HIV Prevention" in *Prescribing HIV Prevention: Bringing Culture into Global Health Communication*, pp. 19-41. © 2015 Left Coast Press, Inc. All rights reserved.

men, intravenous drug abuse, Haitian origin, and hemophilia (Curran and Jaffe 2011). These risk categories were also crudely referred to as the "4H's"— homosexuals, heroine users, Haitians and hemophiliacs—linking identity or disease condition to risk behaviors.

According to the timeline of AIDS put together by AIDS.gov (2012), an information collective managed by the U.S. Department of Health and Human Services, by 1986, the first cases of HIV had been reported in most African countries, China, Russia, and India. By 1988, UNAIDS reported that in sub-Saharan Africa the number of women living with HIV/AIDS outnumbered men. By 1992, AIDS had become the number one cause of death for U.S. men ages 25-44 years. In 1994 and 1995, AIDS became the leading cause of death for all Americans ages 25-44 years. AIDS remained the leading cause of death among African Americans within this age group in 1996. In 2002, AIDS was the leading cause of death worldwide among people aged 15-59 years. AIDS is currently the leading cause of death among women of reproductive age and remains the leading cause of death in Africa (UNAIDS 2012).

Since the 1980s, the global effort to stem the tide of HIV has moved through various phases of multilateral, bilateral, nongovernmental, voluntary, and private programs and initiatives. The World Health Organization (WHO) started the Global Programme on AIDS in 1987, the first global institutionalized effort to contain HIV. Realizing the complex nature of the pandemic, in 1994, UNAIDS, a joint body of six UN organizations, was formed to provide a more comprehensive, complete, and coordinated global response. Even so, for much of the first two decades of HIV, there was a general lack of cohesiveness and clarity in the direction of global planning. This failing has been attributed to difficulties in worldwide data collection, diverse cultural interpretations of HIV, complacency and lack of effective leadership in many countries, scarcity of funds for sustaining long-term programs, inordinate allocation of available funding to expensive drug treatment research, inter-organizational confusion about the scope of each unit's work, an overall fuzzy picture of worldwide AIDS, and an inability or unwillingness to accept the sheer magnitude and spread of the disease (Christakis 1989; Mann, Tarantola, and Netter 1992; Mann, Tarantola, and Global AIDS Policy Coalition 1996).

Global and national policies reflect the disjointed responses to the epidemic. For example, in the US, the media and health professionals increasingly came to use the term GRID, or gay-related immune deficiency, relating sexuality to disease risk, as opposed to the specific risk behavior (male-anal sex), as initial fear and panic led to the identification of 'risk groups' rather than risk behaviors. Some countries implemented repressive policies to prevent the spread of disease such as Cuba's segregating *sidatorios* (O'Connor 1991) and Russia's and the US' tight immigration controls

(Kraft 1994). Resistance to the idea that HIV posed a significant global threat to human health took the form of governmental denial and lack of commitment towards policy development (Bonacci 1992).

In June 2001, the General Assembly of the United Nations held its first ever gathering aimed at discussing the future of the disease. Issues of fund allocation for treatment and prevention efforts, as well as issues of 'culture,' were the focus of attention. The meeting concluded on the note that any future global action needed to be respectful of the different cultural traditions in many parts of the world, which included the use of culturally appropriate language and culturally sensitive management of issues such as homosexuality, commercial sex work, intravenous drug use, and condom use. These directives did not suggest a need to engage with local cultural groups to define or develop effective interventions relative to the social, political, and economic context. Instead, the revised agenda continued to regard the established global interventions as generally applicable across the world, in a cohesive and universal structure to correct the fragmented approaches of the past. Slight modifications were expected at the community and country level to respond to the nuanced values and beliefs of particular social situations. Then Secretary General Kofi Annan endorsed a grassroots, culture-specific approach by emphasizing that women and nongovernmental organizations needed to be at the helm of the global preventive initiative (Harris 2001). In spite of this desire, the meeting solidified commitments from national governments to work with a *global* blueprint that set specific overarching policy and preventive action goals for the years 2003 and 2005, as opposed to unique plans generated by communities to take account of their distinct contexts.

Kofi Annan's desires to develop a new approach to addressing the HIV pandemic led to the creation of the Global Fund to Fight AIDS, Tuberculosis, and Malaria. The Geneva-based multi-billion-dollar health agency was launched in 2002, shortly after the first UN General Assembly Special Session on AIDS. The Global Fund has been hailed as a transparent, efficient aid machine delivering the elements of the AIDS prevention and treatment package prescribed by the UN General Assembly, including HIV testing services, condoms, and antiretroviral drugs for AIDS treatment. It receives only voluntary contributions from governments and private philanthropists, billing itself as an "innovative approach to international health funding." Funding is controlled by local actors, including officials from government and nongovernmental organizations. Countries implement their own programs based on their priorities, and the Global Fund provides financing on the condition that verifiable results are achieved. Despite this unique model of country ownership coupled with performance-based funding, which aims to avoid the inevitable politicization of bilateral programs like USAID and the bureaucracy of UN agencies, the Global Fund has been investigating allegations of corruption in many countries. This situation has resulted in the temporary suspension of payments to the fund from major government contributors (The Global Fund 2010, 2011).

In 2003, U.S. President G. W. Bush announced PEPFAR, the President's Emergency Plan for AIDS Relief. PEPFAR was initially a five-year, 15 billion USD initiative to address HIV/AIDS, tuberculosis, and malaria primarily in the worst affected countries. Despite contributing funds to UNAIDS and the Global Fund, U.S. government administration officials in the early 2000s did not care for the focus of these organizations. They pressed the UN to spend most of the United States' funding contributions on disease prevention rather than treatment. In an extreme attempt to justify this stance, the United States Agency for International Development (USAID) administrator, Andrew Natsios, argued that sending antiretroviral drugs to African countries would be ineffective due to the lack of trained doctors, limited infrastructure, and the inability of Africans to follow a complicated treatment regimen because of their insufficient knowledge of clocks and Western notions of time.[2] The authorizing U.S. legislation stipulated that at least a third of all prevention funds of PEPFAR be spent to promote sexual abstinence and faithfulness, and that faith-based organizations should be allowed to reject strategies they considered objectionable, such as condom distribution. In spite of Natsios' comments, treatment ultimately came to constitute roughly half of the PEPFAR budget.

In recent years there have been some promising movements in global HIV statistics as a direct result of the extensive government and private responses, and rapid advancements in HIV-related knowledge, biomedical technologies, and pharmacology. New infections have decreased by 33 percent since 2001, the number of children with new HIV infections has declined by 52 percent, and AIDS-related deaths have dropped by 30 percent since 2005. Even so, the fourth decade of HIV is faced with many challenges. Though oral antiretroviral drug therapy is considered "one of the most remarkable achievements in recent public health history" (UNAIDS 2012, 50),[3] expensive antiretroviral drugs remain a distant dream for many infected with HIV. Under the 2013 WHO treatment guidelines, HIV treatment coverage in low- and middle-income countries represented only 34 percent of the 28.6 million people eligible (UNAIDS 2013). Furthermore, treatments are not cures, but rather ways of prolonging life. Recently there has been much enthusiasm regarding antiretroviral oral pharmaceuticals as a prevention strategy for people not infected, pre-exposure prophylactic (PrEP). However, structural limitations, acceptance, and ethical considerations pose significant barriers to the full implementation of such an approach in both high- and low-income countries

(Kenworthy and Bulled 2013)[4]. Topical microbicide vaginal gels have so far proven to have mixed results in preventing HIV infection in women (Abdool Karim et al. 2010; Van Damme and Szpir 2012; VOICE [MTN-003] 2011; Ramjee et al. 2007). Similarly, voluntary medical male circumcision, though effective in randomized control trials in preventing HIV infection among men (Auvert et al. 2005; Bailey et al. 2007; Gray, Kigozi, et al. 2007), has not received the desired level of in-country scale-up (to 80 percent of male population) determined necessary for reductions in HIV prevalence (Gray, Li, et al. 2007; Kahn, Marseille, and Auvert 2006; Nagelkerke et al. 2007; Njeuhmeli et al. 2011). Last, countless complexities surround vaccine development as a biomedical prevention strategy (Nabel 2001, Stephenson 2001). Consequently, preventive behaviors remain the only known method for checking the spread of HIV.

HIV Communication

> The goalposts have shifted. It is time for us to regroup and re-strategize. Our redirection must focus on two goals. First, leveraging the AIDS movement as a force for transformation in global health, development and environmental sustainability. Second…mobilizing a prevention revolution.
>
> *Michel Sidibé, Executive Director, UNAIDS (2009)*

In December of 2009, Michel Sidibé called for the mobilization of a prevention revolution. He stressed that with adequate monetary investments today for educational and treatment-based prevention initiatives, the number of new infections could be halved by 2015, claiming "2.3 million new infections can be averted and 12.5 billion USD in treatment costs saved" (UNAIDS 2009a). The 2012 World AIDS Day events embraced Sidibé's calls to action under the theme "Getting to Zero"—Zero new HIV infections. Zero discrimination. Zero AIDS-related deaths. The UNAIDS strategy for 2011–2015, adopted by the Programme Coordinating Board in December 2010 aims to advance global progress in achieving *universal* access to HIV prevention, treatment, care, and support (UNAIDS 2010a).

Global health programs have focused HIV prevention efforts on decreasing an individual's risk for disease through surveillance, personal behavioral changes, and clinically driven care and treatment. This approach has developed out of a long history of knowledge-based health communication campaigns. In the 1960s and 1970s, health-promotion campaigns in developing countries emphasized the transmission of information on healthy lifestyles for the prevention of non-communicable diseases. In the 1970s, public health initiatives started to use the notion of empowerment and self-help to link unhealthy lifestyles to the development of preventable disease (WHO 1986). In the 1980s and 1990s, social marketing emerged as a new approach to health information dissemination, influencing social norms and behaviors (Andreasen 1995). Social marketing encourages creative marketing approaches to the analysis of issues and the development of programs to communicate information. However, some view these creative strategies as attempts by private firms, including U.S.-based foundations, government agencies, and international organizations, to adapt commercial marketing methods to promote neoliberal economic schemes of privatization and individual agency (Manoff 1985; Reid 2004).

By the 1990s, the term 'health literacy' emerged in the health scholarship, describing a patient's ability to understand health care providers and the terminology of health care so as to be able to comply with prescribed therapeutic regimens (American Medical Association 1999; Kalichman and Rompa 2000; Kalichman et al. 2000). Functional health literacy is the ability to read, understand and act on health information, including comprehending prescription labels, interpreting appointment slips, completing health insurance forms, following instructions for diagnostic tests, and understanding other essential health-related materials required to adequately function as a patient of biomedicine (American Medical Association 1999; Baker 1995; Giorgianni 1998; Parker et al. 1995). Under the principle of health literacy, the focus of health care shifted from providing for the patient to one requiring patients to be able to advocate for their own health and independently navigate the health care system. The idea of individual agency in health care has been integrated into the WHO's broader definition of health literacy as, "the cognitive and social skills which determine the motivation and ability of individuals to gain access to, understand and use health information in ways which promote and maintain good health" (WHO definition as cited in Nutbeam 2000). Under this definition, health literacy empowers people to effectively maintain and manage health and health care through improved access to health information and advancement of cognitive and social skills to utilize that information.

In studies conducted with HIV patients, psychologist Seth Kalichman and colleagues (2000, 2000) determined that poor health literacy not only creates barriers to fully understanding one's health, illness, and treatments, but also has the potential to endanger others (i.e., through the generation of treatment-resistant strains of HIV due to improper treatment adherence). The studies found that patients with lower health literacy are significantly more likely to visit their doctors, thus overburdening the system, and less likely to view health providers as involving them in the treatment process.

These findings suggest that persons with lower health literacy place a greater demand on the health care system and their health care providers, and do not feel like agents of their own wellbeing, independently making and imposing health-enhancing choices. Consequently, health literacy is a relatively economical strategy, particularly amid growing demands to lower the costs of health care delivery. This perception has a global reach today, often with unexpected and not necessarily healthy consequences.

Given the costs of treatment based HIV prevention initiatives, rational behavior change through knowledge transfer has remained (until quite recently) the central focus, as suggested in the UNAIDS policy document *Intensifying HIV Prevention* (2005a, 23), "(p)romot[ing] widespread knowledge and awareness of how HIV is transmitted and how infection can be averted." The education for prevention strategy aims to elucidate the problem (what constitutes the virus and how it is transmitted) and then explain the solution (how transmission is avoided, including sex education) (Pigg 2001, 483). The message is very simple—a risk exists and here is the prescription for dealing with it.

The United Nations Children's Fund (UNICEF) outlines its components of HIV prevention education as integrated within a larger Life Skills curriculum for youth (see unicef.org/programme/lifeskills). The UNICEF model stresses three components: knowledge, attitudes, and skills. Knowledge regarding transmission routes, means of prevention, personal risk, and prevalence of HIV form the foundations. Attitudes about social rights, gender, cultural norms, and discrimination are subsequently addressed. Skills relating to communication, value analysis, decision-making, and stress management are then developed. The effectiveness of such knowledge-based models is measured in terms of the acquisition of 'sufficient knowledge' (UNICEF 2002). Sufficient knowledge to protect one's self from HIV is defined as knowing three major ways to help prevent transmission (abstain from sex, have one faithful uninfected sexual partner, and use a condom every time sexual intercourse takes place). It also entails correct identification of three major misconceptions about HIV transmission (AIDS is not transmitted by supernatural means, AIDS is not transmitted by mosquito bites, and a healthy looking person can be infected). In this regard, the 'education for prevention' model appears comprehensive, supplying factual biomedical information, addressing attitudes, and developing risk reduction skills. But has this model been effective in reducing engagement in risk behaviors?

The knowledge-based, rational-actor approach addresses risk behaviors as a secondary measure, assuming that rational action naturally follows from knowledge acquisition in line with many behavior change models that focus on the individual. Such a strategy also conforms to neoliberal concepts of good citizenship, whereby knowledgeable subjects are committed to the truth and value of being informed (Barry 2001) and acting on this knowledge in a rational way to reduce individual disease risk. In this light, HIV prevention is premised on having individuals transform what they know (condoms protect you) into disease prevention behaviors or acknowledge the difficult work they must do in order to know (recognizing risk, personalizing it, and understanding it as controllable) (Foucault 1991). This framing presupposes a relationship between the knower and known and assumes the transparency of self-knowledge—the idea that individuals can discover knowledge of personal risk merely through self-reflection and self-recognition because this knowledge is true, real, and waiting to be realized.

A multitude of factors at the levels of the interpersonal network, community, health system, and larger social structure influence individual behaviors, yet many behavior change models, including the UNAIDS model, target the individual as the element of change with explanations for differentials in HIV rates sought at the level of individual variation (Parker 2001). As shown in Figure 1.1, prominent behavior change models, including the Social Cognitive (improving individual self-efficacy), Theories of Reasoned Action and Planned Behavior (altering individual intentions and perceived self-control), Transtheoretical (moving individuals from stages of identifying the need, seeing the benefits, and having the confidence to change behaviors), and Information-Motivation-Behavioral Skills (correct information, combined with sufficient motivation and skills, results in altered behaviors), focus on the individual. These models only occasionally address, sometimes just as a way for the individual to acknowledge, the influence of external factors as barriers (or promoters) to engagement in safer behaviors.

The focus on individual agency and responsibility disguises the social and political origins of illness[5] and disease.[6] It assumes that individuals can freely choose their actions and make rational calculations on how best to behave to maintain their health (Rhodes 1997; Thomas 2008). It also reduces the responsibilities of the state for promoting and maintaining wellbeing. For example, states can promote personal behavior change as an HIV prevention strategy rather than altering structural conditions that perpetuate engagement in risk behaviors, including high unemployment, gender inequalities, and limited access to health care services. Instead of empowering marginalized sectors, this approach requiring rational action of educated individuals is dis-empowering, as individuals can be held responsible for their bodily condition (i.e., HIV infection), which is perceived to be the result of inappropriate lifestyles or 'pathological habits' (Passmore 1972). Biomedicine has historically categorized patients unwilling to 'follow doctors' orders' as 'ignorant,' 'vicious,' 'recalcitrant,' 'non-compliant,' and what is most recently referred to as 'non-adherent' (Lerner 1997).

Factors impacting risk engagement	Current strategies to change risk behaviors
Structural	**Critical Health Communication**
Poverty • Access to services • Political context • Funding • Education curriculum • Public policy/law • Law enforcement	Shifts the focus from the individual to the collective and the structures that drive risk behaviors
Institutional/Health system	**Dynamic Social Systems Model**
Provision of services • Character-istics of providers • Peer advisors • Accessibility of services • Confidentiality/privacy	Positioned to address the interac-tions between individuals and structures at macro, meso, and micro levels (Latkin et al. 2010)
Community	**Network-Individual Resources Model**
Stigma • Social norms • Commu-nity mobilization • Social leaders (religious, cultural, academic, popular) • -isms (racism, sexism, heterosexism) • Gender equity • Cultural norms	Focused at the intersection of individuals and their social net-works, yet recognizing the impact of access to resources (Johnson et al. 2010)
Interpersonal/Network	**Multiple Domain Model**
Relationship dynamics • Social support • Social capital	Recognizing that the behaviors of individuals are influenced by both individual and larger social factors (Zimmerman et al. 2007)
Individual	**Individual-Level Behavior Change Models**
Knowledge • Risk perception • Skills • Self-sufficiency • Moti-vations • Emotions • Intentions • Attitudes • Beliefs • Perceived social norms • Perceived control • Outcome expectations • SES	*Social Cognitive:* improve self-sufficiency • *Theories of Reasoned Action and Planned Behavior:* alter intentions, perceived control and facilitate action • *Transtheoretical:* rational action • *Information-Motivation-Behavioral Skills:* provide correct information, motivation, and develop skills

HIV Risk Behaviors

Figure 1.1. Factors influencing individual engagement in risk behaviors and corresponding behavior change models.

International, nongovernmental, private, and religious organizations continue to inject ideas about personal responsibility for individual health and expectations of rational behaviors, with little consideration for the complexity of the relationship among knowledge, morality, and health. The *education vaccine*, involving either basic education and/or specific HIV information, remains for some intervention strategists the best and only viable means of prevention available against HIV in the foreseeable future (Vandemoortele and Delamonica 2002). Editors of the collection *AIDS Prevention Through Education: A World View* noted "the often repeated dictum that education is the most effective weapon to prevent infection remains valid... [the simple premise remains that] AIDS is completely preventable with adequate information and the adoption of appropriate measures" (Sepulveda, Fineberg, and Mann 1992, 17-18).

Nevertheless, in Africa in particular, policy makers, public health workers, and social scientists are troubled by the lack of connection between peoples' apparent high levels of knowledge of HIV prevention and their continued failure to engage in protective behaviors (Airhihenbuwa, Makinwa, and Obregon 2000; Airhihenbuwa and Obregon 2000; Smith 2003). Studies conducted in several African societies have documented high levels of awareness of HIV, including recognition of sexual intercourse as the primary route of transmission and acknowledgment of the use of condoms as an effective option for infection prevention (Arowujolu et al. 2002; Maharaj 2001; Meekers and Klein 2001). However, studies have also shown frequent engagement in unprotected sex (Amazigo et al. 1997; Kapiga and Lugalla 2002; MacPhail and Campbell 2001) and continuing increases in the incidence of sexually transmitted HIV infection across most southern African countries (UNAIDS 2010b). A meta-analysis of meta-analyses examining programs for health behavior change conducted by Johnson, Scott-Sheldon, and Carey (2010) revealed significant variation in intervention effects. Similarly, Noar's (2008) review of HIV-related meta-analyses suggested significant heterogeneity in efficacy from intervention to intervention or study to study. These analyses suggest that some interventions are highly effective; however, others fail to have any positive effect. A meta-analysis of behavioral interventions to increase condom use and reduce the incidence of sexually transmitted infections by Scott-Sheldon and colleagues (2011) and a comprehensive review of HIV-prevention interventions by Albarracin and colleagues (2005) revealed that developing skills and motivational training prove more effective than focusing on knowledge alone. Additional studies suggest that addressing community factors (i.e., racism and stigma) that influence individual engagement in risk behaviors results in more positive and sustained outcomes (Reid et al. 2014). Though these complex analyses offer important insights, we only need to look at global disease statistics to realize that the currently employed individual-rational-actor message-based model of much HIV prevention education is not an effective one-size-fits-all strategy for reducing risk engagement.

The Health and Social Welfare Minister, Dr. Mphu Ramatlapeng, brought the issue to national attention in Lesotho. She was quoted in a local paper as saying, "Despite relatively high levels of HIV-awareness, the infection rate [in Lesotho] continues unabated" (Matope 2011a, 12). Just prior to the HIV epidemic taking firm hold in Lesotho, anthropologist Nancy Romero-Daza (1994a, b) explored HIV knowledge and risk behavior among women in the rural district of Mokhotlong. She determined that the majority of respondents were aware of HIV and 85.6 percent knew of the sexual transmission route of the virus. Despite seemingly high levels of HIV knowledge and awareness in even the most remote region of the kingdom, HIV prevalence peaked in Lesotho at 26 percent among pregnant women age 20-24 between 2000 and 2003. At the time of Romero-Daza's study, in 1991/92, over a third of women identified the sharing of toilet seats and clothes as HIV transmission routes. Combined with the rise in numbers of infected individuals over the years, Romero-Daza's findings suggest that both the assessment and the perceived power of knowledge to result in rational behavior change can be misleading.

More recent data from the Lesotho Demographic and Health Surveys (DHS) in 2004 and 2009 indicate an increase in general awareness of HIV of about 3 percent in the adult population, from 93 to approximately 96 percent (MoHSW 2005b, 2009). Similarly, knowledge of HIV prevention methods, specifically the use of condoms during sex and the reduction in number of sexual partners,[7] increased during the two time periods by about 10 percent, from high 70 to high 80 percent in women and from high 60 to high 70 percent in men. Finally, comprehensive knowledge of HIV also increased in all individuals, from 24 to 38 percent in women and 19 to 29 percent in men. Nevertheless, HIV prevalence in Lesotho remained at 23 percent during the six-year period.

A general increase in knowledge of HIV, partnered with unabated risk behaviors, calls into question the premise of the education vaccine and behavior change strategies that rely on information motivating risk calculations and safer practices. Certainly, access to knowledge is important for individuals to be able to identify appropriate HIV prevention behaviors and to take advantage of new technologies for risk reduction. People also need to be able to access prevention resources such as condoms and safe male circumcision services. However, in considering HIV-related knowledge, we must ask: Does knowledge have any effect on risk behavior beyond a low threshold of behavior change? Is it possible that emotional, social, economic, and political factors have greater effect on risk reduction behaviors, outweighing any positive impact knowledge may have? Do prevention skills such as how to negotiate condom use, or how to put on a condom have a greater impact on risk reduction than theoretical biomedical knowledge of the virus alone? Do specific types of knowledge or different ways of considering risk have greater impact than general knowledge and awareness of HIV? Are current tools to measure knowledge able to identify which aspects of knowledge are most important? Does one's position relative to knowledge impact one's ability to translate knowledge into action?

Individual focused approaches for behavior change inappropriately assume the neutrality and universality of the information conveyed and consequent reasoned risk behaviors of individuals receiving the knowledge, and fail to consider non-informational barriers to behavioral change. These assumptions became clear to me when, after returning from Lesotho in 2004, I began working with a needle exchange program in the northeastern US. Needle exchange programs are founded on the philosophy of harm reduction. Program consumers are taught the skills necessary to reduce their exposure to blood-borne diseases including HIV and Hepatitis C in a non-judgmental environment. Their engagements in risk behavior (injection drug use) are not the focus of the program's efforts. Utilizing this approach, I could empathize, provide information, develop skills, and distribute supplies. However, my efforts to convey knowledge, to educate for rational action, offered little to address the day-to-day realities of the needle exchange program's participants. Our program had no link to limited and highly sought after drug rehabilitation programs, should a consumer desire help to manage the addiction that drove her risk behaviors. The program also never considered how to address the cultural drivers of injection-related risk behaviors, including the dynamics of trust that are established in sharing injection equipment between single or multiple partners. These drivers were simply accepted as standard aspects of the behaviors of injection drug users. These relationships become even more important with individuals on the fringes of society, risking disease to prove loyalty. Finally, there were the conflicts in political agendas. Program consumers were seen as engaged in criminal activities by the law, with our mobile service becoming one way for law enforcement to identify delinquents. Our agenda of reducing disease prevalence and transmission through education for rational action (and the provision of clean needles and supplies) was frequently overshadowed by political and legal agendas of restraining drug related criminal activity.

In Lesotho, failure of knowledge-based HIV prevention programs to consider non-informational barriers to risk reduction was most evident in youth condom use behaviors. Since my initial engagements in Lesotho in 2004, I have seen considerable changes in both the awareness and acceptance of condoms as a practical HIV prevention device among youth. Nevertheless, between 2010 and 2012 many young adults within my study sample admitted to using condoms inconsistently, yet offering many logical reasons for this risky behavior. For example, the supplies in the college bathrooms were not restocked, the health center was not always open and never at the moment when a condom was needed, the 'corner store' guy charged 50 Lesotho Loti (LSL) for a triple pack and all he had were banana flavored condoms that were sticky to the touch, bright yellow, and smelled funny. They are, of course, designed for purposes other than vaginal sexual intercourse. By focusing on the individual action, with little regard to the contexts that may compel or even rationalize continued involvement in behaviors that increase risk for disease, the message-based approach heightens awareness, but does little to aid rational action.

Individualized approaches also generate distinctions based on knowledge and risk/disease status. If risk is linked to knowledge, then those who engage in risk, or are infected, either do not have the knowledge or choose not to enact what they know in a rational manner that reduces their disease exposure. Throughout Africa, HIV positive individuals have been stigmatized. In Lesotho, judgments regarding HIV status are primarily linked to recalcitrance— knowing the risks but not trying to reduce risk—or to ignorance—not knowing the risks because the information was never presented. Given the lack of information sources in rural areas of Lesotho, rural dwelling individuals are perceived as ignorant of their risks. By contrast, the constant HIV prevention messaging available in the urban areas suggests that urban individuals who are infected with HIV are obstinate in their refusal to behave rationally. I explore these geographical distinctions in greater depth throughout this book.

The message-based, rational-actor approach is also cognitively biased (Dutta-Bergman 2004c, 2005). Cognitive approaches account for individual behavioral choices that result from an active process of information evaluation, attitude formation, and then 'rational' choice. Many individual health-based behaviors such as habits and spur-of-the-moment decisions cannot be understood with such an approach. The hierarchical prioritization of 'at-risk behavior' essentially fragments communities into categories that treat 'risk' behavior as if it were distinct and separate from relationships, and even draws distinctions between different aspects of one's self (i.e., spiritual wellness, physical health, and psychological wellbeing). HIV prevention education strategies should pay more attention to relationships of risk (i.e., marriage partners, mothers and infants), and how in this era of AIDS those relationships might need to be reconceptualized. Does an HIV positive mother put her newborn at risk by breastfeeding, or is the act nurturing and life-saving? Do marriage partners insist on condom use and routine testing, or does this challenge the intimate bond of trust?

Finally, the one-way transfer of information inherent in the individual focused rational-actor approach privileges 'expert' over 'lay' perspectives (Lee and Garvin 2003). For example, the increasing factionalization and specialization of HIV knowledge, along with the use of surveillance practices and specialized biomedical terminology in health education messages, creates distance between the public health professional and the general public (Lupton 1995, Margolis 1996). While developing biomedical understanding, or health literacy, is effective in promoting safer behaviors (Kalichman et al. 2000; Kalichman and Rompa 2000), the approach should not silence alternative perspectives; communication is, and should be, a two-way process.

Prominent social science HIV researchers John Richens and colleagues (2000) and Edward C. Green (2003b; Green and Ruark 2011) have noted the distinction between interventions that focus on the individual and those that target the collective. Though problematic, Richens and Green use the terms 'Western' versus 'traditional' paradigms. The Western model, they argue, treats HIV as a biomedical problem and individuals are expected to rationally utilize medical solutions for prevention, including biomedical education, condoms, clean needles, and treatment. These strategies are, however, not always accessible irrespective of whether individuals know to use them, are motivated to use them, have the skills to use them, and intend to use them. Traditional models, by contrast, view HIV as an indicator of a collective behavioral problem. Traditional strategies for HIV prevention therefore involve altering sexual behavior norms including partner reduction and delaying initial sexual activity through social action. This strategy is more available and less costly (Green 2003a), but as noted above, only works if there is significant motivation by the collective rather than just individuals. For example, Uganda's successful approach to HIV prevention, involving a vocal government movement to reduce stigma and promote behavior change through the 'zero-grazing' initiative to reduce multiple concurrent sexual partnerships "focus[ed] on what individuals themselves can do to change (or maintain) behavior, and thereby avoid or reduce risk of infection…[*and*] tackled the difficult social and institutional problems" (Green 2003a, 6).

Newer behavior change models have been developed and tested that recognize and directly address factors external to the individual as part of the intervention (see Figure 1.1). The Multiple Domain Model (Zimmerman et al. 2007) recognizes that safer sex behaviors are influenced by individual level factors (attitudes, self-efficacy, intentions, skills), as well as contextual or situational factors, social environments influencing perceived behavioral norms, and larger social structures. The Network-Individual-Resource Model (Johnson et al. 2010) recognizes that the exchange of resources between individuals and their networks underlies and sustains HIV-risk behaviors. As a result, interventions must meet the individual and their network's needs and prompt behavior changes that can be sustained by the resources present within the social system. Finally, the Dynamic Social Systems Model (Latkin et al. 2010) lays out a framework of six dynamic and interrelated structural dimensions on macro, meso, and micro levels for HIV prevention interventions to address. The Critical Health Communication approach, discussed in more detail in the subsequent section, suggests altering the focus of interventions altogether. This approach argues that interventions aim to alter the disease constructs and risk behaviors of the collective and address directly the capacities and structures that drive individual risk behaviors.

Critical Health Communication as an Approach to HIV Prevention

In light of these growing quandaries in disease prevention, this book offers an exploration of HIV prevention communication among young adults. Youth are heavily impacted by the HIV epidemic. In 2010, young people age 15-24 years accounted for 42 percent of HIV infections in people of age 15 and older. Among young people living with HIV, nearly 80 percent (4 million) live in sub-Saharan Africa (UNAIDS 2012). I specifically examined in the prevention strategies aimed at youth in Lesotho, a country with one of the highest rates of HIV infection in the world. My study population included students of a teachers training college, the Lesotho College of Education (LCE), situated in both rural and urban settings. As teachers-in-training, these youth are uniquely positioned as both the receivers and the future disseminators of HIV prevention messages.

In this book I view access, assessment, and comprehension of health knowledge, specifically related to HIV, through the framework of critical health communication. Critical health communication emerged as a field of inquiry in recent years in response to the growing social inequities and health disparities of contemporary society (Airhihenbuwa 1995; Airhihenbuwa and Ludwig 1997; Ford and Yep 2003; Lupton 1994b; Morokos and Deetz 1996; Ray 1996).

Critical health communication scholarship pays particular attention to how dominant *ideology* and *hegemony* influence engagement of voices in spaces of discourse. Drawing on the work of Michel Foucault, critical health communication scholars recognize that power is ever present, circulating through all social relationships and at all levels of society. Power is not considered to be simply constraining and limiting but it is also viewed as productive and enabling. For example, the provider-patient relationship occurs in spaces of inequality (i.e., the clinic, the testing facility, the hospital); yet knowledgeable patient-consumers can regain some control over their own bodies. *Ideology* refers to a body of ideas representing a distinct social group. In the context of critical health communication, ideology represents attempts of powerful establishments to fix meanings that maintain and support their worldviews. For example, the biomedical establishment provides meanings associated with health and illness that are presented as universal truths grounded in the objectivity of science. At the same time, such meanings are used to maintain the power profit margins of the biomedical industry while obscuring the social and economic positions of international development and public health workers. Much of current health promotion work, emphasizing individualism, personal choice, cost effectiveness, and the evaluation of measurable effects, adheres to the dominant neoliberal ideology that promotes privatization, structural adjustment programs, and the reduction of state involvement. In the critical health communication framework, "hegemony" refers to the preponderant social influence or authority of historically powerful groups (i.e., health policy makers, ministries of health, global health agencies [WHO/UNAIDS]) over the general population. Critical health communication scholarship challenges local health communicators to refrain from becoming representatives of such hegemony and to intervene in multiple ways to resist oppressive discourses that are linked with biomedical imperatives, in order to improve the quality of life and health environments for everyone.

In this, the critical health communication approach calls for the expansion of the locus of change from the behaviors of individuals to those of the collective and requires attentiveness to capacities, structures, and community (see Figure 1.1). For example, we cannot expect a sex worker to demand that a client use condoms and risk losing business when she is worried about feeding herself or her family (Basu 2010). Critical health communication scholars work to engage the agency of community members in indentifying the structural impediments to health and act as a team to create conditions that support (and sustain) healthy living by addressing social inequities that contribute to health inequality (Camacho et al. 2008).

Within the discipline of critical health communication, scholars who focus on *culture* recognize that health, disease, and illness are products of a range of cultural practices and norms. Culture is conceptualized broadly in the discipline of health communication to include both (a) values, beliefs, attitudes, language, institutions, and structures of power; and (b) a variety of cultural practices such as daily activities, medical products, mass-produced commodities, and consumption patterns (Lupton 1994b). The work of Collins Airhihenbuwa (1990-1991, 1993, 1995; Airhihenbuwa et al. 1992) argued for the centrality of the cultural realities and experiences of the individuals and community members that receive health promotion messages and programs. In addition, Deborah Lupton (1994b), in her seminal piece examining the dominant paradigm of health communication, noted the importance of critically questioning the broader issues of power, ideology, and hegemony when considering cultural constructions of health.

In considering the universalizing or scaling-up of health communication strategies in different cultural contexts, arguably a top-down approach, communication scholars Mohan Dutta and Ambar Basu take the critical health communication perspective one step further. They recognize two approaches to addressing cultural diversity in communication strategies that focus on the collective and in altering the structures perpetuating individual risk behaviors, namely the *culture-centered approach* and the *culturally sensitive approach* (Dutta 2007; Dutta and Basu 2001).

The *culturally sensitive* approach aims to produce health interventions that incorporate the cultural characteristics, values, beliefs, experiences, and norms of the target population (Resnicow et al. 2002). This approach conceptualizes culture as a collection of shared values, beliefs, and practices that are contained within a clearly defined community (Ulrey and Amason 2001; Brislin and Yoshida 1994). Culture is considered to be static, measured as a conglomerate of traits identified by the expert. The goal of the health communicator is to identify the underlying cultural dimensions that require incorporation into the delivery of the health message, such as individualism-collectivism, masculinity-femininity, uncertainty-avoidance, and power-distance (Dutta 2007). The focus is on developing health messages that adapt to the characteristics of a specific culture for the greatest effect (Dennis and Giangreco 1996; Resnicow et al. 2002; Sue and Sue 1999; Ulrey and Amason 2001). Success of culturally sensitive health interventions is based both on the adequate response to cultural variables relevant to the effective delivery of the message and on the fostering of appropriate behavioral change in the target population.

Consequently, being culturally sensitive means offering communication solutions that fit the cultural characteristics considered relevant by the health communicator (Dutta 2007). This approach to health communication aims to ensure that external social and cultural standards resulting in the erasure, devaluation, and annihilation of the culture of less privileged communities are not imposed on target populations (Airhihenbuwa and Obregon 2000). For example, the integration of HIV prevention education into female initiation rites ceremonies offers a culturally appropriate venue for the open discussion of HIV transmission via sexual intercourse as well as a venue to address local perceptions and practices. An attempt of this strategy in Mozambique employed an 'as well' strategy in order to bridge divergent cultural and biomedical paradigms (Kotanyi and Krings-Ney 2009). The approach recognized and openly acknowledged ritual practices of the community, offering the external biomedical strategies as additional alternatives "in order to achieve efficient integration of biomedical and cultural understandings of HIV and AIDS" (Kotanyi and Krings-Ney 2009, 492). In this manner, the status quo is maintained. The neoliberal agenda of biomedicine's rationalized-actors continues to be pushed, not by offering it as a counter to local rituals, but merely offering it as the scientifically validated and thereby socially neutral perspective.

By contrast, the *culture-centered* approach is concerned with the voices of target populations, frequently subaltern groups, in discussions of health, thereby interrogating and resisting the status quo. This approach to health communication aims to build on the notion of centralizing cultural voices in the articulation of health problems and the development of health solutions (Airhihenbuwa 1995; Dutta-Bergman 2004b, 2004c, 2005). The centralization of voice develops from the perspective that human experience is meaningful when articulated within the richness of the original context (Dutta-Bergman 2004b, 2004c). Yet, subaltern scholarship recognizes the absence of marginalized voices from dominant spaces of knowledge (Beverly 2004; Escobar 1995; Guha 1982). Thus the goal of the culture-centered approach recognizes the need to create alternative ways of opening up discursive spaces to marginalized voices, and developing health communication theories and applications from within the culture. This approach acknowledges the complex and dynamic nature of culture, including interactions between continuous components of the culture's history and shifting responses to state, national, and global fluctuations in politics, economics, and communication flows (Dutta 2007). Culture-centered health communication approaches articulate culture in the meanings that are co-constructed by the local target population and the health communicator rather than by the health communications expert alone (Dutta 2007).

The Global Dialogues Trust, established in 1997, employs the ideals of the culture-centered approach (see www.globaldialogues.org). Drawing inspiration from Didier Jayle's and Antonio Ugidos' groundbreaking project "3,000 Scenarios against a Virus," Global Dialogues employs a participatory, multidisciplinary approach to amplify the voices of youth using social change media. Young people are challenged to write a story for a short film on HIV/ AIDS. Premier filmmakers from the continent then bring the winning narratives to life. From 1997–2012, over 150,000 young people from 50 countries took part in the contests conducted by Global Dialogues. Of these, 39 films were produced, made available in up to 29 languages and distributed to reach over 200,000 people every year (available at youtube.com/globaldialogues). This approach engages with youth in their communities and provides a venue through which they can express their perspectives on issues of crucial importance to global public health. The voices of the marginalized become centralized in the discussion. These narratives are currently being systematically studied to gain new insights on the concerns, challenges, and solutions raised by youth to inform policies and programs at multiple levels.

In some instances, culture-centered engagement with local communities might suggest the necessity to develop culturally appropriate health information resources to be utilized by community members. In such situations, the creation of culturally appropriate health information texts helps build the health capacity of the community, and addresses health information structures by making available community-appropriate health information (Dutta 2007). However, for both approaches, Airhihenbuwa (1995, 123-124) warns that "empowerment of and participation by the people a program is intended to benefit must take into account the degree to which individual decisions are mediated by power, politics, class, and cultural understanding of the meaning of participation and empowerment."

The culturally sensitive and culture-centered approaches thereby offer two contrasting perspectives. The culture-centered approach aims to interrogate the dominant hegemonic configurations by drawing attention to unhealthy structures, while the culturally-sensitive approach typically serves the existing hegemonic configurations by focusing on individual-level health behaviors (Dutta 2007). Even so, the culture-centered approach is itself constituted in the privileged position of the health communicator, who has access to mainstream communicative platforms and discursive spaces of knowledge. As Dutta (2007) points out, the meaningfulness of the culture-centered approach lies in its ability to continuously turn a reflexive gaze upon itself. By examining how power, ideology, hegemony, and culture operate, scholars of the culture-centered critical health communication perspective explore ways to limit health disparities. With this charge, this book explores HIV prevention communication strategies among youth in Lesotho, examining the influence of fluctuating power structures, the dominance of particular ideologies, and the effects of the biomedical hegemony.

Outline of Chapters

I contextualize my critical examination of HIV prevention in Lesotho within an historical exploration of knowledge-based health interventions and broader theoretical issues in health communication. To provide a working definition of knowledge for use in the context of this book, I draw on the work of anthropologist Fredik Barth. Barth (2002, 1) defined knowledge as the "feelings (attitudes) as well as information, embodied skills as well as verbal taxonomies and concepts" that structures our understanding of the world and the purposive ways we cope with it. Barth's notion of knowledge has three interacting aspects: the body of information or assertions; the medium of communication; and the social organizations within which the production, transfer, and acquisition of knowledge take place. Knowledge is acquired, Barth argued, from both direct and indirect experiences. Pointing to the 1948 work of philosopher Bertrand Russell, *Human Knowledge: Its Scope and Limits*, Barth argued that knowledge is based on inference. What we know is often derived from the beliefs of others, the presence of objects around us, studies, and text. We accept the beliefs of others to be valid and in doing so extend the scope and reach of our own knowledge. The validity, reasonableness, authority, or truth of knowledge is determined by social organization—"the distribution of knowledge, its conventions of representations, the network of relations of trust and identification, and instituted authority positions of power and disempowerment" (Barth 2002, 3). The validity of knowledge is also influenced by the source through which it is conveyed, with certain voices holding more authority and consequently disseminating more valid knowledge. This perspective infers that there is no de-contextualized, transcendent truth. Rather, knowledge is established through argument and justification, and to 'know' means to be able to give reasons for one's beliefs that are accepted by others as valid (Ceci 2004; May 1993). Knowledge is therefore justified relative to claims a community is willing to take seriously (Anderson 1995), and truth is a matter of collective judgment (Shapin 1994). Finally, knowledge that is clearly defined, bounded, and difficult to acquire generally holds greater weight in society.

To begin my examination of knowledge-based HIV prevention, I examine the use of surveillance as a tool for knowledge production (Chapter 2). I do not offer a critique of statistics of the HIV epidemic in Lesotho; rather, I explore the data to provide a critical view on how the act of surveillance contributes to the failures of HIV prevention campaigns. Surveillance itself is a bureaucratic strategy that guides the development of prevention strategies as viewed from the level of the population. In this, the diversity of individuals, communities, and countries, and the structural factors contributing to disease clustering are disregarded. Individuals also come to *know* disease and their own risk in relation to statistics.

I then build a cartography of health communication messages from the knowledge/message producer (expert), to the message disseminator (well-informed citizen) and finally receiver (lay person). In Chapter 3, I explore knowledge production through an examination of the construction of hierarchies along the flows of communication between global North and South, among national institutions, and between urban and rural, drawing on anthropologist Charles Briggs' biocommunicability perspective, which explores what he refers to as the multiple and shifting biomedical spheres of communication. Briggs (2005) views biomedical information as channeled through processes that are structured by inequities of power and resources. Such inequities include differential access to both communicative technologies and symbolic capital, thereby promoting access for some to the specific forms of knowledge and practices needed to become rational and self-regulating, while withholding access from others. In Lesotho, the rural-urban divide is not limited to the geography of mountainous regions and lowlands. Individuals in urban areas are considered to be more integrated within the global market. Consequently, people in urban areas are perceived to have greater knowledge, and thus are less at risk for HIV infection. By contrast, individuals from rural areas are considered ignorant, continuing to engage in traditional practices that place them at increased risk of infection. This locally established dichotomy calls into the question the impact of HIV knowledge largely disseminated via behavior change programs conceptualized by institutions in the global North as linked to the globally established power/knowledge paradigm. Aligned with the critical culture-centered health communication approach, Briggs suggests that if we overlook the channeling of health communication, we cloud the influences of dominant ideologies and hegemonic structures.

In Chapter 4, I examine the accessibility of avenues for disseminating knowledge, taking into account Lesotho's existing structural and ideological divides as well as the consequences of the multi-vocality on young adults' risk behaviors. In Lesotho, foreign investments, infrastructural development and tourism, and the introduction of new community-based organizations funded by aid agencies such as the Millennium Development Challenge and PEPFAR have resulted in many different government and nongovernment agencies and institutions largely offering externally produced (Western) messages on HIV risk prevention, sexual and reproductive health, as well as behavioral norms of sex and sexuality. Religious institutions, schools, the Internet, and television (local, regional, and international programming) offer contradictory and conflicting ideas. Messages of HIV prevention (i.e., abstain and be faithful) frequently conflict with the ideas of sexual freedom presented by newly accessible Western media (i.e., many lifetime sexual partners, casual sexual relations) (Chikovore et al. 2009; Garner 2000; Mitchell and Smith 2003; Sherman and Bassett 1999). Such conflicts rely on an individual's ability to critically analyze the message of appropriate, normal, or safe behaviors, and its relevance to their contextual situation for the establishment of a personal prevention strategy.

As knowledge is considered the foundation of rational risk reduction, in Chapter 5, I examine knowledge acquisition of youth in Lesotho. I critique current analytical methods to measure HIV-related health knowledge, given their utilization in determining the effectiveness of health communication campaigns. I measure HIV knowledge of youth in Lesotho using alternative methodological approaches—a self-generated question exercise and associated pile sorting. These strategies aim to circumvent limitations of the commonly used knowledge, attitudes, behaviors, and practices surveys by identifying what knowledge is lacking as opposed to what knowledge is held. My findings of youth HIV-knowledge contradict those published in government policy documents, stimulating questions of how we define 'appropriate' knowledge.

Chapter 6 offers a closer examination of the relationship between health communication and education strategies in stimulating rational disease prevention behaviors. I focus specifically on the institution of education as an avenue for HIV communication, given the global utilization of schools as a platform for HIV education and related behavior change, and my study population of teachers-in-training. This chapter explores the capacity for problem solving and the development of what Brazilian educator and theorist Paolo Freire (1972, 1993) termed 'critical consciousness.' Critical consciousness relates directly to comprehension and behavioral implementation of disease prevention messages. In Lesotho, the formal style of education, emulating South African/British and 'international' curricula, promotes a divide between the teacher (the expert) and the student (the lay person). Knowledge is delivered to the student rather than acquired as a joint enterprise between teacher and student. As a result, behavior is *prescribed* rather than communicated or negotiated. This pedagogical approach translates directly to current health and HIV communication strategies, where the internationally formulated message of prevention, namely that of abstinence, faithfulness, and the use of condoms, is delivered to students presumed 'empty' or devoid of preexisting knowledge in a style of message-based rational-actor models. The message of prevention can be regurgitated by students, but as evidenced by the continuing rise in HIV incidence, is not always put into behavioral practice.

Chapter 7 considers the development of the more recent global HIV prevention strategy related to medical male circumcision as an example of opposition to current structures and models of global health communication. Domestic health officials are staking a claim as 'experts,' rejecting the presumed contextual relevance of randomized control trial findings conducted by Western scientists in countries in the region. Male circumcision presents a particularly intriguing example of the importance of the critical culture-centered health communication approach, as the practice is locally considered within the realm of tradition rather than a modern biomedical practice. This example makes clear the need to apply the critical culture-centered communication approach in the development of HIV prevention strategies in that the focus of efforts should be at the level of the collective and structures, rather than the individual. Furthermore, the individuals within a community should be formulating the message of prevention based on their own logics.

Throughout the book, I interweave my personal narrative with discussions and theoretical debates. As someone who has grown up in both the developing and developed world during the AIDS era, I explore my own experiences with education systems and HIV prevention efforts. I discuss how global forces have influenced the continued negotiations of my own identity as a global citizen. I also question how the critical culture-centered health communication approach has led me to interrogate my own social location and my role as a public health practitioner distributing global health communication messages as a means of prescribing HIV prevention.

Surveillance

The World Health Organization defines public health surveillance as:

> The continuous, systematic collection, analysis and interpretation of
> health-related data needed for the planning, implementation, and eval-
> uation of public health practice. Such surveillance can: serve as an early
> warning system for impending public health emergencies; document
> the impact of an intervention, or track progress towards specified goals;
> and monitor and clarify the epidemiology of health problems, to allow
> priorities to be set and to inform public health policy and strategies.[1]

Surveillance activities, identifying disease clusters and risk factors, are positioned as vital to stopping the spread of disease. In describing audit cultures,
anthropologist Marilyn Strathern (2000, 2) writes, "By themselves audit practices [such as disease surveillance] often seem mundane, inevitable parts of
a bureaucratic process. It is when one starts putting together a larger picture
that they take on the contours of a distinct cultural artifact." In the field of
HIV, statistical enumerations of diseased bodies ideally flow 'up'—from individuals to community testing sites to national level departments or ministries
of health and global health bureaucracies. Here statistical enumerations are
processed by experts, to be disseminated back or 'down' to domestic and local
levels. This structural configuration (an artifact of global culture) has a significant impact on how HIV prevention strategies are formulated and deployed,
and their success in reducing disease.

Working as an epidemiologist with the Massachusetts W. A. Hinton State
Laboratory Institute, I managed the collection of serum and data from HIV positive individuals in Massachusetts, including information about testing histories
and risk behaviors, as part of a new national disease surveillance strategy. The
Centers for Disease Control and Prevention (CDC) utilized this data, along with
data from 16 other states and two cities, to develop a new and refined statistical

Nicola Bulled, "Surveillance" in *Prescribing HIV Prevention: Bringing Culture into Global Health Communication*, pp. 43-64. © 2015 Left Coast Press, Inc. All rights reserved.

method to estimate HIV incidence, or new cases of HIV infection, in a surveillance program called Serological Testing Algorithm for Recent HIV Seroconversion (STARHS) (Prejean et al. 2011). While far removed from the intimate transfer of knowledge to individuals, the examination and management of large datasets offers a perspective on the power of enumeration.

Following four years of collecting data, estimates of HIV incidence for the United States and the individual states involved in the STARHS surveillance program were released. At the national level, program overseers were prepared for some amount of public concern and misunderstanding over the release of the new numbers. Estimates of HIV incidence had previously existed; however, the new estimates released were based on a more refined and accurate statistical modeling. It was expected that the new estimates might suggest a greater number of new HIV infections were occurring, and thus HIV prevention initiatives might be seen as having limited effect on curbing the epidemic. On the other hand, should the new estimates indicate a lower HIV incidence than previously suggested, it was feared that HIV prevention initiatives might lose public interest and funding.

Our state estimate suggested a greater number of new infections than previously calculated. As a result, CDC management staff armed all research sites with scripted statements such as, the new approach "provides a more accurate way of estimating...[is] a more sophisticated process...[and] uses more recent data" (see CDC 2011) to assist the public in interpreting the new numbers and offer the estimate as a starting point for more accurate projections rather than a comparison to old estimates. Nevertheless, high ranking officials in my state opted not to release the data. They feared that the HIV positive community and general public would not understand this new approach, view current prevention efforts as failing, and begin to question the continued funding of ineffective strategies. Using well-developed communication strategies, the release of the new disease incidence estimate would likely have gone unnoticed by the broader community, limiting discussions to the stakeholders more intimately connected to HIV efforts. Instead, by not releasing the information, those with the power to distribute the information were denying the HIV community a clearer perspective on the local disease situation. While certainly not to the same extreme, such control over information dissemination is reminiscent of the Soviet system during the disaster in Chernobyl, where hundreds of thousands across multiple generations continue to suffer the health effects of high levels of radiation exposure because officials did not disclose accurate contamination figures (see Petryna 2002). Such cases highlight the important role the distributors of surveillance play in the process of health communication and disease prevention.

In this chapter, I illustrate the growing significance of quantification in HIV prevention. I present statistics of the HIV epidemic in Lesotho and the corresponding responses of international and domestic health agents to control the epidemic. My intention is not to deconstruct statistical data or determine their accuracy. Rather, I am interested in offering a critical perspective on how enumeration serves as an important component of HIV prevention strategies, not only in guiding policy and intervention development but also in altering how individuals categorize themselves within populations 'at-risk.'

HIV in Lesotho

The Kingdom of Lesotho is a small mountainous nation, surrounded by South Africa. Though individuals continue to identify with different traditional clans, the majority of the people of Lesotho share similar cultural values and beliefs, as well as a national vernacular language, Sesotho, with English as the second official language (Ambrose 1976). Moreover, people identify with a single national identity, Basotho, the people of Lesotho. The Basotho clans were initially consolidated into one people in 1818 under King Moeshoeshoe I, to fight off the displaced Zulu clans invading in the east. To the west, the Voortrekkers (Afrikaans people) began a series of wars over traditional Basotho land that extended into the highly fertile farming area that is now the Free State province of South Africa. Weakened from constant attacks in the east and west, King Moeshoeshoe sought British protection from the continued military aggression of the settling Afrikaans farmers (Boers) in South Africa in 1868. At this time, the boundaries of the British protectorate, Basutoland, were defined with a substantial area of lost territory remaining in South African hands. Lesotho gained independence from Britain in 1966 and is now governed by a constitutional monarch.

The kingdom has a population of about 2 million people, living in an area of about 30,000 square kilometers (11,178 square miles or roughly the size of Belgium). The country is very mountainous. Most people are clustered in the lowlands, what is now a narrow crescent of land lying along the western perimeter of the country. Adjacent to the lowlands to the east is the much larger mountain zone. While most of the land in Lesotho is suitable for grazing livestock, including cattle, sheep, and goats, only about 10 percent is arable with fields planted mainly with maize, wheat, and sorghum. The limited land available for food production has been further reduced by severe droughts. Consequently, small-scale sustainable agriculture is a dwindling practice, necessitating the import of food staples for purchase on the market. Current estimates suggest that one fifth of the children are underweight for their age and 13 percent of the population is undernourished (Lesotho Food Security Monitoring System 2011).

Partly as a result of the historical loss of fertile land to South Africa and recent changes in climate patterns reducing national food production capacity, Lesotho is one of the poorest nations in the world. In 2011, it ranked 160 out of 187 countries on the United Nations Development Program's Human Development Index (UNDP 2011). Lesotho's closest neighbors, South Africa, Swaziland, and Botswana, are ranked 123, 140, and 118, respectively. Lesotho's Gross Domestic Product per capita (GDP) is 296 USD (WHO 2009a). About 50 percent of the population live below the poverty line, and 43 percent live on less that 1.25 USD per day. The level of adult unemployment is over 40 percent. As a result, about 13 percent of the adult population migrate for employment both to urban areas within Lesotho and to neighboring South Africa (SAMP 2010). Migrant remittances have remained the major revenue source for Lesotho, increasing from an estimated 157 million USD in 1993 to 255 million USD in 2004. Migrant remittances accounted for 25 percent of GDP in 2006 (SAMP 2010). However, retrenchments from the mining sector in South Africa are ongoing. Furthermore, female employment in Lesotho's domestic textile manufacturing sector is unstable given the recent global credit crisis.

Despite Lesotho's current development situation,[2] recent developments in foreign investment in Lesotho's urban textile industries, rural dam projects, and diamond mines have fostered the establishment of a growing middle class (DFID 2006: Central Bank and Bureau of Statistics 1995). These developments have allowed a certain sector of the population, particularly those in urban areas, to engage with global media and purchase global commodities. However, according to the Gini index, Lesotho is one of the most unequal countries in the world, with a value of 63.2 (where 0 is complete equality and 100 reflects complete inequality) (CIA 2010). This development situation is inextricably tied to disease burden.

Widespread poverty, social dislocation because of migratory labor practices, and gender inequality underlie the HIV epidemic in Lesotho (World Bank 2000; WHO 2005). As a perpetual negative feedback loop, HIV has further exacerbated social, economic, and political upheaval. This bidirectional adverse relationship has resulted in significant consequences over the past quarter century. While the population annual growth rate averaged 2.2 percent from 1970 to 1990, it has dropped to 0.08 percent since that time, the lowest population growth rate in the southern African region (WHO 2009a). Life expectancy has fallen to age 45, 21 years below what it would have been without AIDS (Hassan and Ojo 2002). HIV accounts for 49 percent of total deaths in Lesotho. Even though 36 percent less than in 2005, 13,986 AIDS-re-

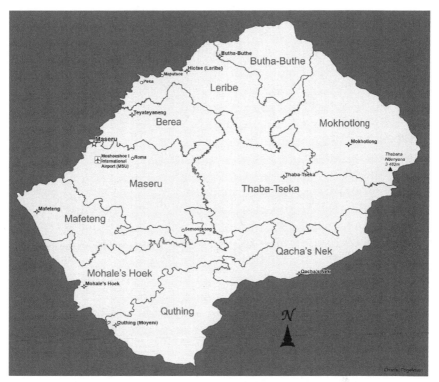

Figure 2.1. A map of Lesotho showing the two sites of the study—Maseru and Thaba-Tseka.

lated deaths were reported in 2011 (UNAIDS 2012). Lesotho also continues to have the highest maternal mortality rate in the southern African region, a statistic shared with Malawi (NAC 2012). At present, 58 percent of the population is under the age of 19 (NAC 2012).

The first case of HIV in Lesotho was identified in 1986, when a medical practitioner from east Africa working in a health clinic in Lesotho's rural Mokhotlong district was diagnosed with HIV. At this time, the first deaths from HIV had already been reported in neighboring South Africa. These deaths were of white homosexual men. The first black South African with AIDS was diagnosed in 1987. HIV prevalence in Lesotho peaked in 2006, reaching 25 percent, and appears to have stabilized in recent years. Currently, adult HIV/AIDS prevalence, or total cases of infection, is at 23.1 percent of people age 15-49, similar to Botswana (23.0 percent) and slightly lower than Swaziland (26.5 percent), the country with the highest HIV prevalence (UNAIDS 2013). The prevalence of HIV in neighboring South Africa is significantly lower at 17.9 percent among adults age 15-49 (UNAIDS 2013,

2010c), although South Africa has the largest total number of people living with HIV in the world. According to the 2013 UNAIDS World AIDS Day Report, approximately 6.1 million people were living with HIV/AIDS in South Africa at the end of 2012. By comparison, there were approximately 320,000 HIV-positive adults (age 15-49) and 38,000 HIV-positive children (age 0-14) in Lesotho in 2012 (UNAIDS 2012). Approximately 17,500 new adult HIV infections occurred in Lesotho in 2011 (NAC 2012), and 3,800 new infections in children (UNAIDS 2012).

Lesotho's National AIDS Prevention and Control Program was formed in 1987 (NAC 2010a). However, due to funding and infrastructural limitations, sentinel surveys among pregnant women and individuals seeking treatment for sexually transmitted infections (STIs) to monitor the spread of HIV were introduced five years later with the assistance of the United Nations. Owing to a lack of funding and technical issues, data collection remained inconsistent until 2000. In 2004, HIV testing was included as part of data collection for the Lesotho Demographic and Health Survey (DHS) (MoHSW 2005b). This allowed for assessment of the magnitude and patterns of infection within the general population of reproductive age, particularly men. Current perspectives of the HIV epidemic in Lesotho are based on the DHS conducted in 2009 (MoHSW 2009).[3]

Immediate causes of HIV infection include unsafe heterosexual intercourse and mother-to-child transmission (NAC 2009c). Prevalence of HIV infection in Lesotho increases with age, with approximately 40 percent of individuals age 30-39 infected. Of individuals age 25-29, 28.1 percent are infected, and of individuals age 20-24, 16.3 percent are infected. This suggests that individuals are likely to be infected in their early to mid-twenties with progression to diagnosable AIDS mounting in subsequent ages. An additional indication of the timing of infection relates to the age of sexual debut. HIV infection in Lesotho is highest among individuals who initiated sexual activity after the age of 19, at 31.9 percent compared to 22.4 percent of individuals with early sexual debut (age <16). There may be two reasons for this counter-intuitive finding. Individuals under the age of 19 are still under the watchful eye of relatives and guardians. As such, though sexual activity may occur, it is likely infrequent as compared to older youth who have greater independence. According to the Lesotho DHS, 25.5 percent of never-married girls age 15-19 had sexual intercourse in the previous 12-months as compared to 57.8 percent of never-married girls age 20-24 (MoHSW 2009). Similarly, 46.6 percent of never-married boys age 15-19 had sex in the previous 12-months as compared to 74.6 percent of never-married boys age 20-24.

While sex may be initiated early by international standards, multiple concurrent sexual partnerships, considered the primary risk factor for heterosexual partnerships, begin in older age groups, similar to increasing frequencies of sexual encounters. The Lesotho DHS reports that 2.1 percent of girls age 15-19 had two or more sexual partners in the previous 12-month period, as compared to 5.9 percent of girls age 20-24 (MoHSW 2009). Among boys age 15-19 and 20-24, the percent reporting two or more sexual partners in the previous 12-months was 13.4 percent and 29.8 percent, respectively. Lesotho DHS (2009) data indicate that *bonyatsi* practices (the culturally sanctioned practice of maintaining many sexual partners) continue beyond the point of marriage, as 6 percent of all women and 22 percent of all men (age 15-49) had two or more sexual partners in the previous 12-months (MoHSW 2009). Among the age group with the highest prevalence of HIV (30-39 year-olds), 9 percent of women and 24.4 percent of men reported two or more sexual partners in the previous 12-months (MoHSW 2009).

Gender differences in the self-reporting of multiple sexual partnerships likely relates to local norms whereby, though culturally sanctioned for both genders, men gain social standing by having multiple partners while women are driven by economic need (Romero-Daza 1994b). Of the individuals testing positive for HIV in Lesotho, 28.9 percent had engaged in multiple concurrent sexual partnerships (MCP), as compared to 25.7 percent who reported no concurrency in the prior 12-month period (only one sexual partner or no sexual partners, 26.2 percent and 21.9 percent, respectively; statistical significance not reported). Recent literature examining the sexual partnership patterns of a community in South Africa found that MCP did not contribute to the spread of HIV (Tanser et al. 2011). These results suggest that MCP as a risk factor for HIV is complex. The relationship may be related more to patterns of sexual networks (Thornton 2008), as well as to a productive immune response resulting from ongoing exposure to the virus (Fowke et al. 1992, Fowke et al. 2000), rather than a simple increase in the probability of disease exposure with a greater number of sexual partners.

Individuals reporting only one lifetime sexual partner were least likely to test positive for HIV. However, lifetime number of sexual partnerships was not equally predictive of risk across genders. Of women who reported 5-9 and greater than 10 lifetime sexual partners, 52.6 and 66.2 percent tested positive for HIV infection. By contrast, of men reporting 5-9 and more than 10 lifetime sexual partners, only 21.9 and 32.8 percent were positive for HIV (MoHSW 2009). These differences by gender indicate both women's increased biological vulnerability to HIV infection, as well as their reduced control over the use of condoms as an HIV prevention strategy.

Overall, HIV prevalence in Lesotho is higher in women than in men (26.7 percent and 18 percent, respectively). This discrepancy is likely the combined result of biological, social, and economic conditions. Women in Lesotho are still socially dependent upon men. Despite significant changes in the legal recognition of the rights and entitlements of women due to constitutional amendments in 1993 granting civil and political rights to all individuals, Lesotho still recognizes customary law. According to customary law, women are legal minors who are dependent upon men (i.e., fathers, husbands, or brothers). This significantly influences women's rights to inheritance, ownership, and equality in marriage and sexual relationships. The government passed a civil law in 2006 that aimed to eliminate discrimination currently imposed by customary law. To date, the new law has had little effect. Lesotho continues to experience high rates of gender-related violence, including rape and domestic abuse (Bureau of Democracy and Human Rights and Labor 2011). Young girls also engage in inter-generational sex that increases their risk of HIV, with 7 percent of women age 15-19 indicating having had sexual relations with a man 10 or more years older within the past 12 months (MoHSW 2009). Payment for sex is also a common risk factor for HIV infection. Men who paid for sex in the past 12 months are much more likely to be HIV positive (31 percent) than men who did not pay for sex during that period (20 percent) (MoHSW 2009).

Although 77 percent of inhabitants live in rural areas, the HIV epidemic in Lesotho is clustered in urban centers (NAC 2011). Despite the urban environment offering greater access to information and risk reduction services and devices (i.e., testing, medical male circumcision, and condoms), HIV prevalence is highest in urban Maseru district (26.5 percent) and lowest in rural Thaba-Tseka district (15.9 percent). National data indicate that 71 percent of urban dwelling, never married, young women age 15-24 used a condom during their last sexual encounter, as compared to 61 percent of young women from rural areas (MoHSW 2009). Similarly, 87 percent of urban dwelling, never married, young men used a condom during their last sexual encounter, as compared to 58 percent of young men in rural areas (MoHSW 2009). Condom-use dynamics are subject to change as relationships become more permanent. Despite these reports of active engagement in prevention practices, higher disease prevalence in urban dwelling residents suggests that some factor unique to the urban environment contributes to risk.

Perceived inequalities with regards to economic and social status may be one factor promoting risky behaviors in the urban area. A recent examination of inequity as a predictive factor in HIV infection in sub-Saharan Africa suggests that in poor regions the rich are most at risk, while in rich regions poor individuals are most at risk (Fox 2009). This disparity may be the result of differential participation in concurrent sexual network structures. In Lesotho, a greater proportion of women in the lowest wealth quintile are likely to engage in multiple concurrent sexual partnerships (MCP) as compared to women in the highest wealth quintile (7.1 and 6.0 percent, respectively) (MoHSW 2009). The situation is reversed in men. A higher proportion of the wealthiest men reported engaging in MCP as compared to men in the lowest wealth quintile (24.2 percent and 20.2 percent, respectively) (MoHSW 2009). For both men and women, a greater proportion of individuals in urban areas reported MCP practices, but differences by geographic environment were not significant. These data draw attention to the significant economic inequality that exists, particularly in urban areas of Lesotho. Individuals, particularly women, migrate to urban areas for low paying jobs, becoming the 'poor' at risk for HIV in the comparatively 'rich' urban area. Their sexual partners are frequently wealthy men who can provide economic support, thus the relatively 'rich' individuals at risk in the 'poor' nation.

These urban-rural, rich-poor, infected-uninfected gendered dynamics are confirmed by national data examining infection status by income level and employment status. In Lesotho, both men and women (age 15-49) with higher income levels (though not the highest quintile) are more likely to be infected with HIV (26.4 percent). HIV infection is higher in employed individuals (27.2 percent compared to 17.6 percent in unemployed). This relation is less predictive in women than in men. For men, 21.8 percent of employed men tested positive, as compared to only 9.4 percent of those unemployed. Given cultural dynamics that place men as the dominant partner, including being the primary financial provider, unemployed men likely have fewer opportunities to attract sexual partners. For women, 21.1 percent of those unemployed tested positive compared to 33.3 percent of those employed. These data suggest that while employment should provide women with financial independence, transactional sexual relations are likely to continue as salaries remain insufficient. In addition, women empowered by economic status may chose to engage with multiple sexual partners. National level data on employment status and HIV status are not further disaggregated by rural or urban location.

Additional gender relations contribute to these disease-distribution dynamics. Men provide physical as well as economic protection for single women, including those women left at home alone while their husband migrates for employment. Women engage in sexual relations not only for economic need and social protection, but also because it is enjoyable (Romero-Daza 1994b), seeking out additional sexual partners when primary sexual partners are not available. Finally, modern lifestyles, including economic success and engaging with modern technologies and global markets, which are becoming more evident in urban areas, may grant women the freedom to behave more 'like men' in that 'modern' women have many different sexual partners throughout their lifetimes (Tawfik and Watkins 2007).

Co-infection with other pathogens (i.e., sexually transmitted infections and tuberculosis) has also been shown to increase vulnerability to HIV infection as well as enhancing disease progression. National sexually transmitted infection (STI) clinic data indicated that the prevalence of HIV among individuals diagnosed with an STI was 54.4 percent in 2009 (NAC 2011). The presence of other STIs further contributes to higher biological vulnerability of women through ulcers, abrasions, and inflammation disrupting the protective epithelial barrier. STIs also affect the immune system, further contributing to co-infections. Embarrassment and poverty conditions limit access to official health care services for STI treatment (Green 1992). HIV co-infections were identified in most individuals diagnosed with tuberculosis (TB). In 2009, 78 percent of individuals diagnosed with TB were tested for HIV; of those 76.5 percent were found HIV positive and 27.6 percent initiated an HIV treatment regime. Malnutrition further increases the negative interactions between TB and HIV in what has been described as a source of "triple trouble" for human well-being (Van Lettow, Fawzi, and Semba 2003). Malnutrition severely impairs immune function, which consequently increases initial susceptibility to HIV and reduces an individual's ability to fight the pathogen (Goldenberg 2003). Good nutritional balance is also required for HIV treatment to function effectively and negate the likelihood of severe side effects of the pharmaceuticals. This issue has led to rumors in the region that HIV treatment is a poison or the cause of HIV-related wasting (Fassin 2007; Himmelgreen et al. 2009; Rödlach 2011; Wierzbicki et al. 2008). In Lesotho, as in other countries in the region, people commonly refer to HIV treatment as "eating" them (Jones 2011: Kalofonos 2010; Kenworthy 2011).

In summary, available data from Lesotho suggest that there are key biomedical, behavioral, social, and structural factors fueling the local HIV epidemic. Biomedical factors include infections with other STIs, TB, and malnutrition. Behavioral factors include the inconsistent use of condoms, and multiple and concurrent sexual partners. Social factors include inter-generational and transactional sex, male dominated gender norms, and sexual and domestic violence. Finally, underlying all other drivers are structural factors including gender and income inequalities that reflect Lesotho's weak position in the global economy.

Domestic Response to HIV

Lesotho's government has demonstrated significant political commitment to HIV interventions in recent years. Figure 2.2 offers a visual overview of Lesotho's response to the HIV epidemic. Yet, national responses to HIV were delayed for the first two decades of the global epidemic. Being initially regarded locally as a foreigners' disease, a full-scale response to the HIV epidemic in Lesotho by the domestic government, local communities, and individuals was

1986	First HIV case identified in Mokhotlong district, male medical doctor from Malawi
	National AIDS Prevention and Control Programme established within MoHSW
1987	Retrovir (AZT) approved as HIV treatment drug by FDA
1990	Lesotho HIV prevalence 1%
1992	Combination HIV therapy released
1995	Lesotho HIV prevalence 15%
1996	Protease inhibitors released
1997	AZT prevents MTCT
2000	King Letsie III declared HIV/AIDS a national disaster
	First national AIDS Strategic Plan developed
	Mbeki publicly denies AIDS, Release of Durban Declaration linking HIV to AIDS
2001	Lesotho HIV prevalence at 26%, PSI Lesotho begins operation
2003	Lesotho AIDS Programme Coordinating Authority established
	Multi-sectoral policy adopted "Turning Crisis into Opportunity"
	International VCT manual released, WHO releases "3x5" initiative
2004	First treatment center opens in Lesotho, Senkatana Clinic, Universal antenatal HIV screening implemented
	UNICEF launches "Life Skills" programs, First generic HIV treatment drug available
2005	UNAIDS launches "Three Ones"
	Lesotho Network of People Living with HIV & AIDS launched
	National AIDS Commission Act passed, establishment of one coordinating agency
2006	"Know your Status" (KYS) universal voluntary HIV counseling and testing begins
	WHO establishes treatment guidelines at 200 cells/µl
	WHO endorses male circumcision
2007	2% of 1.3 million target tested through KYS (Human Rights Watch)
	LPPA opens "Male Clinic" for male circumcision
2008	Lesotho's national "Life Skills" curricula launched
2009	70% target population testing through KYS (MoHSW), Lesotho receives PEPFAR Phase III funding
	WHO alters treatment guidelines at 350 cells/µl, Michael Sidibé calls for the mobilization of a prevention revolution
2010	Lesotho HIV prevalence 24%, decentralization of HIV treatment begins
2011	Plans made for reinvigorated prevention strategy, HIV drama "Kheto ea Ka!" airs on Lesotho TV
2012	KYS-Plus launched, Male circumcision strategy published

Figure 2.2. Overview of the Lesotho HIV epidemic.

slow. Fourteen years after Lesotho's initial case in 1986, the government finally issued the Multisectoral National AIDS Strategic Plan for 2000-2003/2005. The strategic plan was intended to mobilize resources for a coordinated response to HIV, to improve information and communication, and to ensure consistent sentinel surveillance of HIV. Given the threat HIV posed to national development and survival, in 2000, King Letsie III declared HIV a national disaster. These efforts aimed to reduce HIV prevalence by 5 percent, to increase condom use by 50 percent, and provide care for 50 percent of AIDS orphans by 2003. Although HIV prevalence did not rise significantly between 2000 and 2003, efforts did not meet the desired 5 percent reduction in prevalence.

In response, the government committed 2 percent of its budget, an estimated 53.2 million Lesotho Loti (LSL) (about 5.6 million USD) to various government ministry HIV programs until 2009. In 2010, the government committed 5 percent of its national budget towards HIV programs. Donors in Lesotho committed 42.8 million LSL and civil society organizations committed 3.6 million LSL. In total, 99.6 million LSL (10.5 million USD) was set aside for HIV interventions. However, estimates suggested that a minimum of 405 million LSL was necessary annually to effectively implement programs to reduce prevalence, indicating that from 2005 through 2009 a funding gap of 75 percent existed. In 2012, there was an estimated global annual funding gap of almost 5 billion USD, with 18.9 billion USD available for AIDS responses globally, whereas up to 24 billion USD was needed (UNAIDS 2013).

Resources for the national HIV response in Lesotho increased to 724.7 million LSL in 2011, a growth of 630 percent. Growth in funding is largely attributed to significant increases in global development partner contributions from entities such as PEPFAR, the Global Fund, and the Millennium Challenge Corporation (see Figure 2.3 for relative contributions from all sources in 2011). Global development partner contributions have increased by over 400 percent since 2007. The main development partners supporting the HIV response in Lesotho, in addition to the U.S. government, include Irish Aid, the European Union, German Society for International Cooperation (GIC/GIZ, formerly GTZ, DED), the World Bank, and the United Nations. Smaller funders include the Department for International Development (DFID-UK), Japan International Cooperation Agency, USAID, the Centers for Disease Control, Canada Fund for Local Initiatives, the Canadian International Development Agency, Clinton Health Access Initiative (formerly Clinton HIV and AIDS Initiative), the Mennonite Central Committee, the Swiss Development Corporation, the Government of China, and the UK-based Prince's (Harry) Fund. Table 2.1 offers an overview of estimated funding contributions from the different sources from 2006 through 2011, based on the NAC annual partnership forum report 2010 (NAC 2011).

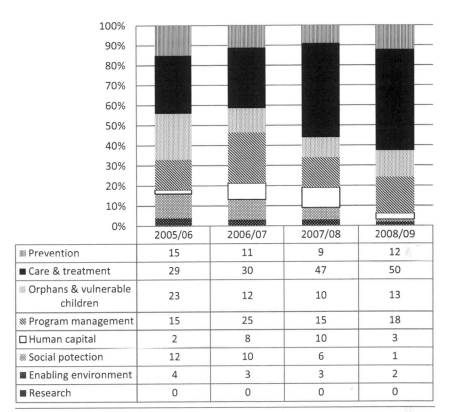

	2005/06	2006/07	2007/08	2008/09
⊪ Prevention	15	11	9	12
■ Care & treatment	29	30	47	50
⊞ Orphans & vulnerable children	23	12	10	13
⊠ Program management	15	25	15	18
□ Human capital	2	8	10	3
⊞ Social potection	12	10	6	1
⊠ Enabling environment	4	3	3	2
■ Research	0	0	0	0

Figure 2.3. Proportional HIV/AIDS expenditures by thematic area.

	2006	2007	2008	2009	2010	2011
Domestic Public	40.2	41.3	41.5	41.5	41.5	49.0
Domestic Private Sector	0	0	0	0.4	0.4	0.4
UN	62.7	60.8	65.8	94.8	162.2	124.8
PEPFAR	2.3	3.4	89.1	35.0	196.0	196.0
Global Fund	13.6	24.9	116.2	179.4	115.8	120.4
Millennium Challenge Corporation	0	0	85.9	147.0	168.0	140.0
Irish Aid	4.8	34.1	56.5	50.0	55.0	60.5
GIZ	1.5	2.4	0.8	1.1	1.7	0.9
EU	0	4.7	24.0	24.0	24.0	25.2
International Private Sector	0	0	0	7.5	7.5	7.5
Total	**125**	**171.5**	**479.8**	**580.6**	**772.1**	**724.7**

Table 2.1. Estimates of monetary resources committed towards HIV initiatives from 2006-2011 in million LSL

According to UNAIDS, in 2012 low- and middle-income countries increased their domestic investment for HIV to an average of 53 percent of all HIV related spending (UNAIDS 2013). In comparison with other low- and middle-income countries in the region and across the globe, however, Lesotho has not made significant increases in domestic investment in HIV. South Africa invested 1.9 billion USD, the highest domestic investment in HIV among all low- and middle-income countries in 2011, a five-fold increase from 2006 (UNAIDS 2012). Similarly, Kenya and Togo doubled their domestic investments for HIV in the last five years (UNAIDS 2012). Brazil, Russia, India, China and South Africa combined contribute to more than half of all domestic spending on HIV in low- and middle-income countries, having increased domestic public spending by more than 122 percent between 2006 and 2011 (UNAIDS 2012).

As a direct consequence of Lesotho's continued reliance on Western donors, the domestic leadership is compelled to modify the national HIV/AIDS strategy to be in accordance with prerogatives set by global health and aid agencies, even if they may not prove suitable for the local economic and social context. The national surveillance program to monitor the domestic epidemic itself poses a huge burden on the national budget. The organization of Lesotho's government sectors to manage the national response to HIV has also followed the framework provided by the global HIV bodies. For example, in response to the UNAIDS release of the "Three Ones" country-level guiding principles (UNAIDS 2005b), the Lesotho AIDS Program Coordinating Authority was abolished and a semi-autonomous National AIDS Commission (NAC) was developed. Lesotho's NAC consists of the National AIDS Secretariat (NAS), the Board of Commissioners and the HIV and AIDS Forum. The "Three Ones" action plan proposes: one national AIDS framework, one national AIDS authority, and one system for monitoring and evaluation. The strategy aims to make optimal use of the limited resources available in response to local HIV epidemics. The Lesotho NAC was removed from the Ministry of Health granting it more independence and authority to work with stakeholders and funders in mobilizing resources, facilitating implementation, monitoring and evaluating programs, and overall managing a coordinated national HIV response outside the government system. As a statutory body, the NAC is also responsible for providing policy guidance to implementing structures. In recent years the separation of the NAC from the Ministry of Health and Social Welfare has resulted in significant tensions and duplication of efforts. As a result, counter to UNAIDS' "Three Ones" principle, the NAC has been reassumed under the Ministry of Health, rather than standing alone.

There is also a moral obligation to make available all HIV-related service, irrespective of the significant financial burden these may pose for the

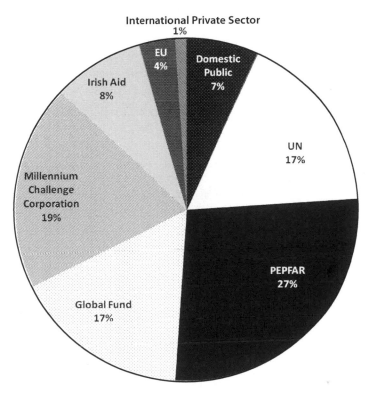

Figure 2.4. Estimated contributions to national HIV response by funding source in 2011.

country. For example, at the end of the third decade of the HIV pandemic, priorities shifted towards biomedical prevention interventions believed to be more effective than strategies that relied heavily on individual risk-reduction through knowledge acquisition and consequent rational behavior change (Granich et al. 2009). In a speech at the National Institute of Health in 2011, U.S. Secretary of State Hillary Clinton reflected on scientific breakthroughs regarding HIV prevention. She noted that a three-pronged approach—eliminating mother-to-child transmission of HIV through the use of nevirapine antiretroviral treatment, scaling up medical male circumcision procedures, and expanding early treatment for people living with HIV—offered a combination prevention strategy that could lead to an "AIDS-free generation" (PlusNews 2011). Despite increasing HIV intervention costs and potential decreases in funding support due to waning interests in HIV and a declining global economy, Lesotho has, for the most part, responded in accordance with directives from global HIV/AIDS institutional bodies for more emphasis on expensive biomedical interventions proven effective in other countries (see Figure 2.4). The proportion of the budget spent on care and treatment in

Lesotho has increased over time, while the proportion spent on prevention through behavior change strategies has decreased, replaced by increases in testing services, prevention of mother-to-child-transmission (PMTCT), and medical male circumcision services (NAC 2010c). The increased demand for such costly biomedical interventions, as directed by global health institution recommendations, will rapidly deplete even expanded national HIV budgets in Lesotho and countries like it in the region.

Though advancements in implementation and delivery have expanded over the years, effectiveness of these mandates from global health institutions is often impeded by limited infrastructural capacity and lack of social demand for such initiatives. For example, mother-to-child transmission of HIV remains a problem in Lesotho. The increased services for PMTCT at the community health center level are not sufficient, given accessibility issues and staffing limitations. As indicated in the annual report from the National AIDS Commission, over 90 percent of pregnant women attending antenatal care services were tested for HIV in 2009. However, many did not return for subsequent visits. These women chose to deliver their babies outside of health facilities, given travel costs, time, and the social stigma that remains attached to HIV (NAC 2009c). Similarly, post-exposure prophylaxis (PEP) services are available across the country. However, they are rarely used because few individuals outside the health profession are aware of the concept of post-exposure prophylaxis and medications used for PEP can only be dispensed by a licensed health professional. Few licensed health professionals are readily available when PEP delivery is most needed, such as when responding to rape victims.

In 2004, driven by global calls for increases in HIV testing, Lesotho launched the "Know Your Status" (KYS) campaign, the world's first attempt to provide universal voluntary counseling and testing (MoHSW 2005a). The campaign aimed to increase HIV testing, raise awareness, and reduce stigma with a campaign slogan of "KNOWLEDGE IS POWER: Know Your Status" (MoHSW 2006). The campaign was founded on data supporting the principle that once individuals are aware of their HIV status, they will engage in greater risk reduction behaviors, having rationalized that either despite their risky behaviors they are HIV-free, or as a consequence of risky behaviors they are infected but now must protect others (Denison et al. 2008). The approach employed the individual-level behavior change in its focus on supplying information, motivating action, and providing access to the service. The approach also attempted to modify the social environment in attempting to reduce stigma. This ambitious campaign aimed to conduct rapid HIV testing on every member of the population over the age of 12 by the end of 2007.

Despite funding from the WHO, Global Fund, Clinton Health Access Initiative, and United Nations Development Program, problems with coordination, resource mobilization, and lack of health care workers significantly hindered the rollout of services. By October 2006, only 720 community volunteers had been recruited to serve as testers, far short of the desired 3,600. Improper training and supervision of testing counselors, inconsistent links between testing and treatment centers, and failures to maintain confidentiality were reported by Human Rights Watch in its investigation of the campaign (2008). Human Rights Watch also claimed that only 2 percent of the targeted 1.3 million people were tested for HIV by August 2007 through the scheme. Nevertheless, according to a report issued in 2010 by the National AIDS Commission of Lesotho, 70 percent of individuals over age 12 had tested for HIV by the end of 2009, thus viewing the KYS campaign as a significant contributor to increases in voluntary testing (NAC 2010c). Discrepancies in the reported outcomes of the program not only influence future intervention planning, but also alter how individuals perceive their responsibility in relation to the epidemic. If the majority of the adult population were tested and know their status (per the NAC report), the people of Lesotho have collectively gained power over the virus. Alternatively, if only 2 percent of the target population was tested under the program (per Human Rights Watch), this finding would indicate a lack of perceived individual responsibility towards the collective interests.

Given the supposed success of the KYS program, KYS-plus, a second round of national voluntary testing, was set to begin in 2012. Tefo Lephowa, Program Officer for Information, Education and Communication at the Lesotho Planned Parenthood Association (LPPA), one of the pioneer organizations in voluntary counseling and testing in Lesotho, believes that KYS was a "good practice," and that KYS-plus will have an even greater positive impact on modifying individual risk behaviors by learning from its predecessor's mistakes.[4] Furthermore, as noted by John Nkonyana, Director of Disease Control at the MoHSW, 58 percent of people who need treatment for HIV do not know their status as they are asymptomatic or just fear testing. He also noted that simply increasing the number of people who are aware of their status will encourage more people to access treatment.[5] In both the reduction of risk as noted by Lephowa and the access of care as identified by Nkonyana, individuals are thought to act rationally in response to knowledge. Neither Mr. Nkonyana nor Mr. Lephowa addressed one of the key failures of the KYS campaign—funding limitations. According to the "Lesotho HIV Prevention Revitalization: Operational Plan 2011" released on October 10, 2011, the roll-out of KYS-plus[6] has been delayed indefinitely as "additional funds [are] needed" (MoHSW 2011b).

An additional complication in initiating the KYS-plus program is the problem of insufficient treatment coverage. Lesotho opened its first public

HIV treatment facility in 2004,[7] 17 years after the first antiretroviral drugs were approved in the US. By 2007, coverage, while limited to a few centralized treatment facilities, had almost met need. However, in 2009, the WHO announced revisions to its 2006 guidelines on treatment initiation (WHO 2009b). Previous recommendations suggested initiating treatment when CD4 cell counts are below 200 cells/μl. New recommendations advise treating anyone with a CD4 cell count at or below 350 cells/μl, following evidence suggesting that reducing the amount of virus present in the body greatly improves life expectancy and reduces viral transmission. Specifically, the average net benefit of providing treatment earlier is 14.5 life years per patient (Johansson, Robberstad, and Norheim 2010). When treatment is initiated at a CD4 cell count of 200-350, 50-199, or less than 50 cells/μl, HIV positive patients can expect to live 4.8, 2.0, and 0.7 life years, respectively. The revised WHO treatment recommendations resulted in a greater number of individuals infected with HIV in Lesotho eligible for treatment. This was not matched by a subsequent increase in service coverage or significant funding. In recent years, HIV treatment delivery has been decentralized to almost 200 health centers in communities across the kingdom, increasing the number of people receiving antiretroviral drugs by 85 percent since 2007. Still, of the 281,000 individuals currently known to be living with HIV in Lesotho, it is estimated that 45 percent are eligible for treatment (CD4 count ≤350 cells/μl per WHO recommendations). Yet, only half of those eligible receive treatment, given limitations in service coverage.

In addition to modeling its national biomedical responses (testing, treatment, and PMTCT) on policy directives from global health institutions, Lesotho has aligned its national 'behavior change' response efforts with the blueprints offered by the WHO and UN organizations. In 2004, UNICEF called for the implementation of life skills as a means of providing young children with knowledge, values, attitudes, and skills vital in psychological development and lifelong learning. A course on "Life Skills" was first introduced at LCE (the national training center for teachers) and the National University of Lesotho (NUL) in 2006. LCE students receive a semester of life skills training during their first year. In contrast, NUL students are taught life skills during a two-day workshop at the end of their final year of study. In 2008, students at select primary and high schools were introduced to a national life skills curriculum. Previously, HIV education had been integrated into health and physical education and biology curricula. This approach focused primarily on factual information dissemination, with very little concern placed on the acquisition of requisite 'life skills' and attitudes for behavior change (Chendi 1999). Chapters 4 and 6 provide a detailed discussion of Lesotho's "Life Skills" curriculum and national implementation.

In 2009, a national operational plan for behavior change communication was developed as part of the revisions to the National Strategic Plan for HIV/AIDS (NAC 2009a). The plan includes the implementation of youth peer education programs, including life skills training in schools, faith-based, and sports-based programs. Lesotho also joined nine southern African countries involved in the 'One Love' initiative that began operations in 2008 to reduce multiple concurrent sexual partnerships. The "One Love" campaign produces posters, flyers, and informational pamphlets about the risks of multiple sex partnerships, and in some countries works with other media outlets (e.g., television) to further promote the message of faithfulness to a single sexual partner. Key stakeholders in Lesotho met in March 2011 to discuss further revitalizing HIV prevention efforts, developing a "coordinated multi-sectoral actionable interventions package building on promising practices and successful interventions" (MoHSW 2011a). This comprehensive "revamped, renewed and visible national response" was launched on World AIDS Day, December 1, 2011 (MoHSW 2011b). There have been numerous suggestions as to what may have prompted these efforts. It appears calls from global health and funding agencies, guided by expert interpretations of domestic and international HIV surveillance, continue to be central in motivating and directing domestic HIV prevention efforts.

The Template of Accepted Facts

The rise of formal global health bureaucracies in the early twentieth century was important for standardization, efficiency, and transregional cooperation in managing disease epidemics. Standardization through statistics and the ensuing practices of classification and categorization has long been critical in the management of population health because it makes evident certain realities on the ground (Foucault 1979). Much work has examined the use of enumeration and statistics in the overall management of nation-states and their citizens, as well as how people come to know themselves and become known politically, socially, and medically through enumeration (Bowker and Starr 1999; Briggs and Mantini-Briggs 2003; Fordyce 2008; Foucault 1977, 1978, 1979; Lorway, Reza-Paul, and Pasha 2009; Porter 1995; Rose 1999; Sangaramoorthy 2012; Sangaramoorthy and Benton 2012; Sangaramoorthy 2014; Strathern 2000).

Numerical knowledge of populations represents ways through which individuals, groups, and nations are rendered as objects and subjects of scrutiny (Rabinow 1999, Rose 2007). The morass of numbers presented here on Lesotho's HIV epidemic has the effect of telling a holistic and authoritative story of a domestic epidemic situated within a global disease pandemic. As a result, we come to see the epidemic as an entity unto itself, greater than the sum of its parts, expanding and contracting over time, unconnected to local lives and communities. In this they leave little room for the recognition of locally specific social and economic factors or consideration of community involvement in the development of disease prevention initiatives. Enumerative practices are therefore critical to the failures of HIV prevention strategies.

It is not the simple presence of numbers that contributes to the failure of HIV prevention initiatives; rather, it is the science of collecting, analyzing, and interpreting numerical data that plays a fundamental role in how diseases and populations come to be known and acted upon. Surveillance establishes an epidemic with risk groups that suggest a particular package of responses whose success or failure can be monitored at the level of the population. Through surveillance, the disease transmission routes, risk behaviors, and corresponding prevention strategies at both the global and domestic levels are highlighted. Surveillance has thereby contributed to the development of what anthropologist Stacey Leah Pigg (2001, 481) argued as "a template of accepted facts"—the presumption that HIV knowledge is well established, systematized, and a unified whole. Following her study of public knowledge of HIV in Nepal in the 1990s, Pigg wrote, "Seen from the receiving end of this knowledge [as developed in 'the West']...from the margins of its production, knowledge about AIDS and AIDS prevention does, however, come rather tightly packaged" (Pigg 2001, 527, n2). In her study of Haitian immigrants in Miami, Florida, anthropologist Thurka" Sangaramoothy (2014, loc 282) revealed, however, that "The landscape of HIV prevention in the US [the West] is highly fragmented, flexible, and deeply contested. Controversies and struggles about how HIV data are interpreted, how funding should be allocated, and how HIV prevention programs are conceived of and translated for various populations in different sites continually occur." Directives from global health institutions that do not consider local structural and contextual variations will continue to compel governments to initiate disease prevention strategies that they have neither the resources for nor the interests to appropriately implement or sustain.

Moreover, dominant groups (i.e., global agencies or local national governments) can also force compliance with their ideologies by controlling the flow of information. Adriana Petryna (2002, 185) offered the phrase "socially constructed nature of the unknown" to explain how states sometimes fudge health statistics and ignore the underlying causes of disease for political reasons. In the case of HIV, certain countries have been accused of releasing false estimates, either reducing or increasing prevalence estimates to show the effectiveness of programs, to booster need-based claims, or to generate a sense of fear and action among the public (Check 2006). In so doing, the dominant can force compliance by controlling what information is disseminated, thereby cementing their own strong positions and deterring any challengers. Those who choose not to participate in the system, based upon the knowledge provided, only become further ostracized and controlled (Petryna 2002).

In examining surveillance as an aspect of the universalized HIV prevention strategy, I am interested in how and why certain numbers and their corresponding meanings travel from the global to the domestic. We should not take this circulation of numbers to be self-evident nor assume that meaning about HIV is simply transmitted (Briggs 2005; Lee and LiPuma 2002; Tsing 2005). Rather, in their very movement, HIV statistics and risk categories become what sociologist Bruno Latour (1987, 227) calls "immutable mobiles," materials meant to flow from one site to another without change. Statistics are more than social data or techniques used to uncover veiled implications of biologies; they play a critical role in how life is both imagined and lived, or what Sangaramoorthy calls "numerical subjectivity" (2014). Through statistics, Sangaramoorthy (2014, loc 666) writes, "we communicate ways of being and belonging, imagining bodies as objects of medical knowledge and numbers as markers of suffering as well as personal triumph and achievement." As I discuss in subsequent chapters, people come to recognize themselves, and others, within the categories of risk defined by statistics (and sometimes contrary to statistics) and adjust their behaviors and perspectives accordingly. Numerical subjectivity thus becomes entangled in enumeration and concepts of risk.

In Summary

The current disease situation in Lesotho suggests that despite evidence revealing the complexity of factors that mediate the structure of HIV risk in each distinct population group, global institutions have established universal expectations regarding appropriate treatments, responsibilities of governments to care for their HIV-positive citizens, and the necessity to implement a variety of specific HIV prevention programs (e.g., life skills lessons, condom promotion campaigns, male circumcision services, PMTCT, and treatment). Although initially slow to respond, the government of Lesotho has shown significant political commitment to HIV prevention, treatment, and care strategies over the past 30 years. The domestic government has implemented strategies that regional or local studies have shown to be effective, specifically altering their provision of HIV related services set out in global directives.

Limitations in resources and occasional cultural barriers have restricted the extent of global HIV prevention and treatment policy implementation and thus reduced the success of certain approaches, including universal test and treat. In addition, financial limitations and the cost of biomedical interventions have compelled significant reliance on donors from the global North. This in turn has perpetuated the implementation of HIV strategies dictated by global public health institutions, guided by expert interpretations of surveillance data, irrespective of their contextual applicability and limited, if any, involvement of local actors. Disease surveillance has not only defined categories of risk behaviors and individuals at-risk, but has also provided a template of accepted facts. These immutable mobiles, both as data and as disease prevention policies and strategies, are circulated from global health bureaucracies to the country level in a top-down fashion. Those receiving the HIV prevention campaigns, or the knowledge of risk-reduction, perceive the message as a constructed whole, a tight package that is not contested or contestable.

The remaining chapters of this book explore how surveillance data are used in HIV knowledge production and dissemination efforts, as Lesotho, and countries like it in the region, try desperately to keep their local epidemics under control.

Knowledge Production

On a cool winter morning in the Lesotho town of Thaba-Tseka, I walked with 12 Life Skills students from the rural campus of the Lesotho College of Education (LCE), the country's teachers training college, to the neighboring secondary school's campus. There was much nervous chatter among the students. Just one week prior, the students had been informed that they would serve as knowledge disseminators by conducting peer education sessions with inmates at the local jail. Given their social position as first year college students, they were unsure what lessons of life they could offer jail inmates with considerable life experience. To their relief, this arrangement had fallen through. Just that morning the assignment had changed and, instead of jail inmates, they were challenged to work with students at the secondary school. Although generally relieved at the sudden change in audience from jail inmates to secondary school students, the LCE teachers-in-training remained nervous. Most had never formally assumed the role of educator or knowledge disseminator before. The LCE teachers-in-training were not sure what to say or how to say it. They were armed only with a booklet newly released by UN-AIDS covering HIV prevention in youth. Without an established lesson plan or script to follow they felt unprepared.

Groups of young students, smartly dressed in their school uniforms, began to emerge from their classrooms as we arrived on the grounds of the secondary school. With no single classroom or school building large enough to accommodate us all, we gathered on an open patch of bare ground. The LCE students huddled together on one side of the open area, watching the secondary school students approach and assemble as a group directly opposite. 'Mme Adel, the Life Skills lecturer and Director of LCE-Thaba-Tseka, led us through the standard lengthy introductions and prayers. The teacher in charge of the secondary school students, and the only teacher I saw on the campus during our four-hour visit, was an LCE student himself. He was

Nicola Bulled, "Knowledge Production" in *Prescribing HIV Prevention: Bringing Culture into Global Health Communication*, pp. 65-91. © 2015 Left Coast Press, Inc. All rights reserved.

completing his second year of training, which involves placement at a school for supervised practical training. After the lengthy introduction routine, the students eagerly dispersed into small groups; four or more secondary students, ranging from 10 to 15 years of age, surrounded each teacher-in-training. Male LCE teachers-in-training met with boys; females with girls.

Once everyone was settled in their small groups the volume of chattering voices in the open field began to subside. The intimate nature of the interactions and the topics (e.g., friendships, love, and romantic attachments) were ideal for the sharing of personal stories, feelings, or reflections on lessons learned. However, no sharing appeared to be happening. The looks of eagerness at being out of class and able to talk with more mature students about non-school related matters had faded. Few of the students looked engaged or even vaguely interested. The conversations did not involve animated back-and-forth chatter between peers, but rather a one-way dialogue. The teachers-in-training spoke of the theoretical, "HIV can be transmitted via sexual fluids and blood," and frequently referenced or even read straight out of the UNAIDS booklets for youth HIV prevention. The association of the booklet with a global HIV organization offered a level of authority that the LCE students could not command on their own. The printed pages of the booklet reminded me of a preacher's bible, the words of an assumed higher entity offering those holding, owning, and referencing it, power and influence. In the case of the LCE teachers-in-training, the booklets also appeared to offer them reassurance in the accuracy and appropriateness of the topics discussed and advice offered. In addition, the formal language within the booklet provided emotional distance and protection from the difficult and sensitive subject matter.

Attempting not to alter the established dynamics of the group, I settled myself down among a collection of boys. The LCE teacher-in-training was trying to persuade the group of obviously bored students that it was inappropriate to engage in romantic relationships with girls at their age. The boys seemed unconvinced, as the LCE teacher-in-training read out of his UNAIDS booklet about increased risk for disease. Given my past interactions with this particular LCE teacher-in-training, I knew that as a student he had had many romantic (though non-sexual) relationships with girls. He had also struggled with his sexuality and had recently begun experimenting in sexual relationships with men. Why did he not offer some of the lessons he had learned in his youth? I knew he had much to offer, as he had frequently reflected on his past with me. I added to the conversation the words of advice I had received from a teacher during my schooling in South Africa, a stern Afrikaans woman who was not opposed to smacking students with a ruler when her authority was tested. She rationalized a delay in romantic attachments by suggesting that they distracted us from our schoolwork and future potentials. Obviously

I had not taken her words to heart as the very next year, free from her watchful eye, I acquired my first boyfriend, though the relationship only involved a coupling for social appearances. Thus, adding a bit of my own perspective I said, "Relationships are sometimes more of a hassle than they are worth. Girls can be demanding. And if things don't work out, people can get hurt. Nicer to be friends with no unnecessary expectations." This advice did not seem to alter the mood of anyone, but the LCE teacher-in-training smiled at me as I winked at him.

Unlike the LCE teachers-in-training, their lecturer, 'Mme Adel, the most senior member of the LCE faculty in Thaba-Tseka and on the verge of retirement, easily engaged with the secondary school students in a maternal yet approachable way. Of all the groups of teachers and students, hers was the only collective engrossed in back-and-forth dialogue. In trying to convince them to abstain from sex until marriage, 'Mme Adel had recognized that they referred to their virginity as "biscuits" (cookies)—a rare, sweet treat. Taking up this word, she kept saying, in her naturally joking manner, "not to share the biscuit," to keep it "locked up tight." Laughing loudly as she made these proclamations. She kept trying to convince them of this by pointing out that when they were married women, they would have plenty of opportunities to share their biscuit with their husbands, adding that it would be a wonderful experience worth waiting for. But, they should wait until they found someone worthy to share the biscuit with, as like a rare treat they would not want to waste it on just anyone.

The contrasting teaching or message delivery styles of the young teachers-in-training and their experienced lecturer is a useful place to begin this discussion of HIV knowledge, education, and prevention. It reflects how understandings of HIV emanate from the lived, as well as mediated, experiences of those directly and indirectly involved in related discourse and information dissemination. The pandemic is as much a social reality as it is a biomedical reality—symbolically and communicatively constructed (Bardhan 2002). However, the peer education situation taking place on a bare patch of ground in rural Lesotho alludes to the privileging and social endorsement of certain views, values, and perspectives that rhetorically and politically shape the future courses of action, policy, and signification (Treichler 1988), in this case, the UNAIDS booklet developed by the global health institutional 'experts' and the abstinence discourse of the wise older parental figure. In exploring HIV prevention education among youth in rural and urban areas of Lesotho, the following chapters offer both a theoretical and an empirical exploration of the power and cultural differentials that mark the various intersecting discourses and knowledges on HIV risk reduction occurring in Lesotho and globally.

Knowledge as Power

Disease outbreaks and epidemics, actual or potential, have over time generated highly specialized, multi-leveled, and globally-connected spheres for biomedical knowledge production, dissemination, and acquisition (Briggs and Hallin 2007). French philosopher Michel Foucault has argued that knowledge is intimately connected to power (Foucault 1977, Foucault and Gordon 1980). Power not only produces knowledge, but power and knowledge also directly implicate one another as "there is no power relation without the correlative constitution of a field of knowledge, nor any knowledge that does not presuppose and constitute at the same time power relations" (Foucault 1977, 27). However, power is not something that a group has or holds, but instead a force that circulates in and among people. If we consider the power of biomedicine, Foucault asserted that the power of the medical gaze is neither embodied by physicians or other health personnel, nor by patients. Instead, the power of biomedical knowledge is related to the discourse participated in by all parties and the structures within which the discourse of knowledge operates.

Structures of knowledge, including universities, research centers, and think tanks, are central to the maintenance of global power differentials. According to noted communication scholar Mohan Dutta (2011, 44), "An entire industry of academic, development, and marketing practices are manufactured to ensure the production and perpetuation of symbolic resources that are at the core of colonialism and neocolonialism...[exploiting] the developing world, under the guise of offering aid and bringing about enlightenment." These institutions of knowledge are situated politically and economically as truth-producing bodies that legitimize the political economy of neocolonialism. Through these positions of power, agents of global health institutions claim 'expertise.'

'Experts' hold specific claim to distinct and defined knowledge (Schutz 1964, 69). Experts attempt to secure legitimacy over knowledge by ensuring that access to their knowledge is limited. In biomedicine, this is evident in the increasingly complex and costly medical school admission process. If obtaining a medical degree were not seen as a challenge accessible to and endured by only the elite few, the public might have less faith in the practitioner's ability to heal (Levi-Strauss 1963). In the case of HIV knowledge, non-local others in the form of NGOs and expatriate contractors have positioned themselves as 'experts' contributing their knowledge systems, practices, and strengths to the local context. It has been argued that funding structures such as the United States Agency for International Development (USAID) and, more recently, the Bill and Melinda Gates Foundation[1] determine the agendas, objectives, and goals of development projects. Networks of 'expert' campaign developers from academe and civil society, as well as the private sector, team up to develop the interventions based on pre-existing problem configurations (see Chapter 7 for an example). Deborah Lupton (1994b, 56) wrote that communication in this model is:

> largely regarded as a 'top-down' and somewhat paternalistic exercise, in which those with the medical or public health knowledge, whether they be physicians, other health care professionals, or health educators, perceive their role as disseminating the 'right' message to the masses for their own good. [These masses] are often regarded…as apathetic and ignorant, needful of persuasion to change their behavior, resistant to change, obstinate, recalcitrant, lacking self-efficacy, chronically uninformed, and 'hard to reach.'

Often, local elites representing government and civil society operate as 'well-informed citizens' (Schutz 1964, 69) and are involved in the development of certain approaches, implementing health intervention messages and managing the intervention process at the local level. They may assist in legitimizing certain knowledge and knowledge structures through periodic evaluations, but mostly members of the local community have a limited involvement in such campaigns. Operating as little more than 'men in the street' (Schutz 1964, 69), local community members passively act as a reserve for data, rather than actively assisting with health education campaign design, development, and implementation.

Such knowledge stratifications generate social hierarchies and inequalities within non-expert sectors of the population. In Venezuela during the cholera epidemic of the early 1990s, for instance, competence as a citizen was measured through the ability of individuals to maintain health or prevent disease (Briggs and Mantini-Briggs 2003). Poor barrio residents, street vendors of food and drink, and indigenous people were most at risk for disease, given their exposure to contaminated water and lack of resources to reduce exposure. Rather than identifying the social, economic, and political barriers to rational disease prevention, these groups were targeted as initiating and perpetuating cholera outbreaks, given their perceived failure to comply with biomedical interventions and systems of hygiene and sanitation. The result was reduced medical provisions and consequently higher rates of disease morbidity and mortality. Hierarchies related to knowledge access have similarly been established in Venda, South Africa. In response to the HIV epidemic, young women in the rural former homeland/*Bantustan* of Venda have become HIV peer educators, procuring competence in biomedical knowledge of HIV in contrast to, and perceived by some as in opposition to, traditional knowledge and authority structures (McNeill 2011). Obtaining biomedical knowledge in this case was not in an effort to limit individual or community disease risk through the public promotion of rational behavior change, but rather to gain personal access to economic opportunities through skilled employment positions in government agencies. As both these examples indicate, knowledge holds symbolic capital (Bourdieu 1991), generating structures within society relative to distribution and access.

In addition, certain forms of knowledge/power are privileged while others are marginalized, an act communications scholar Stanley Deetz (1991) terms "discursive closure." The most common form of discursive closure is disqualification, or the "denial of the right of expression, denying access to speaking forums, the assertion of the need for certain expertise in order to speak, or through rendering the other unable to speak adequately" (Deetz 1991, 187). Discursive closure suppresses potential conflicts as it normalizes who is authorized to speak and when (Murphy et al. 2008). Thus, health policy negotiation, construction, and implementation are communicative processes that involve struggles over meaning among actors with different levels of access to communication spaces and power (Conrad and Jodlowski 2008). By limiting access to realms of communication, the power afforded to knowledge is further increased, with certain individuals securing the rights to control and disseminate specialized forms of knowledge/power. In the U.S. context for example, because middle-class white gay activists generally possessed more symbolic, political, and material capital than women, African Americans, Haitians, or Africans, they were successful in shaping relevant debates in the United States about HIV research, treatment, and representation (Shilts 1987). Their existing social status and political associations afforded gay-activists in the United States "a seat at the communicable table" (Briggs 2005, 284). This social, political, and resulting communicative positioning is regarded as one of the primary reasons for the success of HIV control efforts in the U.S.

In this chapter, I trace the flow of HIV power/knowledge in Lesotho from global public health institutions and funding structures to the local individual level. I show how HIV knowledge (like disease surveillance data) generally flows from the global North (the top) to the domestic sphere (the bottom) by providing a brief overview of the primary global HIV institutions and funders as producers of knowledge (UNAIDS, the Global Fund, PEPFAR). Then I use two knowledge disseminators within the domestic sphere (Population Services International and local newsprint media) to examine the position of 'well-informed citizens.' Through this examination it becomes evident how structures of knowledge production have created and recreated categories of risk and the risky. And, I begin to reveal how the current asymmetrical model of top-down, global North/Western-dominated, communication structures has a profound impact on the HIV risk-reduction behaviors of youth. In doing so, I begin to raise questions related to knowledge production. Who has a voice in establishing HIV prevention knowledge? Who is privileged in this process of knowledge production? Whose agendas are served by this knowledge? What are the underlying ideologies of organizations producing and disseminating knowledge?

The Expert

Global spheres of communication regarding world health were originally established after World War II, when a range of international organizations emerged to manage health problems that transcended national borders, namely cholera, plague, and smallpox. One of the first declarations of the United Nations requested the formation of a single agency responsible for international health cooperation. By 1948, the World Health Organization (WHO) had been formed and the first World Health Assembly had been convened, bringing together representatives from nearly 70 nations. At its formation the WHO set two primary aims that distinguished it from predecessor international health organizations: universal membership and decentralization. As of 2010, 193 countries were included in the member roster, making the WHO a truly global organization. Over the last 65 years, the WHO has played a prominent, though often contentious, role in shaping the landscape of global health.

As discussed in Chapter 2, global public health institutions, such as the WHO, conduct disease surveillance—the collection, aggregation and dissemination of country-level disease data—coupled with informed policy agendas. Standardized, decontextualized biostatistics are circulated locally by national spheres of communication, including ministries of health, local health departments, clinics, doctors, and media. Global institutions frequently call upon the media to help convince heads of state and the public of their positions, thus maintaining their dominance in governing global health affairs. To maintain domestic power and control, health ministries may carefully guard and control the release of biomedical information, particularly during disease outbreaks such as during the 1992-93 cholera epidemic in Venezuela (Briggs and Mantini-Briggs 2003), during the AIDS and SARS epidemics in China, by the allies and axis powers during World War I, and by the Soviets during the nuclear reactor disaster at Chernobyl (Petryna 2002).

The key stakeholders in the global AIDS discourse therefore include global organizations (e.g., the UN and its arm UNAIDS, international NGOs, global media); national organizations (e.g., governments, researchers and policy makers, pharmaceutical companies, insurance companies and other corporate stakeholders, and local media); and community-level organizations (e.g., service-providing organizations, activist groups, local NGOs, and people living with and those at risk for HIV/AIDS). What follows in this section is an examination of the three major global organizations that largely control funding and consequently have historically directed HIV-knowledge production and dissemination: the Joint United Nations Program on HIV/AIDS (UNAIDS); the Global Fund to Fight AIDS, Tuberculosis, and Malaria; and the U.S. President's Emergency Plan for AIDS Relief (PEPFAR). Together they comprised 61 percent of contributions to Lesotho's HIV response in 2011 (with 93 percent of Lesotho's HIV budget being paid for by international donors) (NAC 2011). I offer a brief historical overview of each organization, their guiding principles, and reflections on the consequences of their policies and practices for low-income, heavily disease-burdened countries such as Lesotho.

Joint United Nations Program on HIV/AIDS

The Joint United Nations Program on HIV/AIDS (UNAIDS) was launched in 1996. Unlike many other global programs that develop as a result of intellectual stimulation at conferences or conventions, the creation of UNAIDS was driven by politically-connected activists seeking a stronger response to HIV, a group of bilateral donors (the Organization for Economic Co-operation and Development [OECD]), and a design developed by the United Nations Economic and Social Council (ECOSOC). As emphasized in a report by the Committee of Co-sponsoring Organizations (CCO) to the ECOSOC (UNESC 1995, paragraphs 20-21) outlining features of the new program:

> Because of its urgency and magnitude, because of its complex socioeconomic and cultural roots, because of the denial and complacency still surrounding HIV and the hidden or taboo behaviors through which it spreads, because of the discrimination and human rights violations faced by the people affected...in short, only a special United Nations system program is capable of orchestrating a global response to a fast-growing epidemic of a feared and stigmatized disease whose roots and ramifications extend into virtually all aspects of society.

This mixture of the political and technical resulted in a broad spectrum of expectations for the program. Political advocacy was initially high on UNAIDS' list of priorities. By June 1996, UNAIDS staff had met with political, economic, and social leaders in more than 50 countries to brief them on UNAIDS' mandate and work. Sally Cowal, Director of External Relations at UNAIDS, notes, "as I came to understand more about the epidemic, it became clear to me that the political motivation around it, the need to overcome denial and complacency, were probably as important as anything we could do" (cited in Knight 2008, 48). Awa Coll-Seck, Director of Policy, Strategy and Research, adds that at the time it was not obvious to everyone that AIDS was a problem, that it was killing people and impacting country development (Knight 2008, 49). Consequently, the initial focus of the organization was to heighten awareness of the issue, generate global concern, and ensure political commitment by national leaders.

Currently, UNAIDS is supported by 32 nations, which together provide 270 million USD directly to the fund (UNAIDS 2009b). Over 60 percent of the total budget is covered by the top four contributors—the United States, the Netherlands, Sweden, and Norway. In his message on World AIDS Day, December 1, 2011, United Nations Secretary General, Ban Ki-moon (2011) emphasized the need for a global investment of 24 billion USD annually, claiming that the "results would offset the upfront costs in less than one generation." In June 2011, UNAIDS had set bold new targets for 2015: reduce the sexual transmission of HIV by half, eliminate new infections in children, provide treatment for 15 million people living with HIV, end stigma and discrimination, and close the AIDS funding gap. UNAIDS aims to accomplish these objectives by "build[ing] on the political commitments, investments, energy, activism and determination that have brought us to this turning point" (Ki-moon 2011). The rising scale of HIV over past 40 years suggests that the 2015 targets will be met only through the development of completely new approaches or significant scale-up of existing strategies.

Calls for more funding were largely driven by the significant cost of HIV treatment. Treatment, using a cocktail of antiretroviral drugs, is currently regarded as the most significant contribution to HIV control efforts. Initially low-income countries focused HIV control efforts primarily on behavior change strategies, due both to lack of infrastructure to deliver and the high cost of treatments. Since 2003, via activation of the 3 by 5 WHO initiative (3 million HIV positive people on treatment by 2005) (WHO/UNAIDS 2004), investments in treatment have increased globally. Lesotho's first HIV treatment facility opened in 2004. Now, close to 200 health facilities, including the small primary care clinic on the LCE-Maseru campus, provide anti-retroviral treatment. Treatment costs constitute the largest component of Lesotho's national government's annual HIV budget. UNAIDS policies have also directly impacted the development of Lesotho's National HIV/AIDS Strategy beyond treatment scale-up. For example, in 2009 the national strategy was revised to include monitoring and evaluation strategies as per the UNAIDS "Three Ones" principle (see Chapter 2 for details). This bureaucratic principle requires additional local personnel, skills development, and funding. As a result, more money is spent horizontally, on personnel and facilities, rather than trickling down to individuals the intervention intends to serve (Easterly 2006).[2] Inherent in both these approaches to HIV prevention is a population-level focus driven by analyses of surveillance data with little attention paid to the individuals most impacted by HIV/AIDS. Moreover, such HIV prevention efforts are driven by the UNAIDS experts who determine how monies should be spent, with no involvement of local actors. Given the duplication of efforts, Lesotho has broken from this approach and returned HIV programming control to the Ministry of Health and Social Welfare.

The Global Fund for HIV/AIDS, Tuberculosis, and Malaria

In the spring of 2001, UN secretary-general Kofi Annan put new pressure on world governments by proposing the creation of a Global Fund to Fight AIDS, Tuberculosis, and Malaria. The Geneva-based multi-billion-dollar health agency, Global Fund, was launched in 2002, shortly after the first UN General Assembly Special Session on AIDS. The Fund receives only voluntary contributions from governments and private philanthropists, billing itself as an innovative approach to international health funding (see www.theGlobalFund.org).

The Global Fund has been hailed as a transparent, efficient aid machine that delivers the elements of the AIDS prevention and treatment package prescribed by the UN General Assembly, including HIV testing services, condoms, and antiretroviral drugs for AIDS treatment. Donor governments, including the United States and France (the top two country donors), as well as private foundations, corporations, and organizations such as the Bill and Melinda Gates Foundation, the Global Business Coalition, and (RED), have so far given roughly 23 billion USD to pay for more than 600 programs in 150 countries around the world. The Global Fund works as a partnership between governments, civil society, the private sector, and affected communities. The intention is to offer local actors, including officials from government and nongovernmental organizations, direct control over funding, so that countries implement their own programs based upon their perceived priorities. The Global Fund's only caveat is that it provides financing on the condition that verifiable results are achieved.

Despite the Global Fund's model of country ownership and performance-based funding, which avoid both the inevitable politicization of bilateral programs such as USAID and the bureaucracy of UN agencies, the Fund has not circumvented controversy. At the 21st Board Meeting of the Global Fund held in April 2010, the Finance and Audit Committee released a report announcing the suspension of grants in Mauritania, Zambia, Mali, the Democratic Republic of Congo, Djibouti, and Uganda (The Global Fund 2010).[3] Investigations into allegations of corruption and fraud, and audits on the use of funds are ongoing in other countries, including Cameroon, Cambodia, Dominican Republic, Sri Lanka, Nigeria, Swaziland, South Sudan, Madagascar, Togo, India, and Nigeria (The Global Fund 2011). In total, the Global Fund reports needing to recover up to 19.2 million USD from grants dispersed in eight countries. As a consequence of fund mismanagement, Germany, Ireland, and Sweden temporarily suspended payments to the Fund. Furthermore, in 2011, insufficient donor contributions forced the Global Fund to cancel the funding cycle (Kates et al. 2012; Kaiser Family Foundation Kaiser Daily Global Health Policy Report 2011). Lesotho has not been named in any reports for the mismanagement of funds. Nevertheless, such widespread mismanagement of funds calls into question the approach of the Global Fund. Are local actors competent and honorable enough to propose and manage HIV prevention strategies successfully with finances provided but no other support? Or, is the oversight of costly bureaucratic structures necessary to have a positive effect on disease prevention, given limited local capacity?

Lesotho received its first Global Fund grant of 34 million USD in 2004, to be dispersed over a five-year period. The HIV component of the proposal aimed at scaling-up HIV prevention interventions, providing care and support to people living with HIV/AIDS and impacting mitigation for children orphaned or made vulnerable by HIV/AIDS. The prevention component targeted youth at high risk of HIV infection. Emphasis was placed on expansion of life skills education, peer education programs, access to condoms, and health services. In addition, national efforts for the prevention of mother to-child transmission were expanded in order to limit the number of infants infected at birth. Global Fund money was used to support the launch of anti-retroviral therapy within the public health care system, to expand voluntary counseling and testing services to all districts, and to provide home-care kits. Grant money was also used to provide orphans and vulnerable children with basic services including school bursaries and food packets.

Initially, a number of challenges arose which delayed the disbursement of money from the Global Fund and, thus, the implementation of proposed activities. Lesotho had difficulty meeting the Global Fund requirements for a national monitoring and evaluation system and for procurement and supply management processes. In addition, the establishment of the National AIDS Commission required the renegotiation of implementation arrangements. After the first two-year funding period, Lesotho was informed that it would likely not be awarded funding for a second funding period because of questionable management of grant funds, an unimplemented monitoring and evaluation plan, and complicated and slow disbursement of funds to sub-recipients and partner organizations. Additional funding was eventually approved by the Global Fund Secretariat once Lesotho complied with Global Fund directives.

Lesotho received monies in subsequent funding dispersal periods (i.e., Rounds 5, 6, 7, 8 and 9). In total, the local Global Fund Coordinating Unit has managed over 250 million USD in funds. These funds have been instrumental in developing Lesotho's national systems of prevention, care, and treatment.

With these systems in place, significant advances have occurred in de-stigmatizing HIV (and tuberculosis) and in creating a more supportive environment for individuals, families, and communities to engage with national response efforts. They have also allowed for the development of technical capacity for a national monitoring and evaluation system, and the creation of capacity within various government sectors, NGOs, and private sector partners participating in HIV response efforts. As noted in the Fund's 2009 annual report, "In many ways, the story of the implementation of the [Global Fund] Round 2 grant is really the story of how Lesotho mobilized itself to face two of the most serious challenges to survival and well-being of its people in this period of its modern history as an independent nation" (The Global Fund 2009, 2). The long-term aim of the Global Fund is to enable recipient countries to maintain necessary systems, structures, and policies autonomously. It is unclear, however, if Lesotho, as well as other countries with similar economic situations, will be able to sustain its existing government systems, as developed through funding and guidance of the Global Fund, at their current level without continual external funding. This uncertainty begs the question: Might Lesotho have developed different structures for disease and program surveillance that were more sustainable in the local context?

U.S. President's Emergency Plan for AIDS Relief

In 2003, the administration of George W. Bush launched the President's Emergency Plan for AIDS Relief (PEPFAR), a 15 billion USD five-year program, the largest financial pledge by a single government to a single public health crisis in history. Despite the significant response of the U.S. government on the international stage, PEPFAR has come under scrutiny on several fronts (see Dietrich 2007). I highlight a few relevant concerns here.

Many wonder if PEPFAR was originally developed as another strategy by the Bush administration to boost the U.S. economy, rather than to significantly impact disease burdens internationally. At PEPFAR's start, the administration held that its funds could only be spent on brand-name U.S.-produced drugs, in order to protect patent rights and assure treatment quality. At the time, U.S. drugs were three times more expensive than generic versions and three-in-one combination therapies. In May 2004, the administration altered its policy to permit PEPFAR funding of generics, but only once the drug had U.S. Food and Drug Administration approval through an expedited review process. By 2007, 34 generics had been approved, but in 2006 only 27 percent of PEPFAR-funded purchases were of generic pharmaceuticals. This stipulation ensuring the purchase and distribution of U.S. products quietly pumped billions of dollars into U.S. pharmaceutical and condom production corporations.[4]

A second concern raised about PEPFAR policies involves the restrictive U.S. rules regarding abortion. Long before the inception of PEPFAR, in 1984, U.S. President Ronald Reagan announced the Mexico City Policy, which required NGOs to neither perform nor actively promote abortion as a method of family planning as a condition of their receipt of U.S. funds. Though rescinded by the Clinton administration, President G. W. Bush restored the policy in 2001. During G. W. Bush's presidency, the rule against abortions was relaxed for groups fighting AIDS, but PEPFAR funds had to remain separate from any other funds that might have been spent on abortion-related projects. President B. Obama once again overturned the policy on January 23, 2009.

A third PEPFAR policy igniting global debate includes the U.S. legislative requirement that prohibits funding of any group that does not have an explicit written policy opposing prostitution and sex trafficking. International opposition to the policy was highlighted by the Brazilian government's refusal of 40 million USD in U.S.-PEPFAR assistance, because it felt the requirement inappropriately stigmatized sex workers (a legal occupation in Brazil) and made delivering HIV information and services to this crucial target group difficult. PEPFAR's most recent five-year strategy states that HIV services must be responsive to the public health needs of marginalized communities, which include persons engaged in prostitution. PEPFAR supports governments that engage in targeted prevention, care, and treatment outreach for prostitutes; seek alternatives to prostitution; and work to reduce demand for prostitution. However, countries are still required to sign a pledge opposing prostitution. This constraint continues to generate significant confusion at the national level and has resulted in some countries, including Brazil, being left out of PEPFAR funding streams.

Much greater controversy has surrounded the conservative focus of PEPFAR on the HIV risk-reduction behaviors of abstinence and faithfulness. Initial PEPFAR policy required that at least 33 percent of all funds spent on prevention of HIV from 2006–2008 went to abstinence and fidelity programs.[5] To justify the promotion of abstinence programs, the U.S. administration cited Uganda's successful HIV prevention campaign of the 1980s and early 1990s. However, initial conclusions of Uganda's 'Kinsey' surveys suggested that an increase in condom use, not abstinence nor faithfulness, was responsible for the reduced number of HIV infections (Asiimwe-Okiror et al. 1997). Later, though, a re-analysis of the surveys concluded that a reduction in sexual partners (i.e., faithfulness and delayed sexual onset), under the local "Zero Grazing" agenda, had caused a decline in new HIV infections (Shelton et al. 2004).[6] After examining the research evidence available, USAID researchers (Edward C. Green, Vinand Nantulya, Rand Stoneburner, and

John Stover) strongly supported programs in Uganda that encouraged abstinence, partner reduction, and faithfulness, in addition to condom use (Hogel 2002). This strategy was named by the Bush administration the "ABC" approach for Abstain, Be faithful, and use Condoms. Regardless, PEPFAR funding has heavily promoted abstinence and faithfulness to a single partner over condom use, which may imply promiscuity, and countries that receive PEPFAR funding have been strongly encouraged to do the same.

Anthropologist Edward C. Green attributed the neglect of partner-reduction campaigns like Uganda's "Zero Grazing," in favor of condom promotion strategies, to biomedical hegemony and bureaucratic inertia. In his book *Rethinking AIDS Prevention* (2003b) Green argued that during the 1970s, rich governments poured vast amounts of money into programs to market and distribute contraceptives that would limit a population explosion in developing nations. When HIV began to spread, these pre-packaged approaches were rapidly deployed, much like the pre-structured World Bank's development strategies in Lesotho (see Ferguson 1994). Green's argument, that condoms were just an easy solution and were already available with distribution avenues in place, was vehemently critiqued by other anthropologists working on HIV throughout the world and in the region. Anthropologist Douglas Feldman (2003a, b) asserted that the slowing of HIV in Uganda was more related to an overall recognition and acceptance on behalf of Ugandan society that HIV was a problem that needed a comprehensive, multi-sectoral solution. Douglas Feldman (2003b, 6) argued that significant local involvement and ownership of prevention programs, which included partner reduction and condom use, were responsible for Uganda's success, stating:

> What happened [in Uganda] was a total commitment on the part of the government from President Museveni on down to tackle the epidemic head-on, to destigmatize the disease, to saturate the media with information about AIDS, to bring discussions about AIDS into every home, every workplace, every school, to open the door to aggressively working with WHO on the problem, and to welcome European and North American research.

Contradicting the notion of human agency in altering behavior, anthropologist Robert Thornton (2008) suggested that a slowing of HIV in Uganda was more related to a stabilizing of communities and reduction in migration following the civil war. As soldiers disbanded, sexual units (including polygamous marriages) became more isolated, thereby reducing the size of and interconnections among sexual networks.

The diversity of these three hypotheses of Uganda's success in controlling their HIV epidemic raises clear questions about the nature of global

HIV prevention interventions. Are Western models of AIDS prevention always appropriate for African and other low-resource nations? Have Western donors and researchers been guilty of imposing a one-size-fits-all Western model of AIDS prevention on African nations at the expense of other approaches that might be just as, if not more, effective? Do changes to structures that promote risky behaviors have a greater effect on behavior change than prevention strategies that target individual rational action?

Lesotho was not among the original PEPFAR countries, but has been receiving PEPFAR Phase II funds since 2009. The PEPFAR agreement outlines four ambitious goals to be met by 2014, namely, reducing HIV incidence by 35 percent, reducing morbidity and mortality by providing essential care to people living with or affected by HIV, improving human resource capacity for HIV service delivery, and strengthening health systems (PEPFAR 2010). These goals are almost identical to those set by funding from the Global Fund. This parallel suggests that Lesotho is not ready to operate its established HIV-dedicated systems autonomously, despite the considerable economic investments and expectations of the Global Fund. Lesotho's continued dependence upon international funds ensures that their national response to HIV is driven by top-down approaches developed and largely implemented by global experts, even if agencies such as the Global Fund assume national leaders are setting the local agenda.

The Well-Informed Citizen

Global organizations such as UNAIDS, Global Fund, and PEPFAR operate at a transnational level, providing funding and issuing directives to be implemented by national governments or agencies operating at local levels. The following section discusses domestic disseminators of the largely internationally produced (or at least assembled) knowledge. I highlight specifically international institutions operating domestically[7], using Population Services International (PSI) as an example, and local media. I discuss domestic newspaper media here, as media serves as an important bridge between the international and the domestic, tailoring the message for domestic consumption. While neither media or international institutions operating domestically function strictly as knowledge producers, to some extent they do alter the message in their delivery and thereby function as another layer for knowledge production. Other domestic sources of HIV prevention information are similarly not passive disseminators of knowledge. A critical examination of how they come to frame information for local consumption is therefore necessary. Other sources of HIV knowledge are examined in Chapter 4.

International Organizations operating domestically: Population Services International

Population Services International (PSI)/Lesotho has made significant efforts to address domestic HIV prevention needs, including changing local attitudes towards male and female condoms and, more recently, to medical male circumcision. Using social marketing techniques, including multi-channel media campaigns, a regular schedule of community mobilization events, and targeted interpersonal communication provided by PSI field educators, PSI has introduced the Trust brand of condoms. Advertisements contain images of a happy couple wrapped in each other's arms, indicating that the use of condoms promotes trust in a relationship.[8] PSI also provides a variety of condoms at different costs for different socio-economic groups (Trust, free; Trust Studded, 10 LSL; Lovers Plus, 10 LSL; and Lovers Plus Colored and Flavored, 25 LSL), drawing on concepts of human consumer psychology, which suggests that more costly items are better.

PSI has focused their efforts in urban areas of Lesotho, ensuring that free condoms are available in bathrooms at Maseru's Pioneer Shopping Mall and in local clinics throughout the city. Since PSI/Lesotho began programming in 2001, they have distributed more than 20 million condoms free-of-charge through 130 Ministry of Health and Social Welfare public health clinics, hospitals, and partner organizations nationwide. An additional 12 million condoms were sold under the Trust and Lovers Plus brand labels. In 2010 alone, 10 million condoms were distributed. Recently, PSI/Lesotho has expanded efforts to promote the use of female condoms under the brand name Silk-ee. Commercial distribution was launched in 2012.[9]

In 2010, PSI conducted a study to examine the distribution and accessibility of their condom products (PSI Research & Metrics 2010). It found that national coverage for all condoms had decreased in 2010, likely due to a change in distribution strategy. Coverage in rural, urban, and at-risk areas (e.g., border crossings) was low with only 34 percent of rural, 46 percent of urban, and 39 percent of at-risk outlets having PSI products available at the time of the survey. Vendors also did not meet standards for the presence of promotional materials and adherence to recommended pricing. I asked a student at the LCE-Maseru campus to obtain some condoms, as a way to gauge what products were accessible to students. I expected he would bring back a variety of condoms, some obtained for free at the on campus health center and in the shopping centers and some he had purchased. Two days later he returned with a single three-pack of condoms—PSI's Lovers Plus banana flavored—having spent almost all of the 50 LSL I gave him. I was told by the student that this was the only packet of condoms available from the street corner vendor close to the college campus, where he had purchased them.[10]

This venue was close by, open when perhaps the campus clinic was closed as it frequently was, stocked when campus bathroom condom distributers were frequently empty, and possibly less embarrassing than purchasing condoms at the nearby grocery store. This experiment and my own observations of condom availability confirmed PSI study findings. Although I know experienced researchers in the region will argue with me on this point, it seems clear from my observations and interactions with students that there simply are not enough condoms consistently accessible in the places youth frequent.

With regards to PSI/Lesotho's organizational structuring, the organization should be commended for operating domestically, including hiring local staff and building local capacity (even if management continues to be U.S. citizens). Nevertheless, PSI/Lesotho continued to operate under and perpetuate Western logics—condoms are heavily promoted for all relationships irrespective of local norms that encourage women to become mothers (see Chapter 6); medical male circumcision is encouraged despite the local customs of traditional circumcision (see Chapter 7); and more expensive condoms are promoted, building upon the recent influx of Western consumerism typified in the development of the Pioneer Shopping Mall and a second mall under construction.

The data on condom distribution presented by PSI suggest a pressing need to vastly scale-up condom distribution in the country, but these data may also indicate that condoms are not a particularly effective solution in the Lesotho context. That is to say, condoms may prove to be *one of many* strategies to prevent HIV in Lesotho (the argument of Edward C. Green and even the ABC approach). Consequently, although PSI/Lesotho operates within the local context, it is still driven by the directives from headquarters in Washington, DC. Local considerations and sensitivities are only minimally considered, limited to suggesting ways to implement pre-determined strategies that are adapted for context (the culturally-sensitive approach) rather than developing contextually specific and appropriate strategies (the culture-centered approach). As such, PSI/Lesotho serves as a conduit for pre-packaged Western-developed solutions and strategies of implementation.

Local newsprint media

Local media also serves as a disseminator of knowledge from global spheres to national levels. By virtue of its involvement in developing public opinion (Dearing and Rogers 1996) and its role in disseminating information from the macro to grassroots level, mass media plays a central role in contextualizing, negotiating, shaping, and defining power relationships between stakeholders in the HIV epidemic. In particular, media has a significant impact on contextualizing experiences that are beyond an individual's direct experience, thus acting as a window on the world. The media process frames the social organization of the human experience (Goffman 1974). As a result, the information conveyed by media is highly dependent upon the characteristics of the frame: large or small, many panes or few, opaque or clear glass, facing the street or the backyard (Goffman 1974, 1). In this, media messages may unintentionally or unconsciously provide their audiences with cues concerning which event should be regarded as important through selections, omissions, and interpretations (McCombs 2004). Media messages do so with superficial characteristics including choice of emotive words, images, sources, and style, such as the fear and urgency evoked in the statement "AIDS Kills," which was popular in newsprint press early in the HIV epidemic. Media also frames issues in more fundamental ways, including how questions of life and death, relationships between men and women, sexuality in general, friendships, care-giving, and values such as honesty and openness are articulated (Johnson, Flora, and Rimal 1997, 224). The media thereby puts a 'face' on the issue of HIV, both "mediat[ing] and partially construct[ing] people's understandings of health and health-related issues" (Hodgetts and Chamberlain 2006, 317; Rimal, Johnson, and Flora 1997). As noted by Maxwell McCombs, "The media not only tell us what to think about, but also how to think about [a health issue], and consequently what to think" (1993, 65).

Media portrayals of an issue can be influenced at five different levels: the individual, media routine, organizational, extra-media, and ideological (Shoemaker and Reese 1996). At the individual level, the personal beliefs and values of the reporter, despite professional conditioning, influence decision making. The set routines of information gathering and processing such as reliance on official sources, experts, or other authorities (Gans 1979; Soloski 1989) shape the final product. Structures, policies, rules, and the goals of media organizations form yet another layer of influence. Extra-media influences include the public relations efforts aimed at diverse groups, advertisers, and various forms of government control. The ideological level infuses the entire process with the dominant ideologies of the time and social context.

These influences are evident in feature articles appearing in editions of one of the local private newspapers, *Public Eye*.[11] The first story printed in the February 20, 2009 issue described the hardships of an orphan girl from a rural village (Nyaka 2009a). Lineo came to the capital city of Maseru seeking employment in the textile industries to help support her two younger sisters. After realizing that she still did not earn a sufficient amount to pay for their basic necessities of food, housing, and transportation, she engaged in "night work" (prostitution). The article uses the narrative of Lineo to inform readers of the importance of acquiring biomedical knowledge, noting that Lineo "lacked the skills to resist such temptations, as well as having no knowledge about HIV/AIDS prevention." The narrative serves as the prelude for the article's main objective, the announcement of greater youth involvement in HIV prevention planning by the NAC. The article cites Motlalepula Khobotla, NAC Director of Policy, Strategy, and Communication, stating, "[Youth] engage in sexual relationships without using condoms because they lack the skills and power to negotiate safe sex or to resist an early sexual debut." Despite noting the structural factors that compel youth such as Lineo to engage in risky behaviors (being orphaned at a young age, having a limited social network to provide financial assistance, and low wage employment in the textile industry), the article reveals local judgments about HIV infection, specifically a moral failing to "resist temptations" and ignorance in "having no knowledge." The solution offered is not actually to involve youth in policy development (as the title suggested), but rather to promote rational behavior change through the acquisition of biomedical knowledge inline with Western ideologies of responsible action.

The following month, in the March 6, 2009 edition, the *Public Eye* featured a narrative about 'Makhahliso, a woman in severe pain seeking assistance for labor complications at a hospital in Maseru, written by the same journalist, Libuseng Nyaka[12] (2009b). 'Makhahliso had intended to have the baby at home, but she felt something was wrong and decided to seek professional medical assistance. The hospital staff refused to help her, as she had not tested for HIV prior to her delivery. Although she had been receiving antenatal care, 'Makhahliso explained, "I did not bother to get tested for HIV because my husband had told me not to get tested. I was afraid that if I tested positive I would lose my marriage and be blamed for the infection." The hospital staff held firm despite her reasoning and denied her care. 'Makhahliso's story ends with the authoritative words of the medical provider, 'Mapiers Mohapi, who stated, "Women should stop blaming their husbands for their ignorance. That woman should have gone to the clinic where she would have been properly advised." According to the article, the Lesotho Ministry of Health and Social Welfare launched a policy in 2003 that requires mandatory HIV screening of pregnant women as a means of reducing the transmission of HIV from mother to child. If a pregnant woman is found to be positive, she can immediately begin a treatment course. Delivery can then occur within the health center to ensure minimal viral exposure to the baby at birth, and plans can be made to treat the infant following delivery to reduce the likelihood of infection. However, the article incorrectly represents the 2003 policy. No mandatory screening of pregnant mothers is required. The government put in place opt-out HIV screening as part of routine antenatal care. Any woman seeking antenatal care is counseled on the benefits of HIV screening, both for her and for the child. The journalist represented individuals as free agents, who, when provided knowledge and healthcare services, will rationally engage in health maintenance activities. Mothers who choose not to are portrayed as ignorant and irrational. The journalist also placed authority over health information and rational action within the purview of the biomedicine linked nurses and government policy. Social context is not considered by this journalist as viable justification for avoidance of prenatal HIV screening.

Evident in both stories are the five levels of communication noted by Shoemaker and Reese (1996) that influence how HIV prevention is portrayed by the media. At the level of individual reporter, personal beliefs and values regarding individual agency become central to each story. Particular experts (nurses and medical professionals) and authority figures (government officials) are routinely relied upon in the structuring of the story. Government also serves as an external entity utilizing the media to convey new policy agendas or strategies, including the involvement of youth in policy development and routine maternal HIV screening. The structures and goals of the newspaper are evident in positioning of newspaper's customers/readers as distinct from the individuals portrayed in each story. This division relates also to the ideologies of the time and social context, as the individual reader perceives that in holding knowledge they are empowered to behavior rationally. Accordingly, risky actions are driven by ignorance rather than structural violence.

While the intent of these stories may be to draw attention to the plight of marginalized groups, the framing, word selection, and use of the voice of authority (i.e., biomedicine or government policy) suggest that Lesotho media messages, reflecting the ideologies of their social context, identify risk to be self-determined. The idea of non-compliance with biomedical directives, or simply ignorance of biomedical facts as a risk factor for HIV infection, has pervaded the local Lesotho newsprint media. Individuals are challenged to make rational behavioral choices based upon knowledge acquisition, with little regard for contextual situations. Individuals who do not behave according to the biomedical perspective of rational action are blamed or held accountable for their own circumstances. This attitude is further evident in various headlines: "Ignorance Free Zone: AIDS can kill you too, playa-hater" (*Public Eye*, April 8, 2005); "Education key to HIV/AIDS fight" (*Public Eye*, September 26, 2008).

Blame for infection in Lesotho appears specifically directed at individuals in rural areas, whose limited access to information via media, education, or health institutions logically increases their engagement in risk and consequent likelihood of HIV infection. These perceptions build upon the increasing social distinctions between people who live in urban and rural areas of Lesotho. In Lesotho, rural living is seen as the equivalent of traditional lifestyles of cattle herding and subsistence agriculture. Individuals dwelling in the mountains, growing up as herd boys and attending initiation rituals, are considered to engage with the true Basotho culture. Rural lifestyle is highly valued; as Moeshoeshoe I, the founder of Lesotho, is alleged to have said, "I am Basutoland, only he who honors his roots will achieve greatness" (*Informative*, June 2, 2009). However, Basotho culture as idealized through rural life is vanishing. For many Basotho this change is not seen as a positive consequence of development. As one newsprint opinion piece states, "A nation's culture is the only pride it possesses, hence it always leaves me in tears to see Basotho culture evaporating rapidly.... Girls are dolling themselves up to be as chic as Jennifer Lopez and other foreigners while our culture is gone" (*Public Eye*, November 5, 2004). At the same time, traditional living is ridiculed for being backwards, with statements in the newsprint such as, "Lesotho is rooted in its culture and heritage; the majority of its people dwell in the rural areas where culture, heritage, myths and sometimes superstition are still rife" (*Informative*, June 2, 2009). These statements juxtapose rural 'traditional' living against 'modern' life in urban areas.[13]

By linking rural life to Basotho culture, individuals from rural areas are associated with high risk of HIV infection through one of two interrelated routes: lack of knowledge of HIV transmission and continued engagement in cultural practices associated with HIV transmission. Individuals dwelling in rural areas, although honored for maintaining Basotho heritage, are labeled "ignorant." As Lesotho is a mountainous nation, disseminating knowledge through media and medical services to remote areas is difficult. Newsprint articles frequently claim "the challenge is that most Basotho women, *especially those in rural areas*, still lack information" (*Public Eye*, February 27, 2009, emphasis added). It is presumed that without knowledge, individuals in rural areas are unable to make informed decisions about how to protect themselves from HIV infection.

Without knowledge, individuals in rural areas are unaware that certain cultural practices place them at increased risk for HIV infection. Print media repeatedly draws connections between "culture" and HIV with headlines, including "Culture undermines prevention efforts in Lesotho" (*Public Eye*, September 26, 2003); "Culture threatens HIV transmission program" (*Informative*, June 2, 2009); and "Should we let our cultural beliefs damage our future?" (*Public Eye*, July 21, 2000). Mathoriso Monaheng, former Director of the Lesotho AIDS Program Coordinating Agency (LAPCA) was reported as saying that "social and cultural norms and traditions in Lesotho are hampering efforts to combat the rising HIV/AIDS epidemic" (*Public Eye*, September 26, 2003). She specifically mentioned the sharing of razor blades to shave the head during mourning and to cut foreskin during male circumcision rituals.

Other cultural practices locally considered to contribute to the HIV epidemic include the taboo against speaking with children and youth about sex (*Public Eye*, July 21, 2000; *Public Eye*, April 29, 2001; *Public Eye*, September 10, 2010).

Among the cultural practices of current concern is involvement with multiple concurrent sexual partners (MCP); says Monaheng, "The cultural aspect whereby men are allowed to have mistresses is another problem" (*Public Eye*, September 26, 2003). In Lesotho historically, polygamy was a common practice. Following the arrival of European missionaries in the 1830s, the occurrence of polygamous marriages declined, but MCP continued. Migratory labor further contributed to the practice of multiple sexual partnerships. Throughout the twentieth century, most men engaged in some amount of migratory mine labor (Ferguson 1994). As described in the newspaper article referencing Monaheng, by living "away from their families and the social control of kinship [migrant laborers] are more likely to have multiple sex partners" (*Public Eye*, September 26, 2003). Migration of men for labor contributed to the local practice of *bonyatsi*, whereby women maintain a male lover, for companionship, to ensure safety, and the provision of necessities should remittances from the mines be too little or too slow to arrive (Romero-Daza 1994b). Government statistics released in 2009 indicate that "casual sex with multiple partners accounted for 65 percent of all new infection in Lesotho last year, [in 2008]" (*Public Eye*, January 30, 2009). Individuals living in urban areas do not associate themselves with practices of *bonyatsi* or polygamy.

Tsitsi, a journalist for the *Public Eye* newspaper, explained during a conversation with me that the continued focus on cultural aspects of HIV is not necessarily to place blame on certain individuals, but rather because "culture is relevant to people in Africa." Her statement implied that "culture," or particular behavioral practices, are uniquely African and consequently exotic. The interest of the public or the newspaper readership is, therefore, not to focus on the rather mundane drivers of HIV—poverty and inequality—which directly impact most newspaper readers and, as Tsitsi argues, are "never going to go away," but rather on the fascinating and obscure details of living with HIV which, whether purposeful or not, relate only to certain segments of the population.

A study of public media reports of HIV in Kenya similarly found frequent condemnations of cultural practices (Peters, Kambewa, and Walker 2010). The authors referred to the term "cultural practices" as "a gloss for certain rituals involving sexual intercourse (such as at the end of initiation rites or after the death of a spouse) and customs involving apparently non-voluntary sexual intercourse (such as 'widow inheritance')" (Peters, Kambewa, and Walker 2010, 293). They argued that Kenyan public media appear obsessed with the exotic, with little reference to ordinary sexual relations. Finally, the authors noted that there is a tendency to insert claims of morality, as certain rituals are described as depraved and individuals practicing such rituals as conservative and backward. Mass media in Lesotho similarly frames culture as an entity belonging primarily to rural dwelling individuals. Rural geographic locations limit exposure to modern forms of communication that relay biomedically generated HIV knowledge. Without knowledge, individuals in rural areas are perceived as continuing to engage out of ignorance in the cultural practices that place them at high risk of HIV infection. In most cases, there is no evidence supporting claims that certain cultural practices cause the transmission of HIV.

The media construction of HIV has become inextricably intertwined with matters such as which claims or stakeholders are accorded privilege or credence and the symbolic and ideological content of these claims. The ever-changing interplay between media and social construction has been documented in most parts of the world (Bonacci 1992; Clarke 1992; Grube and Boehme-Deurr 1989; Lester 1992; Lim 1995; Lupton 1993; Netter 1992; Princeton Survey Research Associates 1996; Rogers, Dearing, and Chang 1991; Sabatier 1988; Semetko and Goldberg 1993; Traquina 1996). During the early phase of the global pandemic, global media coverage of HIV was considered scant and marked by fear and ignorance. Given the relative lack of political support from heads of state, media focused instead on identifying 'risk groups' rather than 'risk behaviors.' A second phase of HIV media coverage involved exploration and understanding of the epidemic and an attempt to move beyond labels and blame attribution. There was greater acceptance that HIV has no preferences in whom it infects, shifting focus onto biomedicine and policy (McAllister 1992: Watts 1993). From the 1990s onwards, the focus of media coverage has been on routine events such as World AIDS Day and international conferences. This phase has generated a false sense of security by recasting what remains an urgent issue into a mold of routine (Sepulveda, Fineberg, and Mann 1992). 'Official' sources (Gans 1979) and stakeholders such as biomedical researchers and policymakers (knowledge experts and well-informed citizens) have come to control and shape the contours of the HIV news narrative (Bardhan 2002). Although activists and people living with HIV gained more ground as sources for the media through the 1990s, a significant shift in voice has not occurred (Bardhan 2001; Princeton Survey Research Associates 1996).

In Lesotho, HIV-positive individuals are given a voice in the media, with dedicated newspaper columns. The focus, however, remains on the official voice of biomedical providers and domestic and international government officials, not those suffering from HIV/AIDS. Journalists (not identified by HIV status) focus on rational behavior change through knowledge acquisition. By doing so, the Lesotho print media has established divisions among the public based on their varying access and control over knowledge—authority figures producing, holding, and dispersing knowledge (the experts); individuals who modify behaviors based on received knowledge (the informed citizen); and individuals who either have not acquired knowledge or ignorantly continue to engage in risk despite holding knowledge (the man-on-the-street).

(Re)distributing Blame

The division of populations along lines of expert, well-informed citizen and man-on-the-street as a result of differential access to knowledge, which in Lesotho is intimately connected with rural/urban dwelling, has been termed the "knowledge gap hypothesis" (Tichenor, Donohue, and Olien 1970). Researchers Phillip Tichenor, George Donohue, and Clarice Olien (1970, 159-160) argue that as the infusion of "information into a social system increases, segments of the population with higher socioeconomic status tend to acquire this information at a faster rate than the lower status segments so that the gap in knowledge between these segments tends to increase rather than decrease." Echoing Pierre Bourdieu (1991) and Michel Foucault (1980), Tichenor, Donohue, and Olien (1970) further argue that, given the social capital inherent in knowledge, dispossession of knowledge may lead to relative deprivation of power.

According to the knowledge gap hypothesis a number of underlying factors account for the differential impact upon knowledge distribution and upon consequent social divisions. First, individuals with a higher socioeconomic status tend to have more formal education. This leads to greater reading and comprehension skills, improving their ability to acquire knowledge via newsprint and other sources. Second, prior exposure to a topic and greater awareness enables individuals to develop a better understanding of the idea overall. A study of 15 African countries found that the higher a person's level of formal education and the more often she reads newspapers, the more likely she is to list HIV as an important public problem (Afrobarometer 2004). Third, individuals with a higher socioeconomic status are more likely to discuss public affairs topics with others in their social class, further increasing the knowledge gap between high and low socioeconomic population, and urban and rural dwellers. Fourth, individuals with higher socioeconomic status are exposed to information that is more relevant to them, thus they are more likely to accept and retain that information. Fifth, individuals with higher socioeconomic status are more likely to use media as a source of information, while individuals with a low socioeconomic status are more likely to use media for entertainment purposes (McLeod and Perse 1994). Consequently, higher socioeconomic status individuals gain more knowledge from media than their lower socioeconomic counterparts. Finally, print media is geared more to the interests of individuals with higher socioeconomic status. In Lesotho, individuals with a higher socioeconomic status are those involved in the formal economy and living in urban areas. The intended audience of Lesotho's print media is urban dwellers, identifying the behaviors of "others," namely rural dwelling individuals, as risky.

I do not argue here that media in Lesotho has created a knowledge gap with regard to biomedical knowledge of HIV. Instead, I suggest that print media reflects local perceptions of the existence of a gap in knowledge between urban and rural dwellers, as well as individuals with high and low socioeconomic status. The perception that individuals without access to knowledge are at greater risk of infection is likely the result of international HIV prevention interventions that have narrowly focused on the need to promote knowledge for rational risk reduction (UNAIDS 2005a, 23). Print media in Lesotho indicates that risk groups have been generated based upon knowledge access. Individuals in urban areas engage in self-defined modernized lifestyles as related to their access to information, including knowledge about HIV. By holding knowledge, they consider themselves at lower risk for HIV infection. By contrast, individuals living in rural areas, where access to newsprint is limited, are believed to hold onto cultural practices that biomedicine considers "risky." Traditional cultural beliefs and practices of rural dwelling individuals are perceived as obstacles to appropriate risk-prevention behavior (Pelto and Pelto 1997). As noted by other researchers, local understandings and explanations of HIV that differ from the authoritative biomedical discourse are not addressed in the media or through other educational avenues because these are "misconceptions" that biomedical messages of HIV prevention will readily correct (Eves and Butt 2008; Pigg 2001, 2005). In other words, any belief contradicting biomedical knowledge will simply be displaced by fact. Under this perspective, HIV vulnerability and blame is shifted from those professed to hold the knowledge (urban dwellers) to those with less access to it (rural dwellers).

HIV prevention campaigns developed by large global health institutions spread Western notions of disease etiology and health maintenance through behavior change and self-reliance interventions. More broadly, development communication campaigns are run via mass media to diffuse through the message of enlightenment that is achieved through urbanization, literacy, development of media exposure, greater economic participation, and voting, all of which are treated as markers of modernization in the West. Through the principles of modernization, Western values, particularly those of liberation and independence, are marketed as the universal aspirations for cultures and societies across the globe. Noted Mohan Dutta (2011, 37), "The treatment of these values as secular values, removed from their Western roots and situated more in the context of universal human values, serves to support the agendas of top-down development campaigns." The global-local, urban-rural, modern-traditional binaries in Lesotho result in unequal power-dynamics, wherein individuals from powerful Western nation-states are considered superior. Individuals from urban areas with more direct links or connections to the modern-Western world via access to global media and commodities are considered socially superior to their neighbors in rural areas. Consequently, under the veil of development aid, knowledge dissemination efforts are put into place in developing countries to support the objectives of global organizations and their related transnational hegemony (Dutta 2011, 51).

In Summary

Political Scientist Jeremy Youde (2007, 18) has argued that large global organizations (and their funders) "essentially hold both the intellectual and financial capital to force compliance with [their] ideas and dictates" for better or worse. National governments, NGOs, and private institutions put forth proposals to the funding agency. Funders determine what organizations and initiatives are supported; they establish basic criteria for the proposed initiatives, and they may choose to fund certain elements within the proposals and not others. As mentioned, Lesotho's original 2003 proposal to the Global Fund was not accepted as it did not include a monitoring and evaluation component, and additional funding was withheld until structures were in place that complied with the funding institution's ideals. Lesotho's national HIV infrastructure has been built to comply with global directives, from the establishment of the central overseeing body of the National AIDS Commission to current movements towards service decentralization, irrespective of the local need, applicability, or capacity.

Global agencies dictate interventions and consequently ideologies by employing top-down strategies. These include hiring international employees to manage programs, despite their limited knowledge of local situations and/or ability to speak local languages. Of course, hiring locals and/or individuals who can speak the local language does not ensure that local voices are heard or considered. Funds for international agencies are disbursed directly from agency or country of origin to the countries where the recipient international agency is active. Local stakeholders are frequently not involved in the development of the interventions being funded. Furthermore, while there may be discussions on strategies at the country level, directives on how to operate the intervention are often designed by the funding/recipient international agency (culturally-sensitive approach). Governments, communities, or even individuals who delay or seek other tactics for implementation of such interventions (a culture-centered approach) are often regarded as non-compliant and may have funding delayed or revoked (Eves 2012, Pigg 1996, Youde 2007).

Simultaneously, the distribution of spaces for communication and opportunities to participate in these spaces are unequally distributed, with increasing gaps in access to communicative infrastructures between the rich and poor, urban and rural, and modern and traditional (Dutta 2008a, 2009; Dutta and Pal 2010; Pal and Dutta 2008a, b). These disparities have been observed within local spaces, nation states, and across various sectors of the globe. Of particular concern is the increasing marginalization of the poorest sectors of the globe, whose limited access to material resources prevents their gaining access to platforms from which to articulate their voices (Dutta 2008a, 2009; Dutta-Bergman 2004b, cb; Pal and Dutta 2008a, b).

4

Knowledge Dissemination

One chilly May day in 2011, I arrived on the LCE-Maseru campus to attend the Life Skills lesson. I had come to observe this particular class as this was the single lecture of the semester dedicated specifically to the topic of HIV. 'Mme Mabitle, the instructor, informed me that another American was joining us and would be delivering "the message" for the day. The guest lecturer was associated with the U.S.-based Evangelical organization True Love Waits. This organization's primary aim is to persuade youth to abstain from sexual activities until marriage through the formation of peer pledge groups. Youth publically pledge their commitment to abstain and, through the support and pressure of peers in their accountability group, resist the temptation of pre-marital sexual relations. The True Love Waits program was initiated in the United States in 1993 as part of the Christian Sex Education project. It was introduced in Africa shortly afterwards, first in Uganda in 1994 and in South Africa the following year.

There have been extensive analyses of various abstinence promotion programs such as the True Love Waits program. In May of 2001, the National Campaign to Prevent Teen Pregnancy published a thorough review of programs designed to delay the initiation of sex, increase condom or contraceptive use, and reduce teen pregnancy (Kirby 2001). The review showed that "the evidence is not conclusive about the impact of abstinence-only programs," and that "there [did] not currently exist any abstinence-only programs with reasonably strong evidence that they actually delay the initiation of sex or reduce its frequency." Contradictory conclusions were reported in a separate review of abstinence-education programs conducted by the Heritage Foundation (Rector 2002). In particular, the Heritage report suggests that "abstinence education programs for youth have been proven to be effective in reducing early sexual activity," and the paper identified 10 studies that, it said, demonstrated that abstinence-only programs can reduce sexual activity among

Nicola Bulled, "Knowledge Dissemination" in *Prescribing HIV Prevention: Bringing Culture into Global Health Communication*, pp. 93-127. © 2015 Left Coast Press, Inc. All rights reserved.

youth. To evaluate the contradiction in findings, the National Campaign to Prevent Teen Pregnancy re-examined the 10 studies identified by the Heritage Foundation paper as evidence of reduced early sexual activity (Kirby 2002). Nine of the studies/programs failed to provide evidence that they delayed the initiation of sex or reduced the frequency of sex (the single effective program: Doniger et al. 2001, the nine ineffective programs: Bearman and Bruckner 2001; Borawski et al. 2001; Howard and McCabe 1990; Jorgensen, Potts, and Camp 1993; Resnick et al. 1997; Weed, 1995, 2001; Weed et al. 1992; Weed, Prigmore, and Tanas 2002). While taking an abstinence pledge may delay the initiation of sex among some groups of youth and under certain conditions, it may also decrease the use of contraception when sex is initiated, given concerns over morality of behaviors and shame.

Upon seeing the older white woman enter the classroom the students at LCE, some sharing chairs or seated on broken desks, quickly settled down. The students were already familiar with me, so my presence did little to disturb their chatter. 'Mme Mabitle introduced the guest, "an American (from Virginia), who would be leading today's lesson on HIV." The guest introduced herself as 'Mme Matabo (an assumed Sesotho name) and launched into her interactive two-hour presentation. She noted that the presentation usually required more time, but that she would move through the topics quickly to accommodate the academic schedule.

She began by establishing a contextual frame. She asked students what they idealized as a family unit, their "dream family." They offered the ideas of peaceful situations, with supportive relations, shared respect, unity between family members, and love. 'Mme Matabo recontextualized their statements around the concept of a nuclear family—one mother, one father, and children, though not too many. Few children in Lesotho experience such a family structure growing up. Grandparents, aunts and uncles, distant relatives, or unrelated community members with sufficient resources generally serve as primary providers and caregivers.

Realizing that the "dream family" structure was not part of these students' realities, 'Mme Matabo moved on to directly address current realities of extended family structures, single-parent and child-headed households, making clear the discord that exists between real and ideal and establishing a causal link between behaviors and family structures. She began asking a barrage of questions: *What percentage of youth have sex before marriage?* "None," "Half" responded different students across the room. *What is the average age of sexual debut first in girls?* "15-10-13" yelled out more voices, all female. *What about boys?* "17-12-15" students responded, again all female voices. *How many sexual partners do youth have before they get married?* "None-2-3-5" offered the girls. "10" yelled out a boy. I looked around at the other boys (outnumbered by girls two-to-one at LCE), most were smiling. "Hai no!" responded the girls in disbelief, followed by collective muted laughter. 'Mme Matabo was establishing the argument that the "dream family," idealized as peaceful, respectful relationships, required a nuclear family structure and that this structure is placed at risk by early sexual onset, sexual relations before marriage, and sexual relations with multiple partners.

Next, 'Mme Matabo began to address HIV. Two students were selected from the class, one male and one female. 'Mme Matabo identified them as 'Adam' and 'Eve.' She asked each of them to take a drink of water from separate cups and spit it into a single cup. This seemed harmless enough, but the rising giggles in the class suggested that the onlooking students knew what was coming. The students had seen this, or similar presentations before. I myself had conducted a similar learning exercise with the LCE students in 2004. That particular pedagogical exercise was a bit more visual, as iodine was used to reveal the infected "fluid" that was consumed by all those who drank from a particular cup. 'Mme Matabo began pouring the remnant water/spit mixtures of Adam and Eve back and forth between the cups. The on looking students openly expressed their disgust at this process. Adam and Eve looked nervous. Was she going to make them drink the mixture? The odd look on 'Mme Matabo's face made me think she just might. After substantial, exaggerated pouring back and forth, back and forth, 'Mme Matabo started explaining that the "fluids" mixed in the cup symbolized the shared sexual fluids of Adam and Eve, the class's representative nuclear sexual partnership. The students collectively groaned to indicate their disgust; Adam and Eve blushed.

Adam and Eve were made to remain in the front of the classroom with 'Mme Matabo as she continued with the next part of the lesson—the dangers of having multiple lifetime sexual partners. She started calling up students at random, handing them numbers, 1-2-3-4-5-6-7-8. The girls were told to stand behind Adam, snaking into a longer and longer line. These, 'Mme Matabo explained, were Adam's sexual partners. Would they have to drink from the spit cup? The lengthy line of girls behind Adam offered a striking visual portrayal of just how much fluid exchange could take place inside Adam's body. The message was nothing new to the students in the room, and they enthusiastically assisted 'Mme Matabo to complete her intended lesson—if one of the girls in the line had HIV, any subsequent sexual partner of Adam would also be infected. My iodine visualization offered a similar message. We had constructed sexual networks, all with multiple females for each male, given the unequal gender distribution of students. Individuals within each network had spat into the shared cup, and the iodine had revealed which sexual node carried the infection. Having clearly convinced the majority, 'Mme Matabo quickly moved on to the next section of her presentation.

She proceeded with series of stories and scare tactics warning the students away from the false security offered by condoms. 'Mme Matabo described the case of a sexually transmitted infection causing cancer in a man in Wales that resulted in the amputation of his penis. She pulled out a bag of naartjies (Citrus unshiu, tangerine) and injected one with a red fluid, which she identified as "a poison." Replacing the now infected naartjie, she mixed up the bag of fruit and began offering the naartjies to the students. No one accepted. Her lesson clear, she smiled and clarified that just because the outside looks healthy you do not know what "poison" might exist inside. HIV, she explained, is just such a poison; you cannot tell if it is in someone or not. The image of my former students came into my mind. They had had similar looks of anguish and concern, of fear and helplessness, upon seeing the iodine drops hitting the cups of clear fluid in front of them and the fluid turning, seemingly at random, shades of red. The red revealed an infected cup, and the point at which the infection had entered the sexual network (the shared spitting cup). While I had stressed the importance of condoms as an effect means of HIV prevention, 'Mme Matabo began to preach against the use of condoms as a useful tool to protect against this invisible disease. Although she acknowledge that condoms do offer protection against disease, she stressed that the primary purpose of condoms is "family planning" by "responsible adults," not disease prevention for those who are not yet married.

'Mme Matabo followed the Adam and Eve and poisoned fruit lessons with a sermon of Bible stories, focusing on the importance of remaining true to a single sexual partner. She drew on Proverbs 5:15-18[1] explaining that sex is a good thing, but there is "dirty sex" that brings disease. Using the story of Sodom and Gomorrah from Jude 1: 7, she noted that God warns against sexual immorality and reminds us of the punishment afforded people who engage in illicit behaviors. 'Mme Matabo even revealed that both she and her husband had delayed sexual relations until marriage and had been faithful to each other ever since. During the three occasions when I observed her presentation, this personal revelation always resulted in much chatter among the students. Were students surprised that anyone would be able to, or interested in, limiting their sexual experiences to a single person? Or was their surprise more related to local conventions wherein an elder's open discussion of her sexual habits is considered inappropriate? Did such a personal revelation alter their perspectives of 'Mme Matabo and their evaluation of her message?

The presentation closed with 'Mme Matabo urging students to generate pledge groups in order to assist each other in the development of disease-free dream families by being accountable to others for their behaviors. Before dismissing the students, 'Mme Mabitle, the Life Skills lecturer, took over at the front of the room to offer her gratitude to 'Mme Matabo for delivering such an important message. The lecturer then reiterated 'Mme Matabo's primary points, noting that multiple sexual partners before marriage has a dulling effect, stimulating comparisons with past relationships that cause conflict and criticisms and limiting the powerful experience of love that a faithful partnership can foster. Having been formally dismissed, the students filed out of the classroom in a rush of excitement.

True Love Waits never established pledge groups at LCE during my two year tenure on the campus.

The contradictory results of studies evaluating abstinence-only programs, mentioned at the opening of this chapter, do not suggest that such an approach is ineffective. Rather, they indicate that, given the great diversity of abstinence-only programs combined with very few rigorous studies of their impact, there is simply too little evidence to know whether abstinence-only programs delay the initiation of sex or promote safer sex behaviors in the long-run (Kirby 2002). I remain skeptical that an abstinence-only program can be translated or adapted, or is even appropriate in the Lesotho context where so many youth are forced into sexual relations or who use sex as a way of survival or social mobility (see Chapter 6).

Medium of Knowledge

As is evident in the classroom situation just described, messages about HIV prevention are often in conflict. The True Love Waits' moralistic religious claims promote abstinence over condom use, in contrast to the objective discourse of biomedicine favoring the promotion of condoms and routine testing. Both approaches continue to depend on rational action, though in religious discourse motivations include concerns over morality. Recent research has identified and analyzed characteristics of different sources of HIV information (Blumenreich and Siegel 2006; Chikovore et al. 2009; Eves 2012; Garner 2000, Kotanyi and Krings-Ney 2009; Maluleke 2003a; Mitchell and Smith 2003; Sherman and Bassett 1999; Seidel 1993; Thege 2009). Biomedical HIV knowledge, largely produced in the global North, is disseminated as a 'template of facts' via government agencies, private organizations, popular media, and religion-based HIV prevention campaigns. Knowledge is further contextualized within local situations through news coverage, public policy statements, health initiatives, and even in children's books (Carter and Watney 1989). However, there has been little appreciation of the multiple and often contested discourses around HIV or of how conflicting messages and ideologies intertwine within single knowledge sources, generating confusion, rumors, and social divisions (Treichler 1999; Watney 1991).

In this chapter, I report the results of a survey of 496 first and third year students attending both the Maseru (urban) and Thaba-Tseka (rural) LCE campuses. The self-administered survey measured multiple factors including sources of HIV knowledge, held HIV knowledge, HIV risk and prevention behaviors, and student demographics. I catalogue the sources of HIV knowledge available to and used by the LCE students with whom I engaged between 2010 and 2012, and I present an overview of each of the primary sources of HIV knowledge accessible to youth in Lesotho. I then offer an analytical examination of that medium, including the theoretical foundation or evidence that suggests its effectiveness as a means of risk-reduction knowledge communication. A critical examination of each knowledge source is important, as it is not just message content but also the construct of the source that influences how the message is received and acted upon. Sources of HIV knowledge not only differ in their message content, but they also promote distinct ideologies and hold different social value (Briggs 2003, 2005; Briggs and Hallin 2007). The more the source is valued, the greater the actor buy-in. Sources increase their value further if access is limited.

Figure 4.1 displays the various sources of HIV knowledge accessible to youth in Lesotho. The sources are arranged based on the level at which they are positioned relative to the individual receiving the message from the close interpersonal network to the more distant global structure. Sources vary in print style to indicate the value and utilization of the source by youth (darker type equals more valued, lighter equals less valued). Finally, the value of each source within the global communication structure is categorized within the groups of producer-expert, disseminator-well informed citizen, and message receiver.

The avenues used to transmit HIV knowledge to youth in Lesotho can be grouped into five categories—schools, religions, social networks, medical facilities, and media. These avenues include, but are not limited to the following: radio, television, newspapers, informational pamphlets, health centers, teachers, religious leaders, parents, and friends. The survey results suggest that the primary medium of HIV knowledge changed over the life course: among third year students, a greater proportion identified obtaining knowledge from friends (and family) than first year students, and a smaller proportion identified schools as a source of knowledge. This shift from schools to friends as a primary source of HIV-related knowledge highlights the impact of the college environment, whereby advanced students are acting independently with limited involvement of formerly respected social elders (teachers), living and engaging frequently with peers and beginning to experience romantic and sexual partnerships. While sex is a taboo topic for open discussion in Lesotho (and other ethnic groups in the region), particularly with unmarried

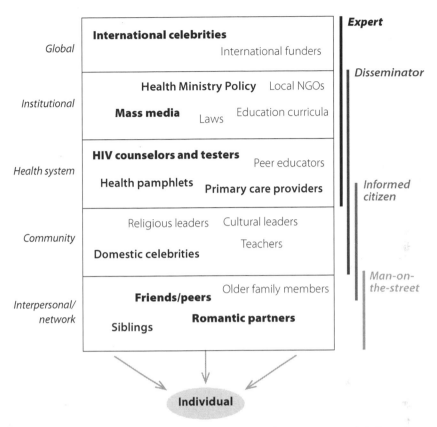

Figure 4.1. Model for HIV prevention communication among youth in Lesotho, representing knowledge sources utilization and value, relative distance from message receiver, and position within the global structure of communication.

youth who are considered too young to have initiated sexual activity (Maluleke 2003b; Romero-Daza 1994a; Setel 1999; Thetela 2002), youth do openly share intimate details with age mates and with romantic and sexual partners. Concerning factual biomedical information, health centers, testing clinics, and other medical facilities are regarded as providing the most accurate information. In Lesotho, certain sources of knowledge (e.g., global media, the Internet, and newspapers) are accessible only in the rapidly modernizing urban environment. However, as shown in Table 4.1, the use of different knowledge sources by LCE students did not differ by urban or rural geographies. Consequently, this chapter explores in greater detail the five primary HIV knowledge sources, given that this student population has relatively equal access to each source.

	School	Social Network	Medical	Media	Total	Chi-Square
Campus						
Meseru	44 (12.43)	67 (18.93)	99 (27.97)	142 (40.11)	354	0.220
Thaba-Tseka	22 (16.06)	17 (12.41)	47 (34.31)	51 (37.23)	137	
Home Environment						
Urban	24 (12.50)	35 (18.23)	62 (32.29)	69 (35.94)	192	0.271
Rural	42 (14.05)	49 (16.39)	84 (28.09)	124 (41.47)	299	
Year of Enrollment						
First Year	40 (18.18)	20 (9.09)	67 (30.45)	92 (41.82)	220	<0.001*
Third Year	26 (9.59)	64 (23.62)	79 (29.15)	101 (37.27)	271	
Total	66 (13.44)	84 (17.11)	146 (29.74)	193 (39.31)	491	

*Significance at $\alpha<0.05$

Table 4.1. Comparison of LCE students (percentages) using various avenues as their primary source of HIV prevention knowledge, by campus, area of origin, and year of enrollment

Schools

School-based HIV/AIDS prevention programs are widely and consistently recommended as an appropriate avenue to target young people (WHO 2006). The Population and Family Development curriculum of the 1990s was Lesotho's first attempt at delivering school-based HIV prevention messages. As in other countries in the region, including South Africa and Zimbabwe, communities did not like the material taught, arguing it promoted youth sexuality (Chikovore et al. 2009; Mgomezulu and Kruger 2011). In discussing this matter with 'Mme Mabitle, the former Population and Family Development instructor at LCE and current Life Skills lecturer on the LCE-Maseru campus, she agreed that the material originally taught was not always appropriate for each intended age group. She explained that information was sometimes too explicit for younger students, or too abstract for older students. Primary school classrooms in Lesotho often contain a wide age-range of students as pupils are advanced based on abilities not age. Consequently, older students in need of more explicit sexual education messages may not receive it. In addition, due to Lesotho's cultural taboo in discussing sex, proposed school-based youth education about reproduction was considered obscene and inappropriate (see Thetela 2002 for discussion of sex discourses and social constructions among Basotho).

Integrative approaches, in addition to specific HIV/AIDS lessons and sex education courses, were also used to convey HIV-awareness messages in schools. This strategy involved the incorporation or integration of HIV prevention and stigma-reduction messages into existing lessons of health, physical education, and biology. However, not all the courses into which these HIV messages were integrated were compulsory, and thus the integration approach was considered by both national and international reviewers as inadequate at a population level (Chendi 1999; Gachuhi 1999; NAC 2009b).

Beginning in 2004, the Population and Family Development, HIV, and Sexual Education lecturers at LCE began to work collaboratively to develop a Life Skills curriculum to instruct their education students how to appropriately teach issues of sexuality and HIV prevention in the classroom. The idea was to combine the elements of sexual education, HIV knowledge and prevention, problem solving, and critical analysis into a single course that increased students' critical awareness of the HIV crisis. The Life Skills course at LCE became compulsory in 2006 for all first year students.

A national Life Skills curriculum for primary and secondary schools in Lesotho now exists. Initially piloted in 2006 and 2007, primary and secondary schools began implementing the curriculum in 2008. Topics addressed include conflict resolution, self-awareness, and confidence, as well as relationships and sex in accordance with age and sexual maturity. The curriculum was originally designed in an effort to broaden skills in problem solving, communication, and negotiation, with much less emphasis placed on biomedical HIV knowledge dissemination. In addition, the curriculum does not directly address taboo topics such as sex and substance abuse. Curriculum developers were sensitive to the local concerns of teachers in being explicit about HIV prevention strategies, primarily the negotiation and use of condoms. As explained by Mpho Maketela,[2] who is in charge of Life Skills at the National Curriculum Development Center of the Ministry of Education, the national curriculum developers perceived that HIV would not be a primary concern for youth in Lesotho in the near future. As a result, schools were encouraged to collaborate with NGOs such as Kick4Life,[3] Population Services International, Lesotho Planned Parenthood Association, and Phela Health and Development Communication[4] to ensure that students received a complete set of skills and messages that complemented rather than contradicted each other. For example, Maketela suggested NGOs could offer condom demonstrations or discuss sexually transmitted infections in a more open manner, filling the void left by the national curriculum and state teachers. Many NGO workers in Lesotho are not Basotho and those that are do not have the same established relationships with the school children that their teachers do, making it easier and more appropriate to have explicit conversations. The student reactions to 'Mme Matabo's explicitness suggests that regardless of who engages in the discourse of sex education it remains an uncomfortable and awkward conversation. The national curriculum is currently being revised to address HIV and related topics more directly and was to be piloted in 2013.

Although school-based HIV prevention programs are encouraged by the global community, and teachers in general believe that HIV/AIDS is an important topic that should be taught in schools at all grade levels (Ballard, White, and Glascoff 1990; Boscarino and DiClemente 1996; Dawson et al. 2001), there is little evidence of the effectiveness of such interventions especially in low- and middle-income countries (Kaaya et al. 2002; Kirby, Laris, and Rolleri 2007; WHO 2006). One possible reason for the limited effectiveness may relate to the frequency and consistency with which the source is used to deliver HIV prevention messages. The Lesotho National AIDS Commission (NAC) believes Life Skills courses to be an underperforming HIV prevention measure, as the target population across all districts is not consistently reached (NAC 2009c). According to Maketela at the National Curriculum Development Center, an internal study conducted by the Ministry of Education in 2010 revealed that, although most primary schools report that they are teaching the subject of Life Skills, only about half of all secondary schools do. Many teachers feel it is not a necessary subject, as they believe more time should be devoted to subjects that have national examinations. These standardized national examinations are used as a measure of a student's academic performance and future potential as he/she advances to subsequence academic institutions.

Another possible explanation for the lack of effectiveness of existing school-based interventions is that they are not implemented with sufficient fidelity (James et al. 2006; Mukoma et al. 2009; Visser, Shoeman, and Perold 2004). In the region, pedagogical autonomy on the part of the teacher is valued, with such autonomy characteristic of excellent teachers (Helleve et al. 2011). Such autonomy, though aligned with the culture-centered communication approach, may reduce the fidelity of the intervention's implementation by failing to address or inappropriately addressing disease prevention knowledge and skills. Maketela of Lesotho's Curriculum Development Center noted that teachers often have the national curriculum books, but do not reference them. Following her routine observations of LCE student teachers during their teaching practice year, the Maseru-based Life Skills lecturer, 'Mme Mabitle, similarly observed the limited use of the national Life Skills curriculum. She regarded the student teachers as either "incompetent or over confident." If they followed the curriculum at all, she observed that they often skipped ahead to more difficult yet not necessarily age appropriate content.

Of the two LCE Life Skills lecturers (one based in Maseru, the other in Thaba-Tseka), I found that neither followed, nor referenced, the national curriculum in her own class. Few students were aware that a standardized Life Skills curriculum even existed. There were no copies of the national curriculum available for reference in either of the campus libraries. Both lecturers at LCE have established their own unique curriculum that aims to teach life skills to their education students. Neither frames her instruction in a way that provides students with the skills to teach Life Skills. Their courses could be structured to conscientiously work through the established national curriculum, examining the lesson plans as developed and negotiating age-appropriate activities and learning goals. In establishing their own curriculum they not only set a bad precedence for their students, but also left out important learning elements based on their own personal perspectives and interests. For instance, the lecturer at LCE-Thaba-Tseka, though very good at discussing issues regarding human relationships and love in an age appropriate manner with her LCE students, was uncomfortable discussing the topic of HIV. She requested that the Maseru-based lecturer or visiting lecturers (including me) handle the HIV aspects of the Life Skills course. Should another lecturer be unable to make it to LCE-Thaba-Tseka in a given semester, then class discussions specifically related to HIV were not conducted.

This LCE lecturer was not alone in being uncomfortable talking about HIV. An assessment of the utilization of Life Skills curricula in public schools throughout Lesotho revealed that few teachers feel comfortable discussing the subject matter (Kolosoa and Makhakhane 2010). Evaluations of school-based HIV-prevention programs in South Africa found that a subset of teachers believed that certain aspects of the interventions addressing sexuality contradicted their own values and beliefs, and that they preferred talking about abstinence instead of safer sex practices (Ahmed et al. 2009; Mukoma et al. 2009). In this, schools serve as the site of collisions of competing views of sexuality, health and illness, modern and traditional norms, sources of authoritative knowledge and morality, and child and adult relations (Adams and Pigg 2005; Silin 1995; Treichler 1999; Weeks 1999). Teachers commonly report feeling uncomfortable or unprepared to teach HIV/AIDS and sexuality (Hausman and Ruzek 1995; Prater and Serna 1993). Specifically, teachers regularly report feeling least prepared to address topics related to social, emotional, and societal issues and most comfortable or prepared to discuss factual information on topics such as HIV transmission (Levenson Gingiss and Basen-Engquist 1994; Levenson Gingiss and Hamilton 1989a). Additionally, teachers report discomfort with particular teaching strategies, such as role-playing, problem-solving, and small-group discussions (Haignere et al. 1996). Studies have also consistently found that teachers have limited in-service and pre-service training in HIV and sexuality education (Kerr, Allensworth, and Gayle 1989), and that teacher preparation programs do not sufficiently address HIV and sexuality education (Rodriguez et al. 1995; Shripak and Summerfield 1996).

Several studies show gains in teachers' knowledge and confidence after participation in in-service or pre-service training programs and courses (Levenson Gingiss and Hamilton 1989b; Remafedi 1993). For example, a study conducted among 8th and 9th grade Life Skills teachers in South Africa and 5th and 7th grade science teachers in public schools in Tanzania found that confidence in teaching on the subject matter significantly improved with formal training (Helleve, Flisher, Onya, Kaaya, et al. 2009; Helleve, Flisher, Onya, Mukoma, et al. 2009). Confidence also increased relative to the number of years teaching HIV/AIDS and sexuality, experience discussing the topic with others, and school policy and priority given to teaching HIV prevention at school.

When assessing schools as a source of HIV knowledge it is, therefore, critical that we examine the process of how knowledge is delivered, including the perceptions and challenges of those delivering the message and the interpersonal context in which delivery takes place. We must also consider that pedagogical styles preferring direct transfers of objective information, as opposed to development of subjective problem-solving skills, represent larger societal and global inequities in power distribution (see Chapter 6).

Religion

Religious ideologies play an important role in the lives of many Basotho. Over 80 percent of Basotho identify as Christian, attending Catholic, Lutheran, Methodist, and Pentagon church services regularly (CIA 2010). This trait is shared with neighboring South Africa, which Robert Garner (2000, 46) called "one of the most 'churchy' countries in the world," noting that half of the population attends church once a week or more.

The LCE campus hosts at least five different churches' services every Saturday and Sunday for students and members of the neighboring community. Additional religious institutions transport students to and from off-site churches on a weekly basis. Students are also involved in church-affiliated youth groups wherein gender roles, love, faithfulness, and abstinence are discussed. Youth also develop close relationships with their pastors, to whom they turn when in need of someone to discuss relationship concerns, including matters of HIV risk.

When I was last in Lesotho in 2012, Basotho and South African gospel music was still very popular among youth, and performing artists often expressly addressed issues related to HIV. For youth who did not attend church services regularly, HIV teachings were accessible via religious-affiliated radio stations (e.g., Harvest FM) and programs, television broadcastings, and Christian-based magazine advice columns. It was therefore not surprising that some element of Christian faith should enter into local discourse of HIV. As Alex de Waal states, the "language of sin and morality is perhaps the most pervasive of all in public discourse on AIDS" (2003, 248). HIV has "called attention to moral judgments and their impact on disease as few modern diseases could have" (Brandt and Rozin 1997, 3).

Given the important function that the church plays in Lesotho, the use of religion as a vehicle for sexual socialization is logical (see Billingsley and Morrison-Rodriguez 1998; Garner 2000). However, while religious leaders do offer guidance on related matters such as love, relationships, and marriage, they were generally not regarded as offering knowledge of HIV by LCE students, and certainly not of biomedical knowledge. This perception may relate to source credibility (Gottlieb and Sarel 1991; Ward and McGinnies 1974).

According to Mokete Hlaelae,[5] the Executive Director of the umbrella organization, Lesotho Inter-religious AIDS Consortium (LIRAC), religious leaders continued to preach that HIV was a punishment from God, linking HIV to morality. This message was understood by youth in two primary ways: first, that HIV had been sent to punish all of humanity for being sinners—"[HIV] is from God, maybe we have angered God" (male LCE-Maseru student); and second, that HIV was the punishment for individuals who act in immoral ways, specifically people who have sex outside the confines of marriage—"I cannot enjoy having a lot of girlfriends because that is a sin" (male LCE-Maseru student; interpretation of Jude 1:7 offered by 'Mme Matabo).

Strong religious ideologies ingrained in contemporary Basotho culture significantly impacted other sources of information. For example, both LCE-Life Skills lecturers brought a religious element to their teaching. They quoted passages from the Bible, used religious parables as teaching tools, and exhibited their personal religious connection through the display of rosary beads or the use of prayers. According to the Life Skills lecturer at the Maseru campus, having organizations such as True Love Waits address the students offered an alternative perspective on the HIV epidemic. This comment suggested that the students had been offered other perspectives, had previously engaged in discussions of the scientific evidence of HIV transmission and prevention, and had been challenged to reflect on contradictions existing among scientific, religious, and cultural cosmologies of HIV. Yet, for the particular set of first year students I observed and engaged with, no scientific information was presented during their Life Skills sessions, and, no opportunity was provided to discuss the alternative messages. 'Mme Matabo's abstinence message was delivered during the final scheduled meeting time of the semester-long course, which was the only session exclusively devoted to the topic of HIV. The rosary beads around 'Mme Mabitle's neck and the invitation of a Christian-based abstinence prevention program clearly indicated the close link between the secular educational institution's ideologies and religious teachings of morality.

The moralizing language and continued focus on abstinence as an HIV prevention strategy within the Life Skills lessons offered within the secular educational institution resulted in significant confusion about HIV risk behaviors, as illustrated in the following conversation with a 22-year-old female LCE-Thaba-Tseka student.

> *Student:* Once vaginal intercourse has taken place there will be contact, so there is high risk of infection.
>
> *Interviewer:* When you say high risk, do you mean that if your partner is positive there is 100% likelihood that you will be infected with unprotected sex?
>
> *Student:* Definitely yes.
>
> *Interviewer:* What if I told you that that is incorrect.
>
> *Student:* No. There would be an argument I think. I would disagree with you.
>
> *Interviewer:* That would mean that any time a boy had unprotected sex with a girl they would be infected.
>
> *Student:* Maybe the partners were HIV negative.
>
> *Interviewer:* No, even if they are HIV positive.
>
> *Student:* They will not?
>
> *Interviewer:* They will not necessarily get HIV. The viral load may be low or the person may have a strong immune system. The chance of transmission to someone else is not 100%. There are things that can increase the chance of transmission, like if the viral load is high, if the person has just been infected, or if people have wounds on their private parts due to STI.
>
> *Student:* So it is possible that they cannot infect each other even though the other partner is infected?
>
> *Interviewer:* Yes.

The moralized discourse of HIV contributes to the stigmatization of HIV infection. In Lesotho, HIV remains highly stigmatized, causing low national rates of routine HIV testing, and delayed initiation and maintenance of treatment protocols (NAC 2009b). Such discourse influences students' willingness to test for HIV. As noted by one third year male Maseru-campus student, "I don't want to test because if I find out that I am positive, I will always feel guilty. I am a religious person and believe that when one has sinned God will not forgive you and you will go to hell when you die." HIV has been further marked by stigma as the disease was first identified among men who have sex with men, a morally unacceptable practice in Lesotho (Brown, BeLue, and Airhihenbuwa 2011; Muturia and Soontae 2010; Shilts 1987; Skerritt 2011).

In a study of different Christian churches in KwaZulu-Natal South Africa, Robert Garner (2000) found that engagement in HIV risk behaviors, specifically sexual liberties including pre- and extra-marital affairs, varied relative to church membership. According to Garner, members of Pentecostal churches had significantly reduced risky sexual behaviors as compared to members of other churches. He suggested that these behaviors were related to the Pentecostal churches' provision of a complete social experience that included indoctrination, exclusion, and socialization. It could also be argued that individuals desiring to change their behaviors (perhaps from those locally considered immoral, i.e., infidelity) seek out institutions that require significant personal dedication. As such, an alternative interpretation of Garner's findings implies that reductions in risky sexual behaviors may not be limited to the unique characteristics of the religious institution but may also involve the characteristics of the individual receiving the message.

Medical

Given its association with biomedical institutions, LCE students considered information acquired from health clinics and medical staff to be the most credible of all the HIV knowledge sources available to them. Informational pamphlets produced and distributed via health centers and educational institutions by the local public health communication organization, Phela Health and Development Communication, provided the template of objective, factual information about HIV, transmission routes, ways to prevent infection, and associated diseases and health conditions. Traditional healers were never mentioned as a source of HIV knowledge.

Counseling and testing facilities   Students also acquired comprehensive HIV knowledge when sitting one-on-one with a counselor during the process of HIV testing. Based on the data acquired from LCE students between 2010 and 2012, almost 70 percent of LCE students self-reported a prior HIV test, with 40 percent tested within the prior six months. Testing behavior did not differ significantly by geography (rural or urban) or year of enrollment at LCE. However, significantly more female students had tested than male students ($\chi2$=8.632; p=0.0133). Of the 30 percent of students who had not yet tested, 70 percent noted a desire to test and almost 90 percent indicated knowing where to get tested. When asked why they had not already tested, students often noted that they were "not ready."

In the first week of the 2012 academic year, 25 HIV tests were performed at the LCE-Maseru campus clinic (see Figures 4.2 and 4.3). Contrary to national statistics, which indicate 20 percent prevalence among the 18-24 year age group (NAC 2012), 100 percent of students tested at the LCE campus clinic screened negative for HIV infection. These results and the statements of readiness, suggest that stigma still impacts local testing behaviors. However, the resident HIV counselor and tester at the campus clinic[6] did not believe that perceived likelihood of infection status impacted students' willingness to test. According to the counselor, students who believed they were infected, given their risky behaviors, tested more frequently and those who presumed they were not infected avoided testing. The results of my survey in 2011 and 2012 confirmed the counselor's perceptions. Of students who perceived themselves at high risk of infection (100 percent likelihood of infection), 91 percent had tested for HIV, whereas, of students who perceived themselves to be at no risk of HIV infection (0 percent likelihood of infection), 79 percent had tested. My survey did not ask for and did not measure HIV status. As a result, HIV status of the students relative to perception of risk and testing behaviors was unknown. The contradiction between students' risk perceptions and their HIV test results might indicate an error in risk evaluation. This error may relate back to the excessive warnings about transmission routes and confusion about relative risk of virus exposures. Alternatively, the incongruence between students' calculated risks, testing behaviors, and test results may relate more to the test results than to the inaccurately calculated risk exposure. Students who knew they were HIV positive believed/knew their likelihood of infection to be high, whereas those who knew they were HIV negative believed/knew their likelihood of infection to be low.

While perceptions of risk behaviors and expected test results may or may not have influenced testing behaviors in this population, concerns over the confidentiality of results significantly inhibited testing. Expressing the concern of many of his fellow students, a 26-year-old, male LCE-Maseru student explained that he did not want to test because the testers could not be trusted to keep the results confidential. His own mother was employed as an HIV counselor and tester, indicating his personal experience hearing the HIV status of members of his community. He said, "I don't feel comfortable going. My mother is a tester, working hand-in-hand with hospitals. If you are very close with the people doing the testing, they may tell their friends if a person test-

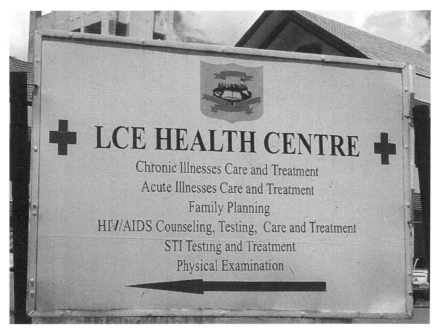

Figure 4.2. Sign for LCE-Maseru Health Center.

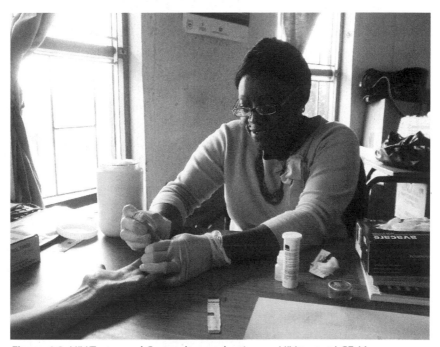

Figure 4.3. HIV Tester and Counselor conducting an HIV test at LCE-Maseru health clinic.

ed positive." Lack of confidentiality of HIV test results is a well-documented problem in Lesotho (see Human Rights Watch & AIDS and Rights Alliance for Southern Africa 2008). Given the socially linked association with immoral behaviors, lack of confidential testing is a serious concern, as it inhibits voluntary testing for fear of lost privacy and future discrimination.

Having played a part in ensuring the establishment of the HIV testing clinic on the LCE Maseru campus, I went through the testing process with the newly hired HIV counselor. Prior to 2012, testing had been conducted by the staff nurses. To begin the session the counselor pulled out a large ledger labeled "HIV counseling and testing," into which she wrote down my full name, the date, my prior testing history, and the test result. This ledger remained on the desk that she shared with another administrative LCE staff member. The office was the site of registering all LCE students seeking health care services and the clinic's waiting room. The other LCE staff member continued to walk in and out of the office, never knocking or requesting entrance as the testing and counseling session continued. I described my various risk behaviors, and my test strip developed on the tabletop.

According to the LCE counselor, the record of names and testing histories was maintained for multiple reasons. First, if people test routinely the ledger served as a record of their testing history. This record was important for determining recent infections for the benefit of the patient, as well as national records. Second, once an individual tested positive he/she was not encouraged to test again. According to the LCE counselor, national policy stipulated that when an individual seeks treatment services the clinicians must call the original testing facility to confirm infection status rather than retesting. This policy was in place (according to the LCE tester) because many individuals attempted to clear HIV from their body using traditional medicines (*muti*) or commercially marketed immune boosters for sale in any supermarket, pharmacy, and street market. These products apparently interfered with the HIV test's chemical processes and caused retests to appear negative. As no formal identification is required to prove identity, clients seeking HIV testing services could offer false names to retain their identity. However, with an established HIV counselor on staff at LCE, this method of maintaining anonymity would become increasingly more difficult with routine testing.

The counseling component of the testing session covered the basics of possible routes of exposure (e.g., sexual, blood contact); ways to prevent infection (e.g., limiting number of sexual partners, using condoms, using gloves when exposed to bodily fluids); routine retesting; and engagement in risk behaviors. I was asked to consider if I had been exposed to HIV and the route of exposure. I listed my potential exposures: occasional grazes from potentially contaminated syringes during my work with the needle exchange in Boston;

multiple lifetime sexual partners; unprotected sex with a marriage partner who had recently tested HIV negative on a required immigration medical clearance exam. Startled either by my frankness or the extent of my varied and unfamiliar exposure routes, the counselor took a moment to collect her thoughts. Taking a deep breath she launched into her much practiced routine. The fact that my sexual relationship is monogamous had no effect on her message, representing the current country and regional surveillance data that suggest marriage is the greatest risk factor for HIV infection in women. She repeatedly stressed that even one unprotected sexual encounter could result in infection and that a partner's HIV status is not indicative of one's own status. She did not refer to my needle-stick exposures. I assume she neglected this aspect for two reasons: the exposure was part of a job I had in the past and was unlikely to be repeated in the future; and injection drug use was uncommon in Lesotho, and therefore the counselor had limited experience with this route of infection and the work involved in a needle exchange program.

After 20-minutes the test result was carefully read and described. If a test indicated a positive HIV status, the counselor would offer details on treatment facilities, including the treatment provided at the LCE campus clinic. If it indicated an HIV-negative result and the client engaged in high risk behaviors, the counselor explained the possibility of a recent infection within the testing "window-period" and encouraged testing again within the next three months. If the test was negative and the client did not engage in high risk behaviors, the counselor would still recommend routine testing every three months.

Though my own counseling session provided few particulars on HIV and HIV prevention, conversations and interviews with students suggested that those who had been tested obtained a better understanding of the biology of the virus, the HIV test design, and risk behaviors. This idea was further confirmed by the findings from my survey, which included a measure of HIV knowledge. Students who tested frequently held greater HIV knowledge than those who had never tested, and had fewer misconceptions regarding local mythology including the virgin cure or transmission by mosquitoes. Students who had tested for HIV identified medical personnel as their primary source of knowledge more frequently than students who had not tested. Moreover, students who identified medical personnel, including HIV counselors and testers, as their primary source of HIV knowledge had the second highest mean HIV knowledge sum scores following individuals who identified schools as their primary source of knowledge.

Yet, not all counselors provided accurate information. Teboho, a popular 23-year-old male student from the Thaba-Tseka campus, offered one example of the inaccurate information relayed by an HIV testing counselor. He described how he prevented HIV infection:

> They are a little bit tricky to practice perfectly, but I know if I make a mistake I may have a chance to get infected. After having sex, I know very well that I am not supposed to get in contact with the CD (condom) because I am supposed to wrap it with toilet paper and use gloves. So I know how to prevent, but I don't always practice it.

Teboho believed that touching the condom itself following use during intercourse could result in infection as the virus from the vaginal fluid and semen on the condom could penetrate through "cuts in your hands and fingers." Consequently, much care had to be taken to remove the condom. As he noted, he knew that he should prevent exposure to the potentially contaminated condom, using a tissue, toilet paper, or gloves to handle it. However, he claimed that he did not always practice the prevention behavior. It was not clear to me whether Teboho did not always use toilet paper to prevent touching the condom, or just did not use condoms consistently because removing them became too much bother. Safe handling of a potentially contaminated condom was stressed upon Teboho by an HIV counselor and tester. Other examples of inaccurate or overly simplified messages included stressing that every sexual encounter is risky, that assisting HIV positive people without gloves is high risk, and that kissing is a transmission route for the virus.

While medical professionals and medical facilities generally provided students with accurate biomedical knowledge, medical practitioners producing and delivering the knowledge (as well as those receiving the information) might imbue personal meanings and interpretations on biomedical facts. The HIV counselors' high position in society, given their connection to the medical realm, impacts the value of the messages they convey. As noted above, students considered information obtained from a biomedicine-affiliated source to be more credible than information acquired from other avenues. Given this assumption, extreme caution should be employed to ensure that the information delivered by HIV counselors is accurate and conveyed in an appropriate manner.

In a critique of the HIV counseling and testing guidelines developed by the US Centers for Disease Control and Prevention, Mattson noted that the process of message delivery is equally as important as the message content. He argued that "current conceptualization and practices of HIV test counseling needs to be reframed in favor of an explicit harm reduction approach that postulates a redistribution of power between the counselor and client toward dialogue that is agency promoting and empowering" (Mattson 2000, 336). As HIV test counseling is an important point of contact with individuals who have likely engaged in unsafe behaviors, the interaction should be utilized to its full potential. Clients are intimately familiar with what is important and relevant to them, and therefore, Mattson argued, the emphasis should be on client discourse and the negotiation of strategies for safer practices that maximize the reduction of harm, rather than a lecture on general risk behaviors.

Peer education   In an effort to address the power differentials noted by Mattson that are inherent in the counseling and testing setting, the peer education model has been established and perpetuated around the globe. The peer education intervention design has been considered one of the most effective strategies for knowledge dissemination and promotion of behavior change (UNAIDS 1999b; Wingood and DiClemente 1996). The approach assumes that peer educators are more approachable, use language that peers understand, know of specific cultural risk behaviors and of the most appropriate and realistic risk-reduction strategies for the community, are considered credible sources of information, and serve as positive role models. In its ideal context and under ideal conditions, peer education is founded on the premise that in contrast to the authority conferred on medical providers as a result of their objectivity and factual knowledge, as noted by Wilson (2000):

> People evaluate changes not on the basis of scientific evidence or authoritative testimony, but by subjective judgments of close, trusted peers who have adopted changes and provide persuasive role models for change.

In a review of the literature, Wolf, Tawfik, and Bond (2000) found that peer education is a cost-effective strategy and that educators address the perceptions of friends' sexual behaviors, which are an influential predictor of sexual behavior particularly among youth. In Africa, HIV peer educators have been used in such diverse populations as dock workers in Nigeria (Ogundare 1998); taxi drivers in Cameroon (Moughtou 1998); truck drivers in Zimbabwe (Mupemba 1999); low- and middle-class individuals in Zambia (Kathuria et al. 1998); factory workers in Zimbabwe (Katzenstein et al. 1998); traditional healers in South Africa (UNAIDS 1999b); female sex workers in Kenya and Zimbabwe (Ngugi et al. 1996); a mining settlement in Tanzania (Mollel et al. 1995); prisoners in Mozambique (Vaz, Gloyd, and Trindale 1996); workers in Botswana (Hope 2003); high school students in The Gambia (Mahe and Travers 1997-1998); and university students in Kenya (Miller et al. 2008). For an account of peer education campaigns in Lesotho with accompanying video see the UNICEF report and video by Tsitsi Singizi (2011). In these various situations, evaluations indicate positive results including significant increases in HIV knowledge acquisition, behavior change, and lower HIV incidence. Nevertheless, peer education programs may fail to meet such outcome expectations as a consequence of improperly trained peer educators, intergroup relations characterized by jealousy and competitiveness, or the underlying assumption of the strategy regarding Western notions of a bounded self.

My work in Lesotho with students at LCE suggested that a limited proportion of students had interacted with and 'acquired knowledge from' specially trained peer educators (9 percent of surveyed population) or undergone training to become peer educators themselves (8 percent of surveyed population). Though potentially effective in improving the knowledge of those actively engaged in the peer education process, peer education campaigns were not considered an important source of HIV knowledge by LCE students who were exposed to this medium of education. For youth in Lesotho, peer educators did not hold positions of social authority, and thus their messages of risk reduction were not highly valued. Moshoeshoe, a male student from LCE-Maseru campus, who held a lay clinic counselor certificate in HIV (a peer educator), explained the problematic position of peer education in Lesotho. He said:

> I need help on how to advise people around here about how to have a
> better future…normally youths do not listen to people of the same age.
> They take me for granted because some of them can't believe I have been
> engaged in these HIV and AIDS campaigns. They think I am telling them
> about things I have no experience with.

These perceptions are supported by research on a peer education programs among similar age groups in Kenya (Miller et al. 2008) and Venda, South Africa (McNeill 2011).

Social network

In the past, social networks were more involved in the sexual socialization of youth in Lesotho than they are today. In many African cultures, elders and authorized members of society ran socially-sanctioned culture or initiation schools wherein, upon reaching puberty, girls and boys would be taught about gender roles and social obligations, including sexual expectations. Parents were not permitted to talk with their children about sexuality. Social elders conducted the coming-of-age ceremonies, schooling youth on appropriate feminine and masculine behaviors and roles (Tamale 2005). Training not only focused on sexuality and gender roles, but also emphasized "chastity, honesty, reliability, courage, humility, and respect for parents, elders and the chief" (Magubane 1998, 108). In addition to providing a socially accepted channel for sexual discourse, initiation rites expressed a universal and consistent message, and established norms of sexual behaviors (Muyinda, Kengeya, and Pool 2001). Puberty rites ceremonies were, or in some communities still are, the only appropriate space for open discussion about sexuality.

As I discovered during my ethnographic work, initiation schools still take place in Lesotho, though more frequently for boys than for girls. However, for the LCE students whom I studied, friends (not formal peer educators, cultural leaders, or initiation trainers) comprised the primary social network members with whom they engaged in discussions of sex and consequently HIV risk behaviors. Many learned about sexual behaviors from observations of, or engagements with, more experienced friends, from whom they found out about when sexual relationships should be initiated and who to have sexual relationships with. The students also learned from their sexual partner(s), who offered ideas about sexual techniques, including the use of condoms. Finally, they observed and emulated the behaviors of older siblings, parents, aunts, uncles, and guardians.

Few LCE students openly discussed matters of sexual behavior with their parents or other family members. Matters of sexual behavior proved very awkward for parents, as they believed their children would laugh at them if they tried to have frank conversations on the topic. A married female LCE-Maseru student described what she perceived as her unique family situation:

> My mother, she is not a stereotypical Mosotho woman. I would sit down when I was still a girl and ask her questions related to sex. But, I didn't just go straight to the point, I tried to say "Do you think I could really be pregnant?" I wanted her to start to break that shyness. Then she would talk, she would tell me everything, but she never mentioned the word sex. After I was married it was then that she told me everything. We would talk a lot, but not about sex. We would talk about affairs, how she wants me to behave, when she wants me to come back home. We would talk about everything, excluding sex.

The taboo against discussing matters of sex, sexuality, and consequently HIV infection included concealing engagements in romantic or sexual relationships from elders. Parents, especially, are not to know if youth have boyfriends or girlfriends, as it is considered inappropriate for young people to have relationships and rude to openly reveal these relationships. During my observations of students at the LCE campuses, I rarely saw couples embrace or hold hands, and I rarely ever saw a male and female student alone together. This secrecy encouraged two HIV-related risk behaviors. First, rather than encouraging public displays of affection such as hand holding, hugging, being in close proximity, and kissing, young couples needed to find secret spaces to be physically close to each other. Secret meetings in private spaces limited the ability of either partner to prevent actions they might not desire, as there were fewer ways to escape politely or to call for help. In addition, secret meetings might foster sexual relations that were rushed and consequently unprotected. Second, when youth were away from home, such as living on the college campus or engaging in migratory labor, they were no longer bound by social obligations to family or extended communities and took liberties to engage in romantic and sexual relationships, often with multiple partners concurrently. According to the Lesotho DHS, among youth of age 15-24, 4.0 percent of females and 20.5 of males had more than two sexual partners in the previous 12-month period (MoHSW 2009). For some LCE students, these multiple relationships functioned as a way of identifying a viable marriage partner, as having more than one partner simultaneously allowed for "side-by-side" comparisons.

Many LCE students expressed a desire to break the barrier of silence that existed between parents and children in discussing romantic relationships, sex, and sexuality. Some wished that their parents had spoken with them more openly when they were living at home, and many said they were determined to speak more openly with their own children. For instance, a 19-year-old, first year, female Maseru-LCE student expressed her desire for more open conversations between parents and children. She said, "I think you [in America] are free to talk with your parents…here it is too much. Basotho respect their culture a lot…I want to be free with [my children]." She referenced traditional Basotho 'culture' as a form of restraint and in opposition to the perceived freedom of open conversation she imagines exists in the US. In this she expressed the commonly shared sentiment among urban youth in Lesotho that modern lifestyles, ways, and technologies are better.

The movement towards urbanization, modernization, and a focus on formal education introduced both physical and time constraints on holding prolonged ceremonies that had served as the primary root for sex-education in Lesotho and surrounding countries (Chakanza 1998; Jules-Rosette 1980; Kotanyi and Krings-Ney 2009; Magubane 1998; Maluleke 2003a, b; Maluleke and Troskie 2003; Pearsons 1990; Phiri 1998; Rasing 1995, 1999, 2001; Richards 1982; Shorter 1991; Turner 1957). Despite the previously important roles these ceremonies served in society, the performance of initiation rites in Lesotho has declined. Even so, research indicates that traditional authorities, including existing practitioners and initiation rites counselors, continue to hold significant influence over people's behaviors (Bukali de Graca 2004; Green 1999; Sitholi 2001; Wolf 2007; Wreford 2008). As a result, initiation rites have been explored as possible avenues for the distribution of biomedical HIV knowledge (Kotanyi and Krings-Ney 2009; Maluleke 2003a; McNeill 2011), based on evidence suggesting that HIV prevention counseling is more effective when connected within culturally based sexual education (a culturally-sensitive approach) (UNAIDS 2000). A study conducted by the Islamic Medical Association of Uganda (1998, 14) found that "individuals are more likely to adopt safer-sex practices if they are perceived as the norm prevailing among their peers and community." These efforts have been further aided by an increasing interest in developing local solutions to HIV, contextualized within the African Renaissance movement. Most notable among these efforts is the resurgence of virginity-testing in communities in Kwa-Zulu Natal, South Africa (a culture-centered approach) (Leclerc-Madlala 2001, 2005; Scorgie 2002).

There have been mixed responses to attempts to utilize the resurgence of tradition, or integration of HIV communication efforts into still-existing culturally based education, as a means of reducing HIV risk behaviors. In an area in South Africa's Limpopo Province, the former Venda *Bantustan*, anthropologist Fraser McNeill (2011, 106) paints an image of conflict and resistance as young female initiates try to bring their modern biomedical knowledge of HIV into the realm dominated by traditional knowledge:

> The only knowledge which was acceptable was that which was shared by the older women.... What did not constitute plausible courses of social action, however, for the senior elderly women who were most dismissive of the girls' references to AIDS, were antiretroviral therapy and the use of condoms. Whilst undoubtedly such things were known to these women, their material existence and physical usage fell outside the core of a lived experience and social milieu shared by old women in rural Venda.

McNeill argues that biomedical knowledge is unlikely to be incorporated into ritual curriculum as it is "currently beyond the boundaries of what should be known and what can be controlled by ritual experts" (2011, 112). In contrast to McNeill's findings in Venda, research in Mozambique suggested that training the ritual experts (rather than the young initiates) in the nuances of biomedical HIV knowledge may facilitate the integration of scientific AIDS education into still existing female initiation ceremonies (Kotanyi and Krings-Ney 2009). Targeting education towards the community elders may limit the threat imposed by biomedical knowledge supplied by the youth on established hierarchical structures of authority.

These cases indicate that re-traditionalization, aimed at strengthening the role that formal social networks have in HIV prevention, has taken two distinct paths. The case of virginity-testing promoting chastity in the name of HIV prevention has embraced biomedical models as a way to reinvent past traditions as modern and relevant. Nevertheless, while the intentions of the biomedical "abstinence" and the virginity-testing "chastity" models overlap, the rationale and logics upon which virginity is determined are not aligned. As a result, virginity testing is an example of the culture-centered approach, as it is a culturally constructed and maintained institution managed under logics and knowledge that lie outside the biomedical frame. In contrast, integration of biomedical knowledge within the puberty rites structures offers an example of the cultur-ally-sensitive approach to health communication. Here, biomedical knowledge finds a culturally appropriate avenue for dissemination but assumes authority over ritual or traditional knowledge. This discord sheds light on the distinctions of the two bodies of knowledge (ritual/traditional and biomedical) and the an-tagonism that can occur as a result of their coexistence. Both are powerful en-tities, and afford those with access and ownership social positions of privilege.

Mass media

Mass media, including television, radio, and newspapers, are routinely used globally as a means of disseminating health information. The majority of stu-dents at LCE reported mass media as their primary source of HIV knowledge (see Table 4.1). Researchers conclude that mass media has been successful in increasing people's general knowledge about HIV transmission (Bertrand et al. 2006; Wilson et al. 2009). Media messages have proved successful in promoting favorable attitudes towards voluntary counseling and testing for HIV, and in offering information on sites for medical and treatment services (Mckee, Bertrand, and Becker-Benton 2004). A recent 10-year review of gen-eral health mass media campaigns by Noar (2006, 21) determined that using media to disseminate health messages can be effective, concluding:

> [T]argeted, well-executed health mass media campaigns can have small to moderate effects not only on health knowledge, beliefs, and attitudes, but on behaviors as well, which can translate into major public health impact given the wide reach of mass media.

In Lesotho, multiple forms of media existed which relayed education messages of HIV. During my research tenure, there were billboards through-out Maseru and other urban areas with phrases such as "God Forgives, AIDS does not," "Let us talk about safe sex," and "Even when you are off duty pro-tect the population, Stop HIV/AIDS" (see Figure 4.4). Unfortunately, these billboards had not changed since I first worked in Lesotho in 2004 and had looked weathered and faded even then. The Internet, which has in recent years become the medium of choice for youth to access health information (Bulled 2011), although available in Lesotho and at both LCE campuses, was expensive and slow. Many students expressed fear about utilizing indepen-dent Internet cafes, given their lack of experience with the medium. They could, however, access the Internet on their cell phones. A growing number were signing on to Facebook® and beginning to develop social network sites with extensive local and international connections.

During my study period, radio remained the medium of choice through-out Lesotho. The most popular and nationally available radio stations were

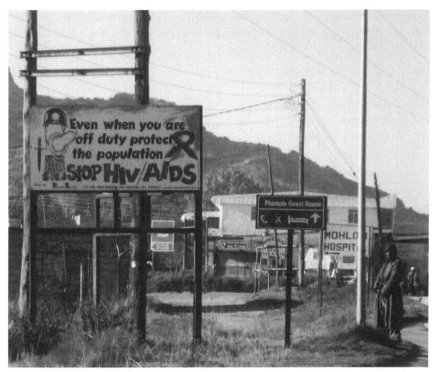

Figure 4.4. Billboard of HIV prevention message in Maseru, Lesotho. (Photo by Stefan Keil, used by permission)

owned by the Lesotho government, including Radio Lesotho and MoAfrika. The remaining stations were associated with religious institutions (e.g., Harvest FM, Joy FM, and Catholic Radio). Consequently, radio dramas and discussions were often slanted towards the ideologies of the station's funding institution (i.e., government or church). Radio slots on national, far-reaching, and widely popular broadcasting stations were set aside for discussion of issues related to HIV. At the time of my research, Radio Lesotho was airing a one-hour HIV-related talk show on Thursday evenings. The broadcasters on this program and others were rarely trained on issues related to HIV and occasionally offered misleading or incorrect information. For example, a male student on the Thaba-Tseka campus told me that a host on Radio Lesotho had described "the signs of a person who is infected [with HIV]." The student explained that people with HIV have "fluffy hair, diarrhea, and their body declines [wasting]." He also noted that "each and every Thursday in urban areas all the people who are positive go to get ARVs." Although the radio host offered symptoms of HIV, perhaps to persuade listeners to test and, if necessary, initiate treatment, this student interpreted the message of the "signs" of

HIV. He may use this knowledge to identify safe and unsafe sexual partners, anticipating HIV infected individuals to congregate at a predetermined space and time. He may even use this 'knowledge' to determine his own status irrespective of confirmatory test results.

According to Bandura's (2001, 285) social cognitive theory, media messages can increase knowledge and promote behavior change through "dual paths of influence" directly through the individual engaged with the media and indirectly as knowledge is shared through social networks. Health-related media messages influence viewers to discuss issues of importance with others in their lives, thereby setting "in motion transactional experiences that further shape the course of change" (Bandura 2001, 285). For example, a study examining the effects of an MTV HIV prevention campaign on interpersonal communication found that respondents who were exposed to the media campaign were more likely to discuss HIV with interpersonal contacts than those who were not exposed (Geary et al. 2007). A BBC Condom Normalization media campaign in India similarly increased acceptance of and talk about condoms (Frank et al. 2012). Other studies indicate that changes in behavior or norms within an individual's social network can influence a person's behavioral intentions even if he/she is not directly exposed to the original media campaign (Valente and Saba 1998, Wakefield, Loken, and Hornik 2010). Media thus works in conjunction with social networks to diffuse ideas about HIV and normalize risk reduction strategies.

Despite the extensive and diverse use of media to convey health education messages, the effectiveness of media-based HIV interventions to disseminate information locally and develop risk-reduction knowledge has been strongly critiqued (see Airhihenbuwa 1989, 1995; Airhihenbuwa, Makinwa, and Obregon 2000; Airhihenbuwa and Obregon 2000; Scalway 2003). A systematic review of 24 mass media interventions on changing HIV-related knowledge, attitudes, and behaviors was carried out by Bertrand and colleagues. Their examination yielded mixed results on the effectiveness of communication strategies to change HIV-related behavior in developing countries (Bertrand et al. 2006). At least half of the studies published between 1990 and 2004 showed a positive impact of communication strategies on reducing high-risk sexual behavior that included transactional sex and multiple sex partners. By contrast, abstinence and condom use showed mixed results or no effects. Among those that did show significant impacts, the effect sizes were typically small to moderate. In Western countries, researchers have found that mass media serves as a major source for both correct and distorted information on HIV (Lupton 1994a; Singhal and Rogers 2003). Mass media often fails to provide the public with complete and accurate information on the epidemic (Lupton 1994a; Nelkin 1991; Singhal et al. 2004; Singhal and Rogers 2003).

There is an increasing acknowledgment that, in addition to spreading basic information, mass media used in health communication campaigns need to address more directly the barriers that prevent the adoption of safer sex behavior (Mckee, Bertrand, and Becker-Benton 2004; UNAIDS 1999a, b). In Lesotho, media served a particularly important role in educating youth about HIV and related sexuality. Families did not offer an open space to discuss sexual behavior, friends offered experience rather than fact, and schools and religious institutions charged their messages on sexual behavior with moralistic discourse. Media therefore offered a venue to explore sex and HIV openly and without judgment or risk.

Entertainment-Education

The use of entertainment platforms such as popular music, radio, television programming, and traveling theatre to diffuse health related knowledge has received considerable attention in recent years (Singhal and Rogers 2001, 2002; Storey et al 1999; Storey et al 1996). Although used widely in other countries in Africa, traveling theatre productions that inform and educate about HIV were not common in Lesotho. A professor at the National University of Lesotho, Charles Duntin, had successfully assisted university students involved in a theatre program to produce HIV dramas. These were recorded and were available for distribution as DVDs. However, none of the students I interviewed spoke of seeing groups of traveling actors conveying HIV messages at school or elsewhere. Furthermore, the DVDs of the taped theatre performances from the National University were not available to students at either LCE campus.

Many students had, however, seen the recently aired, locally produced, four-part television drama series *Kheto ea ka!* (Your Choice). The Lesotho Ministry of Health and Social Welfare (MoHSW) and National AIDS Commission (NAC), in collaboration with Mantsoapo, a private behavior-change communication organization, produced this television series focused on HIV risk behaviors and prevention strategies in the Lesotho context. *Kheto ea ka!* joined the growing list of HIV prevention TV dramas, including the popular long running HIV soap opera series *Soul City* in South Africa, *Twende na Wakati* (Let's Go with the Times) in Tanzania, *Tinka Tinka Sukh* (Happiness Lies in Small Things) in India, *Nshilakamona* (I have Not Seen It) in Zambia, and *Kamisama Mo Sukoshidake* (Please God Just a Little More Time) in Japan. These TV dramas fall within the realm of "entertainment-education," a process of designing and implementing an entertainment program to increase audience members' knowledge about a social issue.

The four part *Kheto ea ka!* in Lesotho was aired on the national television station, Lesotho TV. DVDs of the series were also distributed to major stakeholders and educational institutions throughout Lesotho including LCE. *Kheto ea ka!* used four interwoven narrative portrayals addressing HIV risk behaviors: inter-generational relationships, extra-marital affairs, men who have sex with men, and prisoners. Through the interweaving of these four situations, *Kheto ea ka!* generated a formula of negative, transitional, and positive role models to transmit messages of HIV prevention behaviors.

Negative characters provided models of the consequences of HIV risk behaviors. For example, in *Kheto ea Ka!* two school-age girls develop intimate romantic relationships with older, seemingly successful men. The short-lived economic success of these men, based on a pyramid scheme, in addition to their sexual relationships with school-girls outside wedlock, further painted these men as morally and socially repulsive. The relationships provide the school-girls with the modern commodities they desired, including cell phones, clothes, food, drink, and rides in privately owned cars. One of the girls falls pregnant. Her older male partner is horrified and refuses to see her again. Out of shame, embarrassment, and recognition that she cannot care for a child on her own, the girl has an abortion performed by a traditional healer, an illegal procedure in Lesotho. The final scene of this narrative closed with the girl alone, crouched in a corner of a dark and dirty room, crying as she clutches at her stomach, blood stains evident on her dress.

A positive role model, acting as an opinion leader to provide wise counsel to others, was the grandmother of one of the school-girls. Women in Lesotho are traditionally strong social figures, and their social capital increases with age. However, in contemporary Lesotho, families have become smaller and more nuclear. Elders are no longer family figureheads; they have been replaced by family members who provide monetary support. In this scenario, the primary family provider is the wife, not the husband. The wife works long hours and frequently brings work home. The husband feels challenged in his traditional role as the family provider. As his wife is always busy, he seeks intimacy outside the marriage. The wife begins to insist on the use of condoms during their sexual relations, making evident her suspicions of his extra-marital affairs. Her insistence only heightens the friction between the couple. The positive role model, the grandmother, intervenes by forcing the couple to communicate directly with each other, rather than making insinuations or using other family members to relay their frustration with one another. This is uncharacteristic of older Basotho, who are against open conversations about sexual relations and who continue to regard genders as unequal, with women only acquiring legal status in 2006. Consequently they are unlikely to suggest such a frank discussion between marriage partners. The story closed with the grandmother leaving the couple alone to talk in their stylish living room. The narrative highlighted the challenges faced by families in contemporary Lesotho as traditional gender and age roles are shifting, placing strain on family and marital relations and driving risk behaviors including multiple concurrent sexual relationships.

In contrast to positive and negative characters, transitional characters are key identifiers for the audience, providing self-efficacious models for how to change behavior that audience members can emulate. In *Kheto ea Ka!* one such transitional character appears as the male partner in a newly established heterosexual co-habiting couple. The couple is experiencing difficulties with their relationship as the male partner resists any engagement in sexual relations. The female partner begins to question her sexual appeal and tensions rise between the two. Angry, confused, and hurt the female partner seeks solace at a local bar where she meets a former lover, a married man. Unknown to the female partner, her male partner suffers from post-traumatic stress in response to repeated violent homosexual rapes he endured while imprisoned. Unsure of his HIV status, he has been hesitant to engage in sexual activities. The narrative of this couple closes with the male partner seated in an HIV testing clinic. The male partner in this vignette serves as the transitional character, aiming to inform the audience of how to protect others from possible infection by knowing one's HIV status and limiting risky sexual encounters. It is important to note that his exposure route, forced sexual relations with other men while in prison, portrayed him as the victim. In spite of his past criminality, he is seeking to do the morally, socially, and rationally (based on biomedical evidence) correct thing by resisting sexual relations that may infect his partner. Other characters, including the young pregnant girl, a homosexual couple, and an over ambitious wife, are portrayed as perpetrators who are responsible for their dire circumstances (a risky abortion, known HIV infections, and an adulterous husband).

The entertainment-education strategy capitalizes on the popular appeal of entertainment media to introduce socially relevant themes to the target population, seeking to achieve changes in audience knowledge, attitudes, and behavior, subsequently changing cultural norms and motivating prosocial behaviors (Dutta 2008a). In some context, the strategy also invites community participation, with community members actively engaged in the process of TV drama story development. Through participation, the target population is involved in the process of meaning construction within the local context, picking the story lines and issues addressed (Basu and Dutta 2009; Beltran 1975, 1980; Freire 1972). The entertainment-education strategy has been shown to successfully generate favorable attitudes and changes to overt behaviors (Singhal and Rogers 1999). In relation to HIV risk behaviors, evaluations of entertainment-education programs suggest that the strategy can be highly effective in promoting prevention with measurable effects on changing risk behaviors (Church and Geller 1989; Goldstein et al. 2005; Piotrow et al. 1997; Singhal and Rogers 1999; Valente 1997; Vaughan et al. 2000).

However the entertainment-education approach has been criticized, not only for its assumptions on participatory communication, but also for its trivial approach to significant social issues, the short-lived impact, and expectations of agency on behalf of the audience (Dutta 2008a). LCE students, administrators, and faculty did not perceive the *Kheto ea ka!* series' stories to relate directly to their own lives, though they recognized others and generalizations in the narratives. For example, of the women who are actively employed in the formal business economy in Lesotho, few were more successful than their husbands (if they were still married); few men were likely to dismiss the sexual advances of their female partners; and only a small portion of the population is ever imprisoned. As mentioned earlier in this section, the grandmother figure would be unlikely to intervene in the marital strife of others, and marital partners would rarely discuss their distress. For the students of LCE, the young girl who becomes pregnant by her wealthy older boyfriend was likely the most relatable character. However, the students did not identify with her. First, she appeared to come from a wealthy family. Second, her choice to have an abortion positioned her as unique from the LCE students' experience. While student pregnancies were common, most were carried to term. Consequently, as Lesotho viewers did not perceive an affinity with a particular character they were unlikely to engage in the desired prosocial behaviors offered by the vignettes of the *Kheto ea ka!* series (Johnson, Flora, and Rimal 1997).

The *Kheto ea ka!* series also embodied the limiting entertainment-education structure of a one-way flow of information. The principal effect of the entertainment-education strategy is to increase interpersonal communication about the educational content (Goldstein et al. 2005; Vaughan et al. 2000). Certainly in Lesotho, the explicit nature of the drama series *Kheto ea ka!*, in revealing sexual assault in prisons and sexual relations among men, stimulated conversations. However, according to Bandura's social cognitive theory (1977, 1986), characters need to be seen performing acts, such that viewers feel capable of engaging in the actions themselves. The stories, while bringing up important issues, do not explicitly show characters successfully negotiating condom use with a partner, discussing infidelity in a marriage, undergoing an HIV test, or obtaining information on how to manage an unwanted pregnancy in a safe way. All the narratives stopped before the positive risk-reducing behavior actually took place. Consequently, the series suggested to the audience what they should be doing, but did not show how to do it.

The entertainment-education approach is also limited in that the episodic nature has been shown to result in marginal, short-lived, unsustainable behavior changes (Dutta 2008a). If not stimulated by repeated showings or new stories, conversations and behavioral changes stimulated by the television series will decrease over time (Vaughan et al. 2000). In their analysis of mass media on fertility changes, Hornik and McAnany (2001) argued that changes in behavior are not directly attributable to media campaigns, and that behavior tends to return to baseline after the media program ends. In the case of *Kheto ea ka!* the series had only four episodes. These episodes were repeatedly aired on national television. Additional TV and radio dramas were scheduled for release in Lesotho, though there was some concern that the content was too explicit for national viewership.

Not only have entertainment-education strategies been criticized for failing to represent local situations, they have also been criticized for universalizing Western values and Western ways of viewing the world (Dutta 2008a, Singhal and Rogers 1999). Despite the involvement of national stakeholders and local elites, the agenda and story line of *Kheto ea ka!* and other entertainment-education TV drama series (Dutta 2008a) reflect largely Western concepts of HIV risk behaviors and strategies to reduce risk that relate back to individual agency rather than social and structural contexts. In an historical overview of the development and deployment of the entertainment-education strategy, Singhal and Rogers (1999) identify Population Communications International (PCI) as one of the early initiators of the entertainment-education model, transferring the soap opera model to India, Kenya, and Tanzania. Subsequently, the Johns Hopkins University Center for Communication Programs employed the strategy in over 30 countries with more than 60 entertainment-education projects. Both organizations are Western-based, developing messages that deeply reflect the values of the Western world. Mohan Dutta (2008a) has also argued that the channels of message conveyance (e.g., TV, radio, recorded music) propagate Western products and ideologies, introduce commercialized and globalized values into the developing world,[7] and perpetuate unhealthy geopolitical structures.[8]

Finally, the entertainment-education approach has been criticized for being conceptualized naively as a panacea to health inequities in the world. Dutta (2008a) warns that the entertainment-education approach trivializes the underlying problems faced by marginalized communities, abdicates the national government's responsibility in solving the critical resource needs faced by the people of the nation, and, by promoting Western ideologies, becomes the machinery for the oppression of already marginalized communities. Dutta (2008a, 36) notes that the theoretical conceptualization of the entertainment-education strategy draws on existing prominent behavior change communication strategies that identify "the locus of the problem [as] the individual, his beliefs, attitudes, cognitions and behavioral intentions."

The linear transmission of information ignores the complexity of the social change processes that require interaction, deliberation, and action (Papa et al. 2000). Furthermore, the strategy fails to consider the contextual and structural factors which seriously impede or promote certain behaviors. Thus, similar to other approaches in health communication, the entertainment-education model is based on the conceptualization of the receiver as a rational actor, reflecting Western biases of health interventions that pay little heed to social structures, community context, and local narratives (Dutta 2008a).

In Summary

Bodies of knowledge, including those related to HIV-prevention, are communicated through various domestic sources. Validity of the avenue through which knowledge is conveyed is determined by social context, including factors related to accessibility, relationship to other trusted institutions, and existing authority (see Figure 4.1). Statements of knowledge thus gain power according to who said them, in what context, and whether others accept them as true. Consequently, certain forms of knowledge are considered by local community members to be more or less valid than others depending on the value placed upon the source.

In examining the different sources of HIV knowledge available in Lesotho, it is evident that conflicting ideas on HIV prevention strategies circulate. The message conveyed is heavily influenced by the characteristics and ideologies of the source. Schools, as a result of their close connection with religious institutions, linked HIV risk with messages of morality. Rather than stressing risk reduction strategies (i.e., condom use and routine testing) and acknowledging the difficulties in remaining abstinent and maintaining a monogamous sexual relationship, teachers and religious leaders rationalized positive HIV status as a punishment for sinful behaviors. The biomedical institution, in its link to 'scientific truth,' held greatest credibility. However, its heavy promotion of condom use contradicted strongly-supported religious views of abstinence and faithfulness. Condoms were viewed as modern Western tools that allow for and condone sex before marriage and infidelity. Individual providers, like teachers, allowed their personal perspectives to alter the biomedical messages that they were charged to convey. For example, disclosing the HIV status of testers to members of the community suggested that even trained testers believe HIV infection to be the consequence of inappropriate actions, be they immoral or simply irrational, and that HIV positive individuals pose a threat to their communities. Finally, social networks and mass media did not always convey accurate biomedical information, but were more highly valued, particularly by youth, in the climate of a modernizing Lesotho.

As this overview of HIV knowledge sources in Lesotho reveals, HIV-prevention programs frequently emphasized the consumption of health by the individual. This focus disregards the sociocultural context within which the behavior is embedded, and places the burden of responsibility for disease-prevention on the individual. In doing so, these knowledge dissemination or behavior change communication approaches ignore the structural elements that fundamentally impede engagement in disease prevention behaviors, and consequently marginalize the individuals and groups that they intend to help (Dutta and Basnyat 2008). When assessing the varied sources of knowledge accessible in high-risk settings, we must examine the full context of the message. This includes the process of how knowledge is delivered, the perceptions of those delivering the message, the interpersonal context in which delivery takes place, the barriers established during delivery, and whether those receiving the message have the capacity to engage critically with the information in order to establish their own viable methods of disease prevention.

5

Knowledge Acquisition

Given the continued focus of global disease prevention campaigns on the acquisition of relevant biomedical knowledge to promote rationalized behavior change, I elected to assess the HIV knowledge of youth in Lesotho. As knowledge is distributed, and not always equally, stock of knowledge can vary greatly among persons. These differences "provide much of the momentum for our social interaction, from gossip to the division of labor" (Barth 2002, 1). Here I focus on generalizations, logical coherence, and consistencies, as knowledge is frequently a conglomeration of disconnected abstract ideas used to interpret a dynamic and complex social and moral world.

Much of the information collected on levels of held HIV knowledge and related sexual behavior in the AIDS era has been obtained through Knowledge, Attitudes, and Practices/Behavior (KAP/B) or demographic and health studies. These data collection strategies employ large populations, survey questions, and statistical analyses.[1]

Such quantitative measures have distinct advantages. For example, they can clearly document the relative frequency and distribution of knowledge, attitudes, and behaviors in different populations with a high level of precision and statistical significance (Gortmaker and Izazola 1992, Warwick 1983b). Quantitative methods also make replication of results possible, which is important in terms of validation of scientific inference (Gortmaker and Izazola 1992). Change can be assessed over time and useful predictions made for future trends. These projections can estimate of the relative effects of social and behavioral influences upon the course of the epidemic. Finally, quantitative methods permit calculations of the relative efficacy and cost-effectiveness of an intervention strategy or policy.

Despite their advantages, a major limitation of surveys or quantitative measures of knowledge, attitudes, and behavior is poor measurement quality. In his analysis of Knowledge Attitudes and Practices/Behaviors (KAP/B) surveys, Mauldin (1965) concluded that many are deficient in that they fail to

Nicola Bulled, "Knowledge Aquisition" in *Prescribing HIV Prevention: Bringing Culture into Global Health Communication*, pp. 129-153. © 2015 Left Coast Press, Inc. All rights reserved.

study the reliability and validity of their own data. One published report indicates that the reliability measure (Crohnbach's alpha) of multi-item scales that measure knowledge and attitudes concerning AIDS ranged from 0.52 to 0.68 (Jill et al. 1987). This level of reliability is considered moderate, yet not ideal. KAP/B surveys are also limited in terms of construct and content validity, or how well the scale actually measures real knowledge, attitudes, and practices. Minor variations in question wording and methods of data gathering can result in different measures and hence differential construct validity (see, for example, Izazola-Licea et al. 1991). Due to the complexity of HIV and the sensitivity surrounding sexual behavior and condom use in different social contexts, there is a need to ask different questions of different populations to measure the same underlying construct. Finally, for satisfactory content validity, when measuring knowledge and attitudes, multiple questions are needed to adequately sample all the relevant areas of knowledge.

In addition to limitations regarding reliability and validity, quantitative measures often fail to adequately assess the intensity of the opinions or attitudes reported (Mauldin 1965). Questions regarding HIV transmission routes may miss assessing relative levels of risk in particular behaviors, for example, oral sex versus vaginal sex. Messages of prevention or transmission may be parroted, or prevention methods such as condoms endorsed without knowing how to use them properly (Crosby et al. 2003). Knowledge is therefore assessed superficially, with no regard for the beliefs underlying the responses (de Bruin et al. 2007). As a result, surveys may fail to tap the knowledge most relevant to the complex behaviors involved in HIV prevention with a specific population. Quantitative rigor cannot encompass the richness of human life and sexuality (Ankrah 1989; Smith 2003), and does not consider the configurations of power that influence people's priorities and constrain rational choices (Blanc and Wolff 2001; Machel 2001; Olayinka et al. 2000; Packard and Epstein 1991; Schoepf 1993, 1996, 1997; Wood and Jewkes 1997). KAP/B surveys assume "a linear association between knowledge and attitudes, on one hand, and behavior change on the other" (Chikovore et al. 2009, 503), ignoring contextual and historical factors that may influence behavior (Kelly, Parker, and Lewis 2001; Vance 1991; Warwick 1983a).

It is important to recognize that even though quantitative measures may be imperfect, policy-relevant findings can be derived by assessing the inaccuracies and by placing limits upon estimates. Critiquing KAP/B surveys does not necessarily mean that "all the findings of KAP surveys are questionable and useless" (Hauser 2001, 68). However, a more critical and analytical approach to the use of surveys is still needed with more sophisticated techniques employed (Chandrasekaran 1966). More flexible qualitative approaches are increasingly being used, often in conjunction with quantitative measures to assess context and illuminate micro-level interactional dynamics in HIV risk knowledge and behaviors (see, for example, Campbell 2000; Gold et al. 1992; MacPhail and Campbell 2001; Mavhu et al. 2011; Nyanzi, Pool, and Kinsman 2001; Power 1996; Sherman and Bassett 1999; Taylor 1995).

Understanding Youths' HIV Knowledge

Rather than using a standard approach of a knowledge test, I used an innovative strategy of self-generated questions as employed by Chikovore and colleagues to assess HIV knowledge.[2] Chikovore, Nystrom, Lindmark and Ahlberg (2009) used the self-generated question methodology as a way to overcome the limitations of KAP/B surveys and circumvent confidentiality concerns, ambiguities in interviewer-generated questions, and additional pitfalls reported in face-to-face interviewing with young people on matters of sexuality (Cowan et al. 2002; Kim, Marangwanda, and Kols 1997; Mavhu et al. 2008). Researchers invited 546 primary and secondary school students (51 percent female, age range 9 to 25 years) in a rural district of Zimbabwe to formulate questions on issues about growing up or questions that they could not ask their parents, teachers, or other adults for fear or shame. The intention of this study of students was to examine how the prohibitions and violence described by adults in a larger study might affect young people in the same context. HIV/AIDS was not specifically mentioned to the students as a topic to address in their questions; however, concerns over HIV were raised by the pupils revealing the power of this approach in allowing youth to voice their concerns.

In my study of youth in Lesotho, I asked the students to each formulate one question related to HIV for which they did not know the answer, but did not feel comfortable asking parents, teachers, or other adults. The method is able to tap into knowledge gaps rather than just identifying the level of knowledge that currently exists, as participants generate their own questions rather than answering questions formulated by researchers. The approach also identifies the knowledge most relevant to the complex behaviors involved in HIV prevention within the specific sociocultural context. For instance, knowing why touching or helping someone with HIV is not risky is important to this study population, while knowing how the virus interacts with the body's immune system or various treatment options is not.

I recruited all first year Lesotho College of Education students, in two successive years, to participate in the self-generated question exercise. The first collection of questions, in 2010, took place during a Life Skills class within the classroom. These students had had some level of exposure to school-based HIV education. The second collection of questions, in 2011, occurred during the LCE's registration process prior to the onset of classes. Students moved from one station to another, filling in forms, collecting keys, and registering for classes, and I manned a private station at the end of the line where each student was asked to write their question related to HIV. Being new LCE students, this second group of students may not have had school-based HIV education in primary or secondary school. No names were collected, but students did indicate their gender and age.[3]

Analysis of the self-generated questions focused on the range of knowledge students possessed and application of that knowledge.[4] The initial descriptive codes were eventually narrowed down to the following nine categories: basics (virus origin and transmission), mother-to-child transmission, misconceptions and myths, prevention, treatment or cure, living with HIV/HIV+ partner, disclosure of status, populations at risk, broader impact of HIV, and testing (see Figure 5.1).

Thematically, the questions posed by the two sets of students (2010-enrolled and 2011-not enrolled in Life Skills) were not significantly different (see Figure 5.1). Students enrolled in the Life Skills course (data collected in 2010) appeared to show more concern about the impact of HIV on economics and education, and posed questions about the populations most at risk of infection. These were topics discussed during the LCE Life Skills course. The abstract nature of these questions and distancing of the issue of HIV from the lived experience is likely in response to the classroom environment, where generalized, theoretical abstract issues are discussed. The second group of students, those who were not currently enrolled in Life Skills and therefore might not have received school-based Life Skills training, posed questions that were more related to direct individual experiences of HIV. They were also more likely to question common misconceptions of HIV that circulate widely in Lesotho, such as:

> If I fall in love with someone suffering from HIV and I want to have children, what am I supposed to do?
> (Female, 28)

> Can a person without AIDS have a child with an infected person?
> (Male, 22)

> Is it true that a virgin can cure AIDS? (Male, 24)

> Can mosquitoes pass or spread AIDS? (Female, 25)

> Can HIV/AIDS be spread from one person to another by kissing?
> (Female, 26)

> Is [HIV] an American idea to destroy sex or God's purpose? (Male, 23)

Collectively, the questions posed by both groups of students revealed the

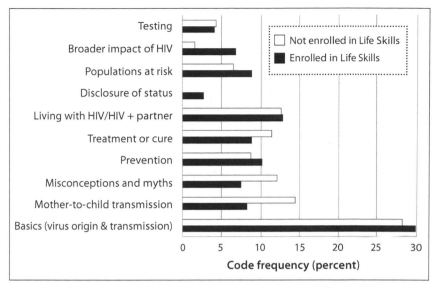

Figure 5.1. Frequency of thematic codes derived from the self-generated question exercise.

difficulty in applying basic factual HIV information to specific lived experiences. HIV transmission routes and means of prevention have been at the center of most educational campaigns for the past 25 years. However, students' questions indicated a lack of understanding of the virus' life cycle and the virus' impact on the human immune system, indicating only a superficial understanding or rote memorization of the virus' transmission routes, as illustrated here:

> I want to know if HIV is inside the sperm because the affected person can make a new born baby without having HIV? Is HIV in blood or inside sperm? (Female, 25)

> We are being taught much about HIV/AIDS and they said HIV cannot be transmitted through kissing, especially with somebody without sores on their lips. How can you guarantee that? (Female, 24)

> I heard about a couple, when tested for HIV one partner was negative and the other was positive. I just want to know if that is possible. (Female, 33)

> Then how is AIDS spread using razor blades if it does not survive when outside the human body? Because what I know is that HIV virus takes crystal form and does not die when outside the body. It survives immediately. (Female, 21)

Without a clear biological understanding of the virus, students revealed an inability to determine what behaviors are constituted as "high risk" and thus how to reduce their risk of infection. For instance, students understood that unprotected sex is a transmission route, but not that it is a more likely route of transmission than kissing, sharing of toothbrushes, the re-use of unsterilized razor blades by a traditional healer, or the care of an HIV infected relative, as exemplified here:

> Is safe sex 100% in protecting a person to get HIV? (Female, 23)
> [This statement references the use of a condom during sexual intercourse to prevent HIV infection.]

> Is it true that wet sex does not cause HIV/AIDS, even having sex with infected person without using a condom? (Male, 20)
> ["Wet sex" here refers to sex wherein the female has not made an effort to dry her vagina by wiping with a cloth or using herbs, in order to increase friction.]

> Why is it that people with many partners are not likely to have HIV/AIDS but the one with one partner are the one who gets HIV/AIDS easily? (Female, 20)
> [This comment relates to personal observations of individuals who appear to have many sexual partners, yet are not infected with HIV. Repetitive, continuous exposure to pathogens may stimulate an immune response that reduces risk of infection (Fowke et al. 1992, Fowke et al. 2000). This is counter to HIV-prevention messages that claim that having many sexual partners increases risk of infection.]

In addition, unclear understandings of the virus and its long incubation period resulted in uncertainty in identifying infection status, as, for example:

> How long does it take to get infected by HIV and AIDS? (Female, 25)

> What are the signs and symptoms of HIV before one can know his/her status? (Female, 21)

> How do I know if one is infected with HIV? (Female, 22)

Without a more complete biomedicine-based understanding of the pathogen and its actions in and out of the human body, students were unable to calculate relative levels of risk in different situations of pathogen exposure. For example, they had been taught that HIV is transmitted through body fluids. As a result, students conceptualized 'fluids' to involve the saliva exchanged through kissing; contact with mucus, vomit, excrement, blood from nosebleeds (frequent in Lesotho's high altitude and dry climate); the sharing of toilet seats; and beliefs about HIV transmission via blood-sucking mosquitoes. Furthermore, by providing only simplified biomedical knowledge, HIV education campaigns may have unintentionally generated misunderstandings. For example, oral tests for HIV generate confusion as it appears saliva is being tested for the presence or absence of HIV. In reality, oral HIV tests determine if oral mucosal transudate contains HIV antibodies. In fact, it is likely that pedagogical strategies to explain HIV transmission such as those employed by 'Mme Matabo and myself involving the drinking of water and spitting into a single cup further contribute to this misconception. In addition, the local perception that every encounter with every person is risky, particularly as individuals do not always project any outward indications of their HIV infection status, could result in the consequent rationalization that there is little point in taking any precautions.[5]

Finally, questions highlighted how HIV is integrated into and impacts daily life. The questions showed a sense of fear related to HIV infection, specifically regarding stigma and reduced future potentials as lovers, marital partners, and parents. The questions also suggested a sense of acceptance that HIV has become part of the health landscape. Students were conflicted in their negotiations of their own disease prevention measures as well as in caring for and living with individuals who are infected, revealing the importance of deliberate engagement with interpersonal networks in HIV communication strategies. These conflicts also included important emotional and moral issues, as for example:

> If I find myself HIV positive, is it wise to tell my partner or not? (Female, 20)

> If I am positive, how can I be proud to tell my parents friends and other people whom I trust? (Female, 22)

> How can I continue to have relationships with HIV positive partner? Is it wrong to leave her? (Male, 22)

> What can I do if my partner is HIV positive and I am not and I love him and want to marry him? (Female, 21)

The overall thematic breakdown of the questions revealed limitations in understandings of the basic biology of the virus life cycle. Rather than there being a disconnect between high levels of knowledge and high levels of risk, knowledge was sometimes faulty, overly simplistic, or irrelevant to personal situations experienced in this specific social context.

To further evaluate the student-posed questions, I paired the collection and analysis of the self-generated questions with free pile sorting of the most commonly occurring questions (see Figure 5.2a and b). Pile sorts are used as

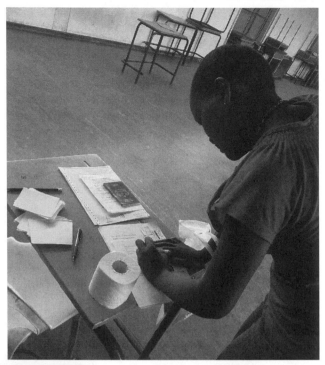

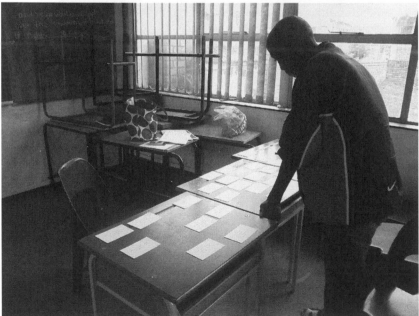

Figure 5.2 (a and b). LCE students completing the self-generated question and pile sort data collection strategies.

a qualitative data collection technique in both the social sciences (Bernard, Ryan, and Borgatti 2009; Ryan and Bernard 2000; Singer et al. 2011; Trotter and Potter 1993) and in several health disciplines (Morse and Field 1995). This research technique enables researchers to gain information about the conceptual dimensions study participants use to appraise their own social experience (Nastasi and Berg 1999; Spradley 1979). In addition to being easy to administer, the results of pile sort data, using sample sizes between 30 and 40, generally reach reliabilities above 0.90 (Weller and Romney 1988). Furthermore, a study by Romney and colleagues (1979) demonstrated a high degree of stability across four replications.

In a pile sort task, informants are asked to sort cards, each containing an item (e.g., image, name, or in my study a question), into piles so that items in any one pile are more similar to each other than they are to items in the other piles. In the unconstrained version of the task, as employed here, subjects can make as few or as many piles as they wish. Subjects are asked to group items according to their similarity, without reference to specific criteria. The informant, rather than the researcher, decides what criteria are most salient and determines similarity. Consequently, the study population, rather than the researcher derives emergent themes. As my study participants sorted the questions that students themselves had posed on the topic of HIV, they identified thematic gaps in knowledge of HIV. These thematic groups were later compared to my thematic grouping of the student-posed questions as outlined above.

I compiled and transcribed onto note cards a list of the students' HIV-related questions that occurred two or more times (45 questions in total).[6] Students were instructed to sort the 45 questions into piles based on perceived similarities in order to uncover site-specific domains of HIV knowledge. Once the student was satisfied with the piles produced, each item in the pile was recorded along with a rationale describing what the questions in each pile had in common.

Consensus analysis revealed that, despite individual differences, students shared a single conceptualization of HIV (Eigenvalue=50.016; Eigenratio=17.932; Average Competence=0.8089). Cluster analysis revealed six major categories or piles of questions (see Figure 5.3 and the corresponding list of questions in Table 5.1). The clusters included questions related to the origins of HIV, life with HIV, prevention of HIV, transmission of HIV, and impact of HIV on Lesotho. A single question relating to how long the virus can survive outside the body remained an outlier.

Fourteen rationales for why particular questions/cards were piled together were mentioned by at least 20 percent of students (see Table 5.2). Most students identified the basic elements of HIV education campaigns, namely prevention (94.4 percent) and transmission (91.5 percent) of HIV. Students also identified questions related to HIV status, symptoms, treatment (antiretroviral therapy, or ARVs), and a cure. They noted concerns about life with HIV, including sero-discordant couples, mother-to-child transmission (MTCT), and helping others who are infected. The category of 'Lesotho' was frequently identified by students, as specific questions were included that directly related to the impact of HIV in Lesotho.

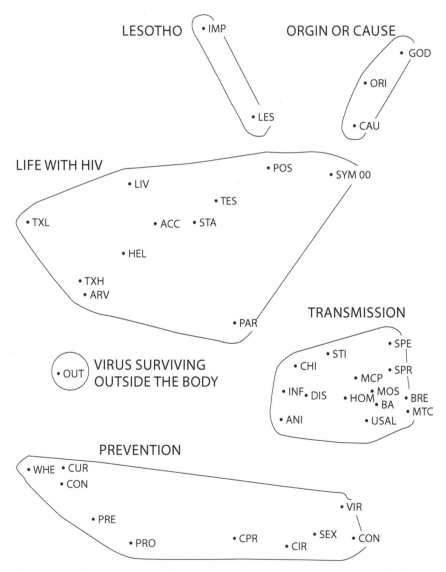

Figure 5.3. Cluster analysis of the 45 self-generated questions included in the pile sorting exercise.

Table 5.1. HIV-related questions extracted from the self-generated question exercise

Label	Question
TXL	How long can someone taking ARVs live?
HEL	How can we help people living with HIV/AIDS?
PRE	What can we do to prevent HIV?
VIR	Can having sex with a virgin cure HIV/AIDS?
MOS	Can mosquitoes pass or spread HIV?
CIR	Does circumcision protect a man from HIV infection?
IMP	How does HIV impact our country?
KIS	Can HIV/AIDS be transmitted through kissing?
WHE	When will HIV/AIDS be cured?
CAU	What causes HIV/AIDS?
MTC	Can an HIV-positive mother transmit HIV to her baby?
CHI	Can someone who is HIV-negative have a child with someone who is HIV-positive?
OUT	How long does the HIV virus survive outside the body?
LOO	What does an HIV-positive person look like?
CON	Is there any risk of getting HIV/AIDS if having sex with a condom?
HOM	Can homosexual people (i.e., men who have sex with men) get HIV through sexual intercourse?
STI	Does having STI (STD) increase the risk of HIV-infection?
TOO	Can you get HIV by sharing a toothbrush with many people?
LES	How many people in Lesotho are infected with HIV?
UTE	Is it possible to get HIV by sharing utensils or plates?
SYM	What are the symptoms of HIV/AIDS?
ANI	Can animals be infected with HIV?
INF	Is it possible that an HIV-infected person can have sexual intercourse with another person without infecting them?
DIS	Can a husband be HIV-positive and the wife HIV-negative even when they have unprotected sex?
SAL	Can HIV be transmitted through saliva?
ORI	Where does HIV come from?
SPR	How does HIV/AIDS spread?
LIV	How long will a person with HIV/AIDS live?
GOD	Is HIV/AIDS a punishment from God for being bad?
POS	How do I know if I am HIV-positive?
TES	How long does it take for an HIV/AIDS test to confirm HIV status?

(Continued on following page)

Table 5.1. (*Continued*)

SEX	Is there any risk of getting HIV/AIDS if I have protected sex (i.e., use condoms)?
ARV	When does an HIV-infected person start to take ARVs?
TXH	Does a healthy HIV-positive individual need to take ARVs?
CON	Why is HIV/AIDS not controlled or cured with medicines (i.e., ARVs)?
SPE	Is HIV in blood or in sperm?
STA	Is it important to know my HIV status?
CUR	Is there a cure for HIV/AIDS?
PRO	What can I do to protect myself from HIV/AIDS?
PAR	What can I do if my partner is HIV-positive?
MCP	Is it true that multiple sex partners spread HIV/AIDS?
BAB	How does a mother infect a baby with HIV/AIDS during birth?
BRE	Can a mother infect her baby with HIV/AIDS through breastfeeding?
CPR	Do condoms offer 100% protection from HIV/AIDS?
ACC	How can you accept yourself if you have HIV/AIDS?

Table 5.2. Pile sort rationale frequencies by gender, campus, home environment, and year of enrollment at LCE

Item	Freq (%)	Gender		Campus		Home environment		Year of enrollment	
		Females	Males	Maseru	Thaba-Tseka	Rural	Urban	1st Year	3rd Year
Protection/ Prevention	**94.4**	89.2	100.0	91.9	97.1	97.4	90.6	92.1	97.0
Transmission	**91.5**	91.9	91.2	86.5	97.1	89.7	93.8	94.7	87.9
Cause/origin	**85.9**	78.4	94.1	91.9	79.4	82.1	90.6	92.1	78.8
Cure	**80.3**	78.4	82.4	78.4	82.4	74.4	87.5	86.8	72.7
Symptoms	**80.3**	89.2	70.6	81.1	79.4	79.5	81.3	89.5	69.7
Status	**76.1**	70.3	82.4	70.3	82.4	76.9	75.0	73.7	78.8
Antiretroviral therapy, ARVs	**67.6**	73.0	61.8	59.5	76.5	69.2	65.6	65.8	69.7
Living with HIV	**52.1**	45.9	58.8	48.6	55.9	51.3	53.1	60.5	42.4
Lesotho	**52.1**	64.9	38.2	40.5	64.7	59.0	43.8	57.9	45.5
MTCT	**40.8**	43.2	38.2	40.5	41.2	41.0	40.6	47.4	33.3
Misconceptions /myths	**32.4**	37.8	26.5	43.2	20.6	30.8	34.4	18.4	48.5
Helping PLWHA	**25.4**	32.4	17.6	32.4	17.6	17.9	34.4	18.4	33.3
Sero-discordance	**25.4**	18.9	32.4	16.2	35.3	25.6	25.0	26.3	24.2
Condoms	**21.1**	27.0	14.7	29.7	11.8	17.9	25.0	26.3	15.2

The discrepancies between my coding of the student-generated questions and the piles generated by the students fall into the following five thematic areas:

- survival of HIV outside the human body,
- symptoms of HIV,
- condoms as a unique prevention strategy,
- misconceptions about HIV, and
- the origin of HIV

Questioning the ability of *HIV to survive outside the body* offers an indication of the conflict that exists between supplied knowledge of HIV transmission and lived experience. Students have been taught that any unprotected sexual exposure, exposure to blood, or any body fluid (including saliva, human excrement, and vomit) results in HIV infection. Yet, through personal and shared experience, they have come to realize that unprotected sexual encounters, kissing, or direct exposures to blood or other body fluids do not always result in infection. While a review article by Thompson, Boughton, and Dore (2003) suggested that HIV can survive outside the human body for a period of up to several weeks, survival of the virus outside the host depends largely upon the quantity of blood, how much virus is present in the fluid, ambient temperature, and exposure to sunlight and humidity. Thus, it is theoretically possible to become infected when assisting an individual who has HIV, whether a relative in the home, someone who has been hurt in a motor vehicle accident, or a child with a nosebleed; however, the virus will likely die soon after exposure to the elements, prior to contact with the care giver. Moreover, unless a substantial amount of infected body fluid makes contact with a large open wound, the skin functions to provide an effective physical barrier to infection. Coupled with a systemic immune response, the simple hygienic practice of washing exposed body areas considerably reduces likelihood of infection.

Student concerns over *symptoms of HIV infection* offer an indication of the uniqueness of HIV as a disease. Most diseases have recognizable symptoms, for example, a cold makes your nose run and influenza makes your body ache. These symptoms reveal the body's effort to clear the disease agent. Through experience we recognize how to treat or manage the condition relative to the symptoms. For a cold we stay home, consuming fluids, waiting for the symptoms to pass, feeling miserable, yet knowing that health providers rarely offer treatment. In contrast, HIV may induce no symptoms in an infected body for many years. This situation has caused considerable confusion and concern throughout the world, as we do not expect to be sick and infectious if we feel well. The symptoms of HIV are frequently discussed on

Lesotho radio talk shows and in newspaper opinion pieces. Locally, HIV is identified through persistent diarrhea and wasting, the rapid loss in body weight. While these are symptoms of AIDS, the symptoms overlap with many other diseases and health conditions that routinely occur locally, including enteric pathogen infections from contaminated water supplies and improperly stored and prepared food.

For LCE students, recognition of the symptoms of HIV is as much related to identifying their own infection status as to identifying the status of a sexual partner. Testing can be circumvented if serostatus can be detected through recognizable symptoms, or conversely, no symptoms. However, an HIV-infected person can remain asymptomatic for long periods of time while still transmitting the virus. Youth in Lesotho hesitate to test as they fear results will not remain confidential. Despite measures to train testers on the importance of confidentiality and the establishment of measures to protect privacy, there is evidence to suggest that individual testers do share results with others (Human Rights Watch & AIDS and Rights Alliance for Southern Africa 2008). In addition, communities across the world have developed countless ways to determine individual test results, including observing which door a patient uses to exit a testing clinic; how long an individual spends in a clinic; or how the individual appears following a visit to a clinic (see Steinberg 2011), bypassing any deliberate attempts of testing venues to maintain patient confidentiality.

Condoms, as a specific and unique form of HIV prevention, were also identified as a highly relevant topic area by youth, with a fifth of LCE students separating condom-related questions into a distinct pile. Condoms are essentially the most effective tool for HIV prevention and *only* tool accessible to these students. Yet, many students remained concerned about the effectiveness and safety of condoms. The sheer number of questions posed relating to condoms and the identification by students of condoms as a singular issue independent from the broader topic of HIV prevention indicates that condoms as a prevention method remains a point of contestation, conflict, and ambiguity. Different claims made by knowledge disseminators (either for or against condoms) cause confusion and consequently deny people a viable, effective, and cheap prevention method.

The category of *misconceptions* included questions related to ineffective prevention strategies, treatments, and cures. It also included questions about potential routes of HIV transmission that are not biologically effective, routes such as through mosquito bites or the sharing of utensils. There was a notable difference in the frequency of identifying misconceptions by gender, campus, home environment, and year of enrollment at LCE (see Table 5.2). Females were more likely to identify misconceptions than were males, as were students enrolled at the Maseru campus, those from urban areas, and third year students. The greatest distinction in identifying or not identifying a category of misconceptions was between first and third year students (18.4 versus 48.5 percent). As the Life Skills course is offered during the first year at LCE it is possible that students obtain the biomedical basics of HIV at this time and, therefore, are more confident in their abilities to recognize misconceptions once the course is complete. However, other factors may contribute to this difference including age, sexual experience, frequency of testing, and sources of information. Regarding differences between urban-rural, the urban environment may offer more biomedicine-based information through more accessible media and medical services. Alternatively, individuals may adjust to the biomedical perspective, which dominates in urban areas, thereby identifying questions that do not correspond to biomedical 'fact' as 'misconceptions.'

Questions concerning the cause or *origin of HIV* were the third most frequently-identified pile sort category for students, mentioned by over 85 percent of participants. This pile often included the question "Is HIV/AIDS a punishment from God?" The concern for knowing the origin/cause of HIV suggests that the cosmological meaning of HIV/AIDS—why does it infect people now when it didn't in the past and why does it infect some people and not others—remains a salient issue for youth, even though they have grown up with the threat of HIV. Some scientists have argued that exploring the origins of HIV is unimportant, stressing that time and funding resources are better spent developing means of prevention, treatment, or cure. In 1992, a WHO official told *Rolling Stone* magazine that "the origin of the AIDS virus is of no importance to science today" (Curtis 1992). Another scientist stated, "Who cares what the origin of the virus is?…It's distracting, it's non-productive, it's confusing to the public" (Curtis 1992). However, others argue that from a scientific perspective, knowing the origin of the virus is important. Epidemiologist Helen Epstein (2007, 40) noted that if the virus crossed into human populations from primates (the commonly accepted route), then "the only way to prevent other chimp or monkey viruses from doing so again is to know how these transfers occurred in the first place," and subsequently how an individual animal-to-human transmission resulted in the worldwide pandemic. From a layperson's perspective, can knowing the origin of HIV explain why the disease emerged when it did, thus reducing disease related stigma? Can disease origin explain why certain populations and individuals are infected while others are not, thereby improving maintenance of risk reduction behaviors? Do scientific accounts of the origin only further promote the hegemony of biomedicine, marginalizing groups with limited access to scientific accounts or those with different worldviews? Or, can understanding what the evidence suggests about the origins of HIV assist in bridging gaps between global dictates and local perceptions of the disease?[7]

The repeated questioning of the origin(s) of HIV reflects distinctions in perceived etiologies or explanatory models of disease that consequently require different prevention and treatment strategies (Foster 1976). A naturalistic perspective of HIV, whereby disease is the consequence of the naturally occurring viral pathogen, rationalizes that the virus can infect anyone regardless of age, gender, ethnicity, or nationality, should one be exposed to the pathogen in a specific manner. Prevention involves the avoidance of exposure to the pathogen by employing specific behavioral measures (e.g., using a condom when having sexual intercourse, sterilizing cutting instruments, not reusing needles for injection). In contrast, a personalistic perspective of HIV, whereby infection is the result of an active agent within the social sphere, such as God, explains HIV infection as a consequence of behaviors that are considered reprehensible to the powerful entity. For example, in response to sinful or immoral acts God punishes an individual (or community) by infecting him/her with HIV. Similarly, conspiracy theories from the southern African region suggest that the White man is infecting the Black body because he is Black or because of his traditional ways. Under this logic, disease prevention involves ensuring behaviors are in keeping with Christian ideology or the norms of powerful institutions (including biomedicine with its demand for rational action based on health literacy or the White dominated colonial or neocolonial power structures).

Given Western biomedicine's foundation in germ theory—the idea that microorganisms invade the body and cause disease—even the most basic educational messages involve the conceptualization of HIV as an invisible entity, as a virus that causes illness. For individuals to acknowledge and incorporate this idea into their health ideology they first require a naturalistic perspective of disease (or belief in germ theory). Should personalistic medical ideologies be in place—the belief that illness is the consequence of immoral behaviors, the result of witchcraft, an imbalance in humors, a reflection of political conspiracies, or even the harboring of dirt—biomedicine-based educational campaigns will likely have little effect.

Anthropologists have continued to raise this issue of contention between international prescriptions of HIV educational campaigns and local conceptualizations of HIV. Richard Eves notes in regard to knowledge-based HIV prevention interventions in Papua New Guinea that "how such information [on HIV transmission] may be received or understood in implementing this elemental strategy [of HIV prevention] is unclear," (2012, 4-5). Stacy Pigg, in her work in Nepal, noted that adaptations of the simple message of HIV to local contexts assumes the neutrality and universality of the information conveyed, with any beliefs that contradict the authority of biomedical knowledge being displaced by the established 'template of facts' (Pigg 1996, 2005;

see also Patton 1990). Local understanding and explanations that differ from the master discourse of biomedicine are rarely addressed in HIV prevention messages (Eves and Butt 2008; Pigg 1996, 2005).

Moreover, producers and conveyers of knowledge who attempt to simplify the message for consumption by the lay public may unintentionally generate misconceptions. Rumors concerning public health promotions are common and widely reported in Africa, particularly around issues of family planning and more recently HIV (Nichter and Nichter 1996). Anthropologists have argued that rumors are often at the base of important community responses and resistance to health promotions imposed from outside. As Mark Nichter and Mimi Nichter stated, "What is labeled as 'rumors' are often 'social facts' backed by cultural common sense. Rumors consist of health knowledge that runs counter to that propagated by biomedicine and the state health authorities" (1996, 72-75). In her essay *Illness as Metaphor*, Susan Sontag (1979) described how when people do not understand the causes of an illness they tend to imbue these afflictions with moral or metaphysical significance. They may deny the disease's existence, attribute it to dark forces beyond their control, or search the cosmos for answers. Studies in South Africa have found that belief in conspiracy theories negatively impacts testing for HIV (Bogart, Kalichman, and Simbayi 2008; Kalichman 2009; Tun et al. 2010) and engagement in unsafe sex (Grebe and Nattrass 2012). U.S. studies have similarly found strong inverse correlations between AIDS conspiracy theories and condom use (Bogart and Thornburn 2003; 2005; Bogart, Galvan, et al. 2010; Ross, Essien, and Torres 2006), testing for HIV (Bohnert and Latkin 2009), and adherence to antiretroviral treatment (Bogart, Wagner et al. 2010).

Quantifying Youths' HIV Knowledge

In order to further examine the HIV knowledge of youth in Lesotho, I developed a self-administered written survey to pair quantitative and qualitative data. The survey (written in English at a sixth grade reading level) contained a 26-item scale of knowledge. The items were drawn directly from the questions originally posed by students and included in the pile sort exercise. The scale assessed standard areas of HIV knowledge including HIV transmission, HIV prevention, and commonly-mentioned misconceptions. Based on the results of the pile sort exercise, the knowledge scale also included thematic areas identified by students as relevant to understandings of HIV in this youth population, for example, the origins of HIV. Response options were coded as dichotomous (correct=1; incorrect=0). A cumulative score was generated by adding all the correct responses.[8]

The overall knowledge scores ranged from 7 to 24. The scale had a mean of 18.46 (Std dev=2.92) and a standardized Cronbach alpha measure of reliability of 0.53. Scales are generally not considered reliable if alpha values fall below 0.70 (Nunnally and Bernstein 1978).[9] An examination of the Cronbach alpha table, which shows alpha values when items are deleted, revealed that the overall alpha of the initial scale would not be improved by up to 0.05 if any of the items were removed.[10] As the students had generated the questions and as the knowledge constructs included in the original scale were relevant and necessary for a comprehensive understanding of HIV, I decided to retain the original scale. The construct validity of the scale was measured by testing the association between this scale and selected constructs. The results showed that HIV-related knowledge was significantly associated with age (r=-0.16; p=0.0008), year of enrollment at LCE (χ^2=42.00; p=0.0007), and gender (χ^2=34.78; p=0.0066), as observed in the analysis of the pile sort data. The proportion of students who answered the dichotomous (yes/no) statements correctly, with correctness based on current biomedical evidence, is displayed on Table 5.3.

Supporting findings from the self-generated questions and pile sort, students appeared to comprehend or at least have memorized the basics of HIV transmission and prevention (i.e., that HIV is found in blood not saliva, condoms are an effective means of preventing HIV transmission, multiple sexual partners increase HIV risk, HIV is not a result of witchcraft, feeling healthy does not guarantee that you are not HIV-infected, and HIV has no cure). However, understanding HIV transmission to the point of comprehending levels of risk of specific behaviors remained limited. Approximately 70 percent of students believed that HIV can be transmitted when caring for an HIV infected individual without wearing protective gloves. Almost half of students believed HIV can be transmitted by sharing a toothbrush, and that a mother cannot transmit HIV through breastfeeding. Approximately 30 percent believed HIV can be transmitted through kissing or via mosquitoes. In addition, about 30 percent of students remained confused about the scientific claims of the benefits of male circumcision[11] and about the safety of hospitals, and continued to regard HIV as a punishment from God (personalistic perspective) rather than a pathogenic infection of the human body (naturalistic perspective).

Although almost 90 percent of students correctly noted that HIV test results must be confirmed after three months, only 20 percent correctly stipulated that a negative test result is not conclusive. This suggests that most students considered a negative test result as final, and routine retesting does not take place. High-risk behaviors may continue, should an HIV test result be negative, as individuals may interpret the results as an indication that their past behaviors have not been risky or immoral enough to result in infection.

Table 5.3. Correct responses to HIV-related knowledge questions (frequency), where "correctness" was based on current biomedical evidence

HIV Knowledge Questions—Correct Answers based on current scientific evidence	Total	Frequency (%)
There is the same amount of HIV in blood as there is in saliva.	464	93.55
It is possible for a person to be cured of HIV and AIDS.	419	84.48
Almost all babies born to mothers with HIV get HIV/AIDS.	361	72.78
If you feel healthy, you can be sure that you don't have HIV.	393	79.23
A person can get HIV from a mosquito bite.	353	71.17
You can get HIV by caring for someone who is HIV infected without gloves.	148	29.84
People can get HIV from witchcraft.	439	88.51
A mother who has HIV cannot pass the virus to her child by breastfeeding.	284	57.26
There are special medications available to treat someone with HIV.	314	63.31
Sharing a toothbrush can transmit HIV.	245	49.40
It is ok for youth to have more partners. If one disappears they will still be left with someone to be close to.	446	89.92
You can get the HIV from having sex with someone, even if you know everyone they have slept with.	380	76.61
The chance of transmitting HIV sexually is very high during the first 3 weeks of infection.	248	50.00
Condoms are an effective way to prevent HIV infection.	398	80.24
If the HIV test is negative, it means the person is not infected.	98	19.75
You can get infected by tongue kissing with someone who has HIV.	345	69.56
A person with a sexually transmitted disease (STD), such as gonorrhea or syphilis is more likely to get HIV than a person who doesn't have an STD.	402	81.05
A circumcised man's chances of getting HIV from occasional exposure through unprotected sex are lower than a man who has never been circumcised.	351	70.77
HIV was produced in a laboratory.	381	76.81
Scientists have discovered a cure for HIV, but they won't give it to infected people.	400	80.65
People admitted to hospital can get infected with HIV because the hospital is dirty.	371	74.80
If you marry a person who is infected with HIV, you will be infected with HIV.	227	45.77
A person should retest 3 months after having an HIV test to confirm the result.	440	88.71
The symptoms of HIV are the same as the symptoms of sugar diabetes.	437	88.10
HIV is a punishment from God.	367	73.99
Traditional healers can cure HIV/AIDS.	445	89.72

Questions related to multiple concurrent sexual partnership (MCP) practices and marriage revealed the conflict that exists between rational risk reduction based upon biomedical fact, and engagement in risky behaviors as a consequence of social expectations. Although 90 percent of students reported that engaging in MCP practices is inappropriate,[12] a third of students reported having more than one sexual partner in the prior six-month period (perhaps suggesting rapid consecutive partnerships, which are equally risky).[13] Over half of the students indicated that HIV infection was inevitable if you marry an HIV infected individual. This belief is likely related to the important social marker of child-bearing. In Lesotho, there is no access to biomedical measures which can prevent HIV infection while fertilizing and implanting an egg or embryo, thus sero-discordant couples who want to have children run the risk of infecting the HIV negative partner in the process.

On average, female students had higher knowledge scores than male students. Male students were more likely to believe in conspiracy theories including that HIV was produced in a laboratory ($\chi^2=30.94$; $p=0.018$), that scientists have a cure ($\chi^2=5.64$; $p<0.001$), and that condoms are an ineffective prevention tool ($\chi^2=14.04$; $p<0.001$). Male students also believed that they can reduce likelihood of infection by knowing their sexual partners' sexual histories ($\chi^2=14.49$; $p<0.001$) and by not sharing toothbrushes ($\chi^2=4.70$; $p=0.030$). Finally, male students believed that MCP practices are socially acceptable ($\chi^2=20.94$; $p=0.018$), and that HIV transmission between mothers and children is not preventable ($\chi^2=7.22$; $p=0.007$). Males may have consciously forgotten what they know about HIV transmission routes and prevention strategies, or have not taken an interest in learning about HIV because disease prevention strategies ran counter to the behaviors they desired to engage in (e.g., condom-free sex, multiple sexual partnerships). In other words, male LCE students may have employed a form of opportunistic ignorance.

There were few significant differences in knowledge between students from urban and rural environments. Students from rural environments more frequently believed that dirty hospitals transmit HIV ($\chi^2=8.37$; $p=0.005$), and that marrying an HIV-infected person results in HIV infection ($\chi^2=6.39$; $p=0.012$). There were a few significant differences in understandings of HIV that offer an indication of changes in conceptual models of HIV that occur as one moves between environments (i.e., rural students moving to the urban campus and vice-versa). Students from rural areas who remained in rural areas were more likely to believe that HIV is in saliva ($\chi^2=10.27$; $p=0.016$), that HIV has the same symptoms as diabetes ($\chi^2=8.76$; $p=0.030$), that HIV is transmitted in dirty hospitals ($\chi^2=7.90$; $p=0.020$), and that HIV is inevitable with an HIV-positive marriage partner (χ^2=7.90; p=0.040). Students who moved from rural environments to the urban campus held the belief that marrying an HIV-infected partner will result in HIV infection. Students in urban environments, both those who grew up in an urban environment and those attending LCE-Maseru, were more likely to agree that MCP is socially acceptable (χ^2=9.69; p=0.020). These results from urban students suggest that a cosmopolitan, modernized lifestyle was being expressed through sexual liberation and the maintenance of multiple romantic partners.

First year students had higher average knowledge scores than third year students. This finding is particularly intriguing, as first year students completed the survey prior to beginning coursework at LCE and thus had not yet completed the required Life Skills class. All third year students completing the survey had completed the Life Skills course. These results suggest that the Life Skills course contributed little to students' biomedical knowledge of HIV, and discussions in class may even have altered perspectives of the disease or generated more confusion (as discussed in Chapter 4).

To compare knowledge of this youth sample with the national youth sample (MoHSW 2009), I generated a variable for 'comprehensive knowledge' to match with the complex indicator of 'comprehensive knowledge' reported widely by country demographic and health surveys. 'Comprehensive knowledge' is measured by the following: knowing that chance of HIV infection can be reduced through consistent condom use during sexual intercourse (question 1) and having only one uninfected faithful partner (question 2), knowing that a healthy-looking person can have HIV (question 3), and rejecting the two most common local misconceptions about HIV transmission and prevention (questions 4 and 5). The Lesotho Demographic and Health Survey (DHS) adds the two common local misconceptions regarding mosquitoes as a route of infection and HIV transmission through the sharing of food with a person who has HIV. According to the 2009 Lesotho DHS, approximately 40 percent of young women and 30 percent of young men (age 18-24) held comprehensive knowledge of HIV (MoHSW 2009). Globally, 24 percent of young women and 36 percent of young men in low- and middle-income countries responded correctly to these five questions on HIV transmission and prevention (UNAIDS 2013).

Students' comprehensive knowledge[14] of HIV is similar to the national sample of young men and women age 18-24. Overall, only 35 percent of students held comprehensive knowledge, with 38 percent of female and 24 percent of male students correctly answering all relevant questions (χ^2=28.73; p=0.0001). However, in comparison with youth globally, more female LCE students held comprehensive knowledge, whereas, in contrast, fewer male LCE students held comprehensive knowledge. This finding for male students may relate to the conscious ignorance of the male students discussed previously, given that prescribed prevention behaviors do not align with personally desired and socially motivated actions of these young men.

"Mosquitoes as a transmitter of HIV" was the most common incorrect statement, as it is elsewhere in the world. By omitting this question, 74 percent of students correctly answered at least four of the five questions. By including all items on the HIV knowledge scale developed by using the student-posed questions, 66 percent of the surveyed students correctly answered at least 70 percent of the questions (20 of the 26).[15] Given that the more inclusive measure of knowledge suggested that the majority of students hold basic HIV knowledge, the utility of the comprehensive knowledge indicators used by national governments in assessing the relationship between knowledge and risk behavior appears limited.

While these data from students are suggestive of the failures of current HIV education efforts to provide knowledge that can be translated into rational risk reducing behaviors (discussed further in Chapter 6), there are significant limitations in drawing conclusions from LCE students. Students of tertiary level education institutions may not represent the general youth population in Lesotho or in the region. While there has been a significant expansion in tertiary education facilities in Lesotho, with two new private universities opening in the past five years, only between 5 and 9 percent of individuals age 15-35 have beyond a secondary school education (MoHSW 2009). Furthermore, the use of college students in social science research is not without critics (Peterson 2001). The scholastic environment may limit certain data recovery methods because students perceive that they are being tested and answers are predefined as right or wrong. In addition, individuals attending these schools may have higher levels of education than the average person.

Nevertheless, higher levels of general education have not been shown to offer protection from HIV infection (Anderson 2010; Bulled and Sosis 2010; MoHSW 2009). Education may actually increase risk of HIV infection in some social settings, as education connects individuals to the formal economy and through it to industries of modernity. Research in Tanzania (Setel 1999), Nigeria (Obidoa 2010), and South Africa (Ashforth 2005; Leclerc-Madlala 1997, 2001; Posel 2005) indicates that individuals engaging with industries of modernity are involved in riskier sexual behaviors and, consequently, are at higher risk of HIV infection. As stated by Georgia Rakelmann (2001, 36), "Education, sex education and ambitious life concepts in no way shield from AIDS… rather…those who have access to the possibilities of a modern individualized lifestyle are particularly susceptible." Furthermore, the LCE is the only tertiary level education facility in Lesotho offering a diploma in education. Students in the the three-year teacher certification program came from all ten national districts of Lesotho and received a government bursary to cover tuition and living expenses. As such, LCE students represented the country's economic and geographic diversity; were actively engaged in 'labor migration,' which constitutes a locally identified risk factor for HIV transmission; and were greatly influenced by the increasingly available global commodities, which included global messages on HIV prevention and sexual norms.

The Moral Order

With the continued emphasis of international HIV health education campaigns on knowledge-transfer through behavior change communication interventions, and the measurement of HIV knowledge as an indicator of such prevention strategies' success, we can draw the logical conclusion that many funders and policy-makers still believe, despite extensive evidence to the contrary, that knowledge impacts behavior. This perception of knowledge-based rational action and the consequent individual responsibility for health develops out of the relationship between health and morality. Historical and anthropological research suggests that all societies create concepts about what constitutes a well-functioning moral order (Lock 2000) and that these concepts are intimately associated with what is assumed to be the health and well-being of the individuals of that society (Janzen 1981). Being healthy or engaged in healthful behaviors is therefore equivalent to being a 'good' person. In recognizing the profound need of social elites in France to attain purity, perfection, and immortality, Foucault (1998, 18) defined behaviors of self-maintained wellbeing as "technologies of the self" or practices that "permit individuals to effect by their own means or with the help of others a certain number of operations on their own bodies and souls, thoughts, conduct, and ways of being." Sociologist Peter Conrad (1994) argued that "wellness"— the avoidance of disease and illness—has become a "virtue" and for some, a secular path to salvation.

However, the complex relationship of morality and health operates in many ways and often with considerable ambiguity, and new knowledge confers new responsibilities and a set of new moral expectations about health and disease (Brandt and Rozin 1997). For instance, while some may celebrate the positive impact that stigmatizing smoking has had on smoking cessation, others recognize the potential for victim-blaming inherent in such strong moral positions emphasizing personal responsibility. The ongoing contentious debate about the cause(s) of AIDS highlights the moral position in health, with some viewing immorality as the cause of disease and by this logic the perils of violating moral conventions. Under this construct, morality and health are viewed as synonymous (Stephens and Breheny 2008). One need not be concerned about the risk of disease, nor can be held accountable for one's disease state (Sznitman et al. 2009), as long as one engages in the rational behaviors of a moral life. Sociologist Adele Clarke and colleagues (2003) describe this as a shift in focus that is "no longer on illness, disability, and disease as matters of fate, but on health as a matter of ongoing moral self-transformation.... Terms such as 'health maintenance,' 'health promotion,' and 'healthy living' highlight the mandate for work and attention toward attaining and maintaining health." Individuals unable or unwilling to maintain their own health continue to be pushed to social peripheries: smokers are ostracized (Reid 1997; Seiter et al. 2010), obese individuals are ridiculed (Rogge, Greenwald, and Golden 2004), and HIV-positive individuals face stigma (Petros, Airhihenbuwa, and Simbayi 2006).

Current models of knowledge-based health communication fail to fully acknowledge that those who do not acquire the knowledge, or adopt appropriate behaviors, are not necessarily irrational, undisciplined, or immoral. They fail to consider the impact of a social context that compels continued involvement in behaviors that increase risk for disease (Biehl 2007; Das and Das 2005). Individuals or communities may have differing perceptions of the situation or have different theories of disease causation (Eves 2012; Pigg 1996). E. Maxine Ankrah's (1991) and Vicci Tallis' (2000) examinations of social inequities across Africa, and Susanne Leclerc-Madala's (2001) engagements with Zulu youth in South Africa demonstrate that in some contexts there is conscious opposition to expectations of the maintenance of a moral order through rational disease-prevention behavior as people refuse to (or simply cannot) use the knowledge they have acquired to protect themselves against HIV until differentials of power are addressed explicitly.

In Summary

Measures of general knowledge and awareness of HIV on a national level in Lesotho remain low, with fewer than 40 percent of women and 30 percent of men holding what has been defined as 'comprehensive knowledge' of HIV (MoHSW 2009). General awareness of HIV in Lesotho has, however, reached almost 100 percent, and at least 70 percent of the adult population know the primary ways to prevent HIV transmission (MoHSW 2009). While the comprehensive knowledge indicator might suggest greater need for additional educational strategies, it might also prove to be a flawed indicator of knowledge.

Depth and application of knowledge among youth in Lesotho has gone unexamined, and beliefs in misconceptions that do not appear on standard survey tools have not been documented. In this chapter, I examined HIV knowledge of students of LCE using two qualitative research methodologies. Results suggest that, on the whole, youth knew the primary transmission routes of HIV. However, given the complexity of the life cycle of the virus, basic knowledge was not sufficient to drive prevention behaviors during particularly difficult, emotionally intense situations. Moreover, students acquired mis- or incomplete-understandings resulting in the belief that HIV can be transmitted in a seemingly infinite number of different ways. This belief was coupled with a personalistic view of the disease, linking infection with bad behavior rather than a biological imbalance resulting from pathogenic infection. Consequently, simple, yet perhaps undesirable, prevention measures including condoms and male circumcision were perceived to offer little in the way of negating risk.

If a new model of HIV communication is to succeed in developing individuals who can manage their level of disease-exposure independently, as the globalized biomedical model of health care requires, education needs to address local perceptions of HIV. Specifically, ideas about the origins or etiology of HIV need to be acknowledged. The distinct ways in which individuals rationalize HIV infection result in different perceptions on how or whether one can prevent risk. Of course, models of knowledge communication should also acknowledge that the understandings of the origins of HIV and the various conspiracy theories generated are ways of contesting, circumventing, accommodating, or even embracing scientific knowledge regimes, practices, and technologies of global biomedicine, all of which are highly dependent upon specific social and cultural settings and national and local political histories.

Medical authorities, policy makers, and public health workers might do well to seriously reconsider what we know about levels of HIV knowledge, and the methods we use to test knowledge and understanding. The opportunistic ignorance of the male students in this sample of youth, or more generally the continued beliefs in conspiracy theories and personalistic perspectives of disease, suggest that we pick and choose what we want to know based upon whether the knowledge fits with our desires and local ways of understanding.

6

Rational Action

Immediately upon arriving at the LCE-Thaba-Tseka campus, after a grueling six-hour journey tightly packed into 15-passenger taxi van, I was asked by the campus director to teach her Life Skills lesson on HIV. She admitted that she was uncomfortable with the subject matter and had business to attend to off campus. I was eager to assist in any way that I could. The college had been so gracious in hosting me and ensuring that I could conduct my research with limited interruptions and difficulty. Teaching the first year students in Life Skills would also facilitate my entry into their lives and ease future data collection.

Given my understanding of current student knowledge of HIV (see Chapter 5), I established a lesson plan that challenged students to reflect critically on what they knew and the sources from which they obtained their knowledge, rather than presenting them with the Western 'template of facts.' The Life Skills class at LCE-Thaba-Tseka was small, containing no more than 20 students. This was a vastly different situation from LCE-Maseru, where Life Skills was taught either in a lecture hall holding over 200 students or in three separate sections each holding 50 or more students. With 20 students, I could run the class as a seminar engaging students in group work and discussions.

I opened the class by having students describe ways to prevent HIV transmission. My intent was to empower students by revealing to them that they already held considerable 'factual' knowledge of HIV transmission and risk reduction. I hoped that in recognizing their existing knowledge they would feel more comfortable turning a critical gaze upon that knowledge. Next, I presented basic statistics on Lesotho's HIV epidemic. We discussed perceived distinctions between urban and rural settings and how these perceptions translated into ideas of modern-traditional lifestyles, behaviors, and HIV risk. I asked the students to reflect upon their own engagement in what they themselves defined as "modern" and "traditional" values and behaviors, how these associations did or did not impact their own level of HIV risk, and whether

Nicola Bulled, "Rational Action" in *Prescribing HIV Prevention: Bringing Culture into Global Health Communication*, pp. 155-173. © 2015 Left Coast Press, Inc. All rights reserved.

their own behaviors were in concordance with perceptions of geographical-ly-linked risk levels or rather more aligned with national statistics.

Counter to common local perceptions that HIV risk is higher among uneducated/illiterate, rural dwelling individuals who continue to engage in risky cultural practices, latest figures show that HIV prevalence in Lesotho is higher in urban areas than in rural areas (29.1 percent and 21.9 percent, respectively) (NAC 2010c). Recent findings from the Lesotho DHS (MoHSW 2009) further contradict links between high risk behaviors, ignorance, culture, and rural dwelling. Data indicate that sexual intercourse with a non-marital, non-cohabiting partner is not linked to either dwelling area or knowledge. The proportion of individuals reporting MCP within the past 12-months does not differ significantly by rural/urban dwelling area (6.3 percent versus 6.7 percent for women; 21.5 percent versus 22.9 percent for men). In addition, males with no education reported the lowest rates of MCP (18.7 percent), whereas males with secondary or higher levels of education reported the highest rates of MCP (23.5 percent). Women with no education reported higher rates of MCP (8.8 percent), while those with at least a secondary level of education reported the lowest rates of MCP (5.7 percent). These findings suggest that MCP is more closely linked to gendered economic inequalities than to cultural beliefs, rural dwelling, or level of knowledge.

Having set the stage for an open (yet directed) discussion between instructor and students, I broke them into small groups with four or five students per group. I handed each group copies of local newspaper articles about Lesotho's HIV epidemic and asked them to critically consider the message presented. I asked them to reflect specifically upon the following questions: What information about HIV was presented by the journalist of the article? What populations were identified as 'at risk'? What risk behaviors were presented? And, how could HIV be prevented in each situational context? Following discussions with their group members, a representative from each group presented to the class an overview of the article and their critical reflection of the intended message. Each article I had selected for this exercise portrayed individuals in the rural areas of Lesotho as more at risk for infection and more likely to suffer disproportionately from the disease, given limited access to care.

Although each group provided a clear overview of its assigned article, few offered any critical reflection. Being situated as they were in a rural area, the LCE-Thaba-Tseka campus, I challenged them to consider why the journalists might present the rural areas as more risky, and reminded them of the contradicting national statistics. After some time thinking and conversing among themselves they concurred—people in rural areas simply *lack the knowledge* to be able to enact prevention behaviors. Despite being in a rural area, the LCE students did not really consider themselves from 'rural areas' or 'traditional

Basotho.' Being students at a tertiary level education institution, regardless of its location in a rural setting, LCE students perceived themselves as engaged in a rapidly modernizing world. Theirs was a world that no longer dressed in traditional clothes such as animal skins, engaged in traditional subsistence agriculture,[1] or practiced traditional cultural rites, conveyed in the newsprint as 'risk factors.' They were also highly educated.

The students were confused and frustrated by being pushed to consider and reconsider their perspectives, interpretations, and positions on the situations as presented by the newsprint. Although they appeared to enjoy this different approach to teaching—the open conversation, the dialogue exchange among students and between student and teacher—they also appeared dissatisfied. Their notebooks remained open to blank pages, their pens ready to take down notes of facts and ideas that might appear later on an exam. I did not offer them any. There was no finality to my statements, no black and white evidence, no conclusions of right and wrong. I engaged them in an exercise of reconsidering something they had taken for granted, reconsidering a strategy for learning that involved critically evaluating the accuracy of information presented, and reconsidering how student-teacher relationships might be redefined to guide learning and knowledge development.[2]

In this chapter, I apply the concepts of positionality with regards to knowledge (expert, disseminator, lay person) within the realm of educational institutions. I focus here on the institution of education as this is the primary HIV knowledge source of my student population. I critique the divisions that exist between the teacher (the knower/expert) and the student (the learner/man-on-the-street). Finally, I examine the effect that such positionality related to knowledge and the characteristics of health education, and theories of pedagogy in general, have on 'rational' risk reduction behaviors.

Pedagogy of the Oppressed

Brazilian pedagogue and educational theorist Paulo Freire describes one-way transfers of knowledge as the 'banking' form of education. The banking concept of education valorizes the encyclopedic command of existing bodies of knowledge in line with the ideals of scholarship found in literary traditions, which Freire (1972, 45) described as follows:

> The teacher talks about reality as if it were motionless, static, compartmentalized and predictable. Or else he expounds on a topic completely alien to the existential experience of the students. His task is to 'fill' the students with the contents of his narration—contents which are detached from reality, disconnected from the totality that engendered them and could give them significance.

This form of education requires students to memorize mechanically the educational content provided by their teacher. This approach to education favors the prescription of formulaic behaviors, rather than the generation of new knowledge through systematic exploration. Students become containers to be filled by the teacher; the more completely they are filled the better the teacher. The more meek the student, in allowing him/herself to be filled, the more successful they are considered as fulfilling their role as students. Freire's reference to students as "receptacles," corresponds to Jean-Paul Sartre's (1947) "digestive" or "nutritive" concept of education, in which knowledge is "fed" by the teacher to the student to "fill them out." In my own experience this was termed "spoon-feeding" by my parents, drawing on the image of the feeding of knowledge as a *passive process* that requires little engagement and effort on the part of the student.

In this banking style of education, the role of the student extends only as far as the receiving and storing of the deposits. Knowledge is a gift that is bestowed upon those who know nothing by those who consider themselves knowledgeable. The teacher presents himself to his students as their opposite: he possesses the knowledge while they know nothing. By considering the students' ignorance absolute, the teacher secures his status of authority both in the classroom and in the community and in so doing justifies his own existence.

In the banking style of education, people are regarded as adaptable and manageable. The more students work at storing the knowledge deposits entrusted to them, the less they develop a critical consciousness. The more completely they accept the passive role imposed upon them, the more they tend simply to adapt to the world as it is and to the fragmented view of reality deposited in them. Minimizing or annulling the students' creative power indoctrinates them to adapt to their current situations.

I vividly recall this style of education employed during my high school history classes in South Africa. We had no textbook. Our history teacher, a stern Afrikaans man, supplied us with the text he wanted us to learn in neatly typed-out pages of world and South African history. Paging through my notebook, which I have carried with me for over 20 years, my careful highlighting and underlining of important passages filled the page with bright colors. Like many young students, I had left few words untouched, considering each important and in need of my careful attention and memorization. I recall sitting for the mid-year exam, hurrying to write out my teacher's notes verbatim as I responded to each of the essay questions. What I was writing about was forgotten the moment I stepped out of the exam hall.

This memory has been particularly important to me through the years for a number of reasons, and reflects the teacher-student/oppressor-oppressed relationship described by Freire. First, with no standard textbook approved by a national educational oversight committee we were taught only what our instructor wanted us to know. I am not implying here that a textbook presents all information in a non-biased way or that a history textbook approved by the apartheid government would have portrayed history any differently than my teacher's notes. South Africa's history and the history of the world have been misrepresented in many textbooks. Nevertheless, by learning only what our instructor believed was significant, our knowledge of and understanding of both world and South African history was limited to his perspective. We learned the South African history of the White man, the triumph of the British and the Boers over the savage natives, a propaganda that made us believe our position in society over the Black man was justified. At the time we had only two Black students in our class, as integration had only just begun to occur in public schools. We never considered that their view of history was quite different from ours.[3] Second, South African history in our classroom never extended beyond the end of World War II, thus never addressed the rise of the apartheid era in the 1950s. As I mentioned previously, for this reason I was oblivious to the African National Congress' struggles, the imprisoning of political activists, and Lesotho's role in keeping men opposed to the ruling apartheid government party safe. I never reflected on how my education was conditioning me to be an "oppressor," while at the same time conditioning the Black body to be "oppressed." This pedagogical design of "projecting an absolute ignorance onto others, a characteristic of the ideology of oppression, negates education and knowledge as processes of inquiry" (Freire 1972, 46).

Freire (1972, 46) argued that this banking education maintains and even stimulates the oppressor-oppressed relationship through the following attitudes and practices, consequently mirroring oppressive society as a whole:

1. The teacher teaches and the students are taught.
2. The teacher knows everything and the students know nothing.
3. The teacher thinks and the students are thought about.
4. The teacher talks and the students listen meekly.
5. The teacher disciplines and the students are disciplined.
6. The teacher chooses and enforces his choice, and the students comply.
7. The teacher acts and the students have the illusion of acting through the action of the teacher.
8. The teacher chooses the program content, and the students (who were not consulted) adapt to it.
9. The teacher confuses the authority of knowledge with his own professional authority, which he sets in opposition to the freedom of the students.
10. The teacher is the subject of the learning process, which the pupils are mere objects.

Freire (1972) argued that pedagogical styles that do not engage learners in critical thought are designed to define and maintain power differentials. In his examination of the oppressed-oppressor dichotomy, Freire noted the self-deprecating characteristic of the oppressed is driven by their internationalization of the opinions oppressors' hold of them—marginalized or socially dispossessed populations internalize the negative images of themselves that are created and propagated by the oppressors. The oppressed so frequently hear that they are good for nothing, know nothing, and are incapable of learning that they come to believe in their own failings; they "call themselves ignorant and say the 'professor' is the one who has knowledge and to whom they should listen" (Freire 1972, 38). Rarely do the oppressed realize that they also know things learned through their experiences in the world. Consequently, as long as they distrust themselves, the oppressed are reluctant to resist oppression. Furthermore, Freire argued, the oppressed develop a belief that their oppressors are invulnerable and all-powerful and at a certain point they feel an irresistible attraction towards the oppressor and his way of life.

Such shifts in power dynamics through the alteration of behaviors and attitudes have allowed invaders to succeed in cultural conquests in addition to obtaining economic and political control. In cultural invasion it is essential that the oppressed come to view their reality from the outlook of the oppressors, rather than their own. Thus, the oppressor can dominate by molding others to their patterns and ways of life. The more the oppressed mimic the oppressor, the more stable the oppression becomes. As Freire noted, "the more those invaded are alienated from the spirit of their own culture and from themselves, the more the latter want to be like the invaders: to walk like them, dress like them, talk like them" (1972, 122). Obtaining the same lifestyle becomes an overpowering aspiration for the oppressed desiring, at all costs, to resemble their oppressor.

While cultural invasion is on the one hand an instrument of oppression, it is on the other the result of oppression. The cultural action of the oppressor, in addition to being deliberate and planned, is perhaps also simply a product of oppressive reality. Freire draws on the example of the parent-child relationship, arguing that the home environment usually reflects the objective cultural conditions of the surrounding social structure. If the conditions in the home are authoritarian, rigid, and dominating, they increase the climate of oppression, as children internalize parental or elder authority. In Lesotho, this authoritarian relationship between parent and child extends into the classroom.

The banking style of education also relates to the transfer of HIV prevention knowledge. In Lesotho, students are able to regurgitate globally formulated HIV prevention messages of abstinence, faithfulness, and condom use, but have given little thought to why each method might reduce risk, how each method can and should be employed given different circumstances, or if the method is even relevant to their current situations. For example, there is the general perception among youth that one unprotected sexual encounter will result in HIV infection. While intending to promote safer sex behaviors, this oversimplification has potentially dire consequences. First, when an individual does not become infected following an unprotected encounter, the validity of the message is called into question. Second, if any and all unprotected sexual encounters result in HIV infection, then protective behaviors become an unnecessary burden as infection appears inevitable.

When collecting questions on HIV to examine gaps in knowledge, many students said they knew everything there was to know about HIV. When I asked what they meant by "everything," they explained, with sincerity, that they knew the ABC approach and that was the only thing they needed to know. However, as evidenced by the continuing rise in HIV incidence, youth are not necessarily capable of transferring this 'knowledge' of the ABC approach into risk-reducing practices that will truly empower them to overcome their oppressed status. Furthermore, as I realized while teaching the Life Skills course at LCE-Thaba-Tseka, students are unable to reflect critically upon the messages of prevention and the sources supplying the information. This inability supports Freire's argument that in believing they know nothing, or everything, students had no confidence nor reason to question the messages of HIV risk and prevention provided by voices of authority, whether in the classroom or via mass media. In addition, the messages of risk reduction, or safer practices, are not applicable to their situations or desired lifestyles.

In the following section I discuss models of HIV knowledge-communication that have developed through the course of the global HIV epidemic, and show how these models have naturally become more egalitarian in their inclusion of multiple voices as the public becomes more educated about the specifics of the disease. In becoming more involved in the conversation, individuals are more empowered to engage in risk reduction strategies and prevention strategies are targeted more toward unique contextual factors. Nevertheless, knowledge producers (situated mostly in the global North) continue to serve as the voice of authority in dictating policies to be implemented in multiple settings irrespective of their applicability (see Chapter 7).

Dynamics of HIV Communication

Instead of maintaining a vertical approach asserting the dominant voice of the expert, structures of HIV communication *have* changed over the course of the epidemic, via either formal education or more informal media messages and health intervention campaigns, to engage more purposively with the message receiver. Nilanjana Bardhan (2002) suggests that the dynamics of expert/man-on-the-street have shifted overtime as a consequence of shifts in the public's overall understandings of and responses to HIV epidemics. Bardhan offers four models of the inherent power structures that exist between expert/layman of HIV knowledge, which I examine in more detail below: the *press agency* or *publicity model, public information model, two-way asymmetrical model,* and *two-way symmetrical model.* Bardhan suggests that, with greater shared understanding of the disease given more equitable access to the constantly developing global knowledge of HIV, the expert/layman power dynamic has shifted to one that is more balanced.

The communicative phenomena of silence, denial, hype, and distortion of information characteristic of the early days of the HIV epidemic represent the first model. In the press agency/publicity model health information dissemination activities aimed to get the attention of relevant publics often through sensationalism and distortion of fact. The power to initiate communicative action was perceived to be with the information disseminator/expert. As HIV was first being discovered in many parts of the world during the early to mid-1980s, national governments, heads of state, and policymakers were silent. Global organizations, such as the WHO, were struggling to set up a response, being unclear about just how many infections were occurring worldwide (Christakis 1989). In the United States, it was not until October of 1987 that President Ronald Reagan first spoke publically about the disease and the surgeon general offered a report about the epidemic (Rogers, Dearing, and Chang 1991). By the end of that year, the silence had resulted in 59,572 reported AIDS cases and 27,909 AIDS-related deaths in the United States (ACT UP 2012: Bronski 2004; Shilts 1987). Governments in other parts of the world were similarly in denial about AIDS, labeling it as a foreign disease (Bonacci 1992; Sabatier 1988). The fear and uncertainty surrounding the issue resulted in overt stigmatization of people considered at risk and of those infected (Sontag 1988). Discriminatory responses in the United States included labeling AIDS as a 'gay disease' or blaming Haitian immigrants as being the source of the virus (Grmek 1989). Misinformation circulated about how the virus could be contracted, coming from both official and unofficial sources (Fauci 1983). As a result, the relationship between experts and laymen was marked by conflict, uncertainty, blame attribution, and a general lack of cultural sensitivity. Excluding a few prominent activist groups such as the AIDS Coalition for Unleashing Power (ACT UP), the people whose lives were most affected by the virus, the real experts or at least informed citizens, were mostly invisible and powerless in this early rhetoric of the pandemic.

In the latter half of the 1980s, as the heterosexual scare phase mutated into the 'normalization' and 'medicalization' phase (Albert 1989; McAllister 1992;

Nelkin 1991), dissemination of accurate information through the media became a priority. In the second model, the *public information model*, the expert aimed to inform the layman through dissemination of accurate rather than sensationalized information. The power to initiate communication remained with the expert. Governments around the world were paying better attention to the HIV pandemic and their local epidemics, and the globally coordinated response through the formation of disease specific organizations began to take clearer shape (Sepulveda 1992). Biomedical researchers in the West searched for a miracle cure, while policy makers began speaking the language of education and prevention. Although activists, NGOs, and informed citizens were gaining more presence and voice, the more traditional or 'official' voices of authority (Gans 1979) continued to shape the grand discourse of the pandemic (Bardhan 2001). According to a study of the coverage of AIDS by the *Washington Post*, the *New York Times*, the *Los Angeles Times*, and the *Chicago Tribune* between 1983 and 1989, 90 percent of the stories were drawn from mainstream medical journals and publications (Walters and Walters 1996).

With some lessening of social stigma and more open discussions in global and local forums occurring in the 1990s, behavior-based research and persuasive programs aimed at prevention and changing harmful health beliefs and practices became more visible. Nonetheless, theory driven top-down programs (Airhihenbuwa and Obregon 2000) and policies continued to dominate. UNAIDS was formed and international and national level efforts to control HIV intensified. While these communication initiatives were two-way, they were mostly asymmetrical in the sense that feedback was elicited to fit a-priori planning. The third model, the *two-way asymmetrical model*, emphasized feedback from the layman so that the expert could capitalize on his communication activities to systematically and scientifically persuade knowledge-receivers of the message. Although feedback from individuals receiving the information is crucial in this model, the purpose of this feedback is to empower the expert not the layman. With this model of communication, policy makers gained ground as spokespersons, and biomedical authority remained undisturbed (Bardhan 2001). The voices of the public remained muted despite increasing involvement of informed citizens in the form of NGOs and other local grassroots organizations. Being uninvolved in the production or dissemination of knowledge, people most affected by the epidemic had little voice in determining the direction of research and funding, initiating and devising policy and programs, and shaping the content of information disseminated.

The last model, the *two-way symmetrical model*, reconfigured the traditional focus on the expert and emphasized a transactional approach whereby both experts and laymen were open to the ideas of change and mutual adaptation. This model values the diminishing of power differentials as laymen become experts of specialized knowledge or are able to express their under-standing of and expertise in local issues. Conscious adoption of the two-way symmetrical model would be a progressive step towards grassroots empower-ment and involvement, that is, a transfer of power to marginalized communi-ties and community members through increased co-participation in shaping the programs and discourses that affect their lives.

There is recognition that past and current global/local approaches to HIV education programs have defined and maintained power differentials be-tween experts and laymen. In order to develop two-way symmetrical models of health education, local voices need to be encouraged to recognize both that global and national entities are forcing their marginalized situations and that their knowledge in the context of their lived experiences has value in develop-ing local HIV-prevention strategies. Progress towards the local/global/local approach is being made globally (see Chapter 7); however, current HIV dis-course in Lesotho remains asymmetrical. Although information has become more accessible through global media and the Internet, the production and dissemination of HIV knowledge have largely been and remain controlled by Western institutions and the experts affiliated with these institutions.

This situation became evident during my brief early morning conversa-tion with John Nkonyana, Director of Disease Control, HIV/AIDS, Ministry of Health and Social Welfare. It had taken a great deal of effort for me to schedule this interview. He was a busy man. My questioning of the national data his office was responsible for developing and my consequent pushing him to explain the data rather than just recite it clearly annoyed and frustrat-ed him. In an obvious effort to end our brief conversation and have the last word he mused about the current fixation of the international HIV stake-holders on multiple concurrent sexual partnerships (MCP). With a note of anger and aggravation in his voice he stated that his American friends in the United States were *always* having "sex parties," but America was not suffering the same heavy HIV burden. "MCP is *not* the cause of HIV in Lesotho!" he asserted. Ironically, the latest country progress report released by Lesotho in 2012 lists "Multiple and concurrent sexual partnerships" at the top of the list of primary behavioral drivers of the local epidemic (NAC 2012).

This conversation portrayed to me the nature of knowledge-dissemina-tors (e.g., teachers, report writers, national policy makers, and media), who generally view discourse as a challenge to authority. To Mr. Nkonyana I may have been a representation of figures from the West who have historically been unwilling to consider his perspectives or offer him a voice in discussion of national policy. However, as a young woman I also represented what was at the time in Lesotho a socially inferior group. Consequently, my desire to engage in back-and-forth conversation was likely regarded as a challenge to his authority rather than a meeting of equal minds desiring to better understand and address the local HIV crisis. Ultimately, I interpreted Mr. Nkonyana's frustration as evidence of the contradictions and unequal standards that exist in the world. In his view, the oppressor is fixated on controlling the sexuality of the oppressed, using claims of immorality to maintain their level of power, and limiting the voice of dissent. The Western oppressor fails to look beyond the behaviors of individuals to the structural factors of inequality and poverty that not only underlie individual disease risk, but are a direct result of the West's oppressive actions.

In his books, *Pedagogy of the Oppressed* (1972) and *Education for Critical Consciousness* (1993), Freire argues that the goal of education should be to achieve an in-depth understanding of the world and one's place in it—what he terms "reading the world." Learners should question the nature of their historical and social situations, thereby exposing social and political contradictions and heightening awareness of oppression. In so doing, learners can act as subjects in the creation of a democratic society. In relation to HIV knowledge, by questioning sources of HIV information and the information conveyed, learners should feel empowered to challenge the social, cultural, economic, and political contexts that place them at risk for HIV infection, develop contextually appropriate risk-reduction campaigns, and enact risk-reducing behaviors.

In referring to the development of *critical consciousness*, in which thinking and doing becomes intentional, Freire drew upon the work of Alvaro Vieira Pinto, who stated,

> The essence of consciousness is being with the world and this behavior is permanent and unavoidable. Accordingly, consciousness is in essence a 'way towards' something apart from itself, outside itself, which surrounds it and which it apprehends by means of its ideational capacity (Pinto 1960 as cited in Freire 1972, 44).

In this process of learning, both teachers and students are subjects, not only in unveiling their reality and in doing so coming to know it critically, but also in the task of re-creating knowledge. Through communal reflection and action used to attain knowledge, both students and teachers discover themselves as the creators and re-creators of knowledge—as joint experts.

In education, Freire called for intergenerational equity between teachers and students in which both learn, both question, both reflect, and both participate in meaning making. "Liberating education," Freire explained, consists of acts of cognition rather than just transferring information. It is a learning situation in which the cognizable object comes between the cognitive actors, the teacher and the students. Such problem-posing education requires breaking the vertical patterns characteristic of banking education and current HIV prevention communication, with cognitive actors (teachers and students) working and dialoging together. Accordingly, problem-posing education demands a resolution of the teacher–student contradiction. Through active communication, the teacher-student dichotomy ceases to exist. The teacher is no longer just the-one-who-teaches, the expert, but is himself taught by the students, who in turn also teach (Freire 1972). This shift cultivates a symbiotic relationship of learning and redefining positions, relative to knowledge.

Consequently, while banking education anesthetizes and inhibits creative power, submersing consciousness, problem-posing education involves a constant unveiling, critical reflection, and intervention in reality. Teachers serve the role of advisors rather than voices of authority, encouraging students to take personal responsibility and empowerment, to learn through experience, problem-solving, and critical reflection. This new model takes the claim of expertise away from teachers, removing them from their valued positions of authority in the classroom and the larger society. Nevertheless, this style of education represents the practice of freedom, for both teacher and student, as it offers an opportunity for all to be considered part of the world.

With this approach, HIV knowledge-delivery depends less upon the content of the message (though this remains important) and more upon the process of educational delivery and its ultimate aim. Transcending the classroom walls into the realm of policy development, I argue that it is not the role of international experts or global media to speak to the people, imposing upon them a certain view of the world, but rather to dialogue with the people about different views. We must realize that our distinct views of the world, manifested in our diverse behaviors, reflect our contextual situations. Educational, developmental, and political action that is not critically aware of this situation runs the risk either of 'banking' or of preaching in the desert (Freire 1972, 68). In the banking style of education, the educator gives the globally marginalized 'knowledge' or imposes upon them the Western model of the 'good man,' a global citizen, contained in a program whose content he or she has organized. Consequently, many political and educational plans fail because their authors designed them according to their own personal views of reality, never once taking into account (except as mere objects of their action) the men towards whom their program was directed.

As evident from my conversation with Mr. Nkonyana, even local individuals with both specialized biomedical and local knowledge are expected to succumb to the prescriptions for HIV prevention provided by the global institutions. His aggravation towards me reflected his frustrations in trying to direct local HIV policies, yet being muted by voices of greater authority, specifically the voices of funders and global health institutions situated in the global North. His experience remained a two-way *asymmetrical* model of communication, as international organizations expected his office to provide data they considered relevant and in the formats they determined while imposing Western logics in their interpretations of the local data. I discuss this dynamic further in the following chapter, which explores newly imposed global health institution policies to scale-up medical male circumcision services as an HIV prevention strategy, despite Lesotho's national data suggesting it is an ineffective strategy in the local context.

The Man-on-the-Street

To examine how HIV knowledge is conceptualized and acted upon by individuals, within a larger framework of distinct social and geographic settings, I offer the narratives of two LCE students. These students provide a general indication of the access and use of HIV knowledge in Lesotho. Yet, Senate and Letsie also offer voices that are specific to this generation: a self-confident young woman challenging her traditional passive, dependent female role; and a young man questioning his sexuality and desires to freely express his sexual preference within the confines of a conservative, religious society. These are voices that many in Lesotho are not eager to hear. Their stories offer evidence of youth drawing upon the different sources of knowledge to resist hegemonic structures that attempt to control their sexuality, sexual conduct, and even development as adults with their persistent messages of abstinence and limited sexual partners (Ahlberg 1994; Castells 2010; Dilger 2003; Mahdavi 2008; Setel 1999).

Senate's story

> With only three months left before her final exams, Senate was starting to worry about finding a permanent teaching position. Although apprehensive, she was eager to put the role of student behind her. As a teacher she would be respected by her students, her community would see her as financially successful, and she would no longer be a burden on her single mother. She also recognized that with her schooling completed she could consider settling down and starting a family. This would further promote her social standing. Unmarried and childless women were considered one in the same and referred to as *ousi,* sister or small one, regardless of age, career, or economic success. Women with children received the revered title of *'Mme,* mother or madam.
>
> When we met, *ousi* Senate was in search of "true love" and a single life partner, noting, "The time will come when I meet the man of my dreams." Western media had instilled in her the romantic perspective

that a single partner could satisfy all her desired criteria (i.e., looks, intelligence, wealth, romance, conversation, emotional support). As her time at LCE quickly drew to a close and she looked towards her future, *ousi* Senate's anxiety in finding a suitable life-partner increased. Like many of her contemporaries, Senate was the product of a single headed household. Her parents had legally divorced. Her father had left the family, providing no financial support. Given the stark contrast between the idealized Hollywood view of relationships and the reality of her parents' relationship, Senate was beginning to acknowledge that identifying a 'perfect' single life-partner was difficult.

Senate had not considered that her parents were faced with the same difficulties in finding the 'right' partner. During her parents' generation, marriages were still arranged by family members, limiting the choice of potential partners. One solution to the problem of having too many options, coupled with the feeling that her optimum marriageable age was coming to a close, was to have multiple romantic partners, sometimes overlapping. Senate explained that with multiple partners she could choose the correct one by comparing them side-by-side. Having many boyfriends simultaneously had become part of the urban custom. In addition to being vetted as potential life partners, boyfriends in the urban context were recognized as viable sources of the commodities necessary for a modern lifestyle. "Girls have many boyfriends. [They have a boyfriend] that can spoil them with money, [another for] clothes, [or] whatever. They call them 'ministers'—Minister of Finance, Minister of air time."[4]

Ousi Senate had experienced a series of unsuitable boyfriends while she was at LCE-Maseru. The last boyfriend was a policeman, whom Senate described as a respectable person with a steady job and an income. However, Senate had come to realize that they were not compatible as a couple. He liked to party, she did not. He liked to drink alcohol, she did not. He liked to have sex without a condom, she did not. Negotiating condom use proved to be a precarious task. She feared provoking violence or termination of the relationship. At times she even convinced herself that she would like to conceive. Being unable to negotiate condom use when her boyfriend was intoxicated, Senate feared that she was infected with HIV. Senate had tested for HIV. To her relief, she had tested negative; however, as she noted, "The worst part was that my boyfriend did not like testing and I wondered why. I shared my results with him and he was impressed. He told me that if I am negative, he is also negative, therefore there is no need for him to test." Senate's relationship with the policeman came to its inevitable end. However, upon hearing from a mutual friend that her now ex-boyfriend was unwell and had lost weight, she feared that she might be infected with HIV in spite of her negative test results.

The uncertainty of her HIV status added to her anxiety about her exams and job prospects. She planned to return to the clinic to retest, but could not face a possible positive result until her final exams were completed. Regardless of the test result she intended to continue to test routinely such that if she were to test positive she could receive treatment quickly and remain healthy to achieve her life goals. In addition, Senate expressed feeling an increased pressure to become a mother as she was about to assume her new role in society—no longer a student but a working adult. While she was not in an established relationship, she was routinely being propositioned by men. For young women in Lesotho, propositions from men were constant. Taxi drivers offered free rides; vendors offered free food; even instructors provided or denied grades for sexual favors. Senate described her propositions as follows:

One of my classmates requested me to visit him so that we could have sex. He is not only married but also old.... During Independence holidays I met a man who proposed to me. I did not agree to his proposal because I know his background. He drinks beer too much and he has many partners already. I don't love the guy because I never thought of having a partner who is not educated.... I have a friend at TY, he is my ex-boyfriend, but now he is married. He always tells me that he still loves me, but I told him that I am a girl, he is a man, hence I can't be involved with him anymore. He always calls and tells me that he is missing to kiss me.

These propositions, the threat of violence, and societal pressures to assume a new role as woman/mother provided justification for Senate's occasional unprotected sexual relations. As Senate expressed, she was "still a girl" and according to Basotho culture would remain a girl until she had children of her own, regardless of her education, employment, or marital status. On the verge of completing her diploma and looking to the future, Senate confessed, "I feel like I am old enough to have a child." If she were not able to find the man of her dreams, Senate was content to be a single mother and assume her position as a woman in Basotho society without a husband, revealing, "I sometimes have unprotected sex believing that I will conceive." Though this practice placed her at risk of HIV, she was willing to take the risk, societal expectations holding greater weight in her decision making process than her own individual disease status. Senate compromised these competing societal and individual (and one might argue, global) agendas by engaging in routine HIV screening.

Letsie's story

Like Senate, Letsie grew up in a single-headed household with his dad and his older brother. His mom died when he was young and a beloved older sister died shortly afterwards, during the birth to her first child. Consequently, a happy and loving family situation suddenly became disjointed, lonely, and even abusive. His dad made Letsie and his older brother feel guilty for the loss of their mother, venting his pain by yelling at and hitting them. At times, the young boys would seek safe haven at an aunt's home, where they could play as children with their cousins. Despite the imperfect situation at home, Letsie was provided with a quality education at one of the most prestigious and expensive high schools in Maseru. The family was not wealthy, sharing a two-room house on the outskirts of the city; however, money was set aside to pay for Letsie's school fees and school uniform. Letsie was even able to spend much of the year between high school and college at home watching television, instead of working to bring in a small amount of money to assist the family's financial situation.

To distance himself from his abusive father, on admission to LCE Letsie requested to be placed at the rural LCE campus in Thaba-Tseka. He romanticized the rural countryside as quiet and calming, noting, "I like the outskirts, the mountainous places, cool, and secluded." Letsie felt that the rural towns were the true Lesotho and was proud to reconnect with the spirit of his homeland. While he enjoyed the simplicity of the rural campus, Letsie was also comfortable in the urban space of Maseru. He shopped at the newly-built mall, used the library in town, had his own Facebook page, travelled to South Africa to stay with family, and even spent a few evenings with friends at a newly opened, very discrete, gay bar in town.

Letsie rarely told anyone about his sexual preferences for fear of the consequences. He explained:

For a long time I have known that I am a bisexual person, but I was just trying to fit in with everyone else. I have done a really good job of keeping this from people for fear of being ridiculed by society. Us Blacks especially, it is quite a taboo. It is something we don't talk about. I don't know what I would do if my family found out about it.

In the past, he had had relationships with girls, many girls, sometimes having multiple relationships at the same time, sometimes dating a girl and seeing a boy at the same time. Despite these relationships, he considered himself sexually inexperienced. He had only rarely had sex with his girlfriends. He offered this inexperience as a reason for his inconsistent condom use, explaining, "I guess we were just young and naïve. Things just happen all too quickly. I am not really a sexual person; I don't do it all the time."

Shortly after his arrival at the Thaba-Tseka campus, he started experimenting sexually with men. At times he seemed unhappy, even disgusted with himself. He had been given a New Testament bible by a campus church group looking to recruit new members on his first day at LCE and carried it around with him for weeks. He was determined to find evidence in this text that his homosexual desires were evil and against the will of God, as common Christian perceptions in Lesotho suggested. Letsie's determination to find confirmation within the New Testament bible was short lived. His first sexual encounter with a man happened within the first few months of his arrival at LCE-Thaba-Tseka, with a male lecturer. Although ashamed that an older man with authority had seduced him, Letsie seemed relieved that some feared barrier had finally been crossed. Letsie described the lecturer's advances as persistent and psychologically wearing, much like the propositioning experienced by Senate. Even so, it was a short-lived affair.

Despite his sexual preference, which in the United States tends to heighten awareness of HIV, Letsie admitted that he rarely considered HIV. He, like many Basotho youth, appeared to accept HIV as a part of his health landscape, viewing it as nothing unique or overly concerning. As he did not consider HIV to be a major threat, he had not bothered to test for HIV. He said:

Even though I hear that HIV kills a lot of people, personally I don't know all that many people with HIV, at least they don't disclose their status. (considering again) I know a couple of people, my relatives, my uncle passed away a couple of years ago from AIDS, and my neighbors and whatever. But it really isn't that much a pandemic in my circle. It is like a foreign idea for me.

The narratives of Senate and Letsie reveal distinct perceptions of risk relative to gender, social status (as new student or future teacher), and sexuality. Senate projected to her future as she completed her tertiary education and prepared to enter into the workforce. In doing so, she became increasingly aware of social expectations of women to marry and have children. Given the difficulty of finding a suitable marriage partner, she had altered her approach to confirming her womanhood by settling on conception without a marriage partner. Although not socially acceptable, single parenthood is a social norm, with grandparents frequently serving as primary caregivers and parents providing monetary support. By contrast, as a new student, Letsie was more engaged in exploring his adult identity within the parameters of his new freedoms from parental oversight. His concerns were directed towards developing relationships that confirmed his sexual identity, not in conforming to social norms given the strong opposition towards homosexuality by the predominant Christian belief structures in Lesotho.

Both students, like many others in Lesotho, transitioned frequently between rural and urban geographies and sensibilities, suggesting that there are no defined 'urban' and 'rural' risk categories or knowledge bases even though individuals locally perceive these to be distinct categories. Neither individual lacked the knowledge of HIV transmission. Both appeared to be aware of what constituted risk behaviors. Both engaged in risk; neither appeared to be doing so irrationally. As mentioned previously, the rationale employed by both Senate (to become pregnant) and Letsie (to confirm identity) were logically considered. However, neither individual's logic aligned with those offered by global HIV prevention programs, revealing that the top-down directives of global organizations and the Western hegemony of existing knowledge structures are not accounting for local rationales that perpetuate exposure to disease.

In Summary

In articulating what it means to know the world, including acceptable tools for knowing and applications of knowledge, dominant knowledge structures validate, privilege, and foreground certain forms of knowledge that continue to celebrate the dominance of Western institutions and ideologies over others (Dutta 2011). In contemporary discursive spaces, the interests of knowledge structures are interwoven with the interests of modernity, whereby knowledge is intrinsically linked to the mercenary interests of the dominant institutions of capitalism. People in developing countries, through historical colonial legacies, their pedagogical styles, 'democratic' structures and, more recently, health and development initiatives and global media, come to believe that their behaviors are backwards and dangerous. They view themselves as ignorant in being unable to develop and implement effective health strategies and tainted in that they will always be diseased. Only by engaging in Western biomedical practices (and other modern activities) will their inferiority be overcome. As Freire noted, the oppressed desire nothing more than to resemble their oppressor. Consequently, international development, health, and donor programs establish and maintain binary social divisions, the global-local, modern-traditional, the urban-rural, the rich-poor, and the infected-uninfected. Power differentials are continuously maintained in the realm of who comes to know the world and who gets to be scripted 'expert' and 'man-on-the-street.'

Structures have ensured that marginalized communities have been kept out of communicative platforms, spaces, processes, and resources (Dutta 2008a, b, c). Once learners are liberated from images of their inferiority and are empowered to evaluate critically their social, economic, and political positions, marginalized individuals can end a culture of silence that keeps them in inferior positions. The presence of marginalized voices, and their alternative and multiple logics, in spaces where global campaigns are negotiated offers an opportunity for social change by transforming structural inequities. As Freire noted, "If the structure does not permit dialogue the structure must be changed."

Freire's argument is central to the recognition of power differentials that constitute the tension of human existence—a struggle between the oppressor and the oppressed that is articulated and negotiated through dialogic opportunities (Dutta and Pal 2010). Freire suggests that only dialogic encounters entail the process of achieving social change that offers freedom and equality. In processes of social change, dialogic opportunities engage the oppressor and the oppressed, the teacher-student, expert-lay person, continually creating spaces for reworking the identities, roles, and relationships of the expert with the target community. In developing new models of HIV education, attempts should be made to ensure that marginalized communities can compete more fairly in the production of knowledge or be more purposively involved. In the following chapter, I examine how Lesotho's well-informed citizens are beginning to challenge the oppressive relationship with the global public health institution 'experts' by resisting calls to scale-up national medical male circumcision services.

Biomedical Shift:
Medical Male Circumcision

In recent years, global public health institutions have invested more heavily in and supported biomedical approaches to HIV prevention including routine testing, treatment (both for infected and uninfected individuals), and medical male circumcision (MMC). The link between male circumcision and HIV prevention was first hypothesized in 1986 as a possible factor in elevated rates of female-to-male HIV transmission among certain populations (Alcena 1986; Cameron et al. 1989; Fink 1986). The primary cause for elevated rates of HIV transmission through heterosexual contact was demonstrated to be the presence of genital ulcer diseases (Caldwell 1995; Caldwell and Caldwell 1993; 1994; 1996; Plummer, Moses, and Ndinya-Achola 1991). Differences in frequencies of certain genital ulcer diseases provided the general background for why parts of Africa have a raging heterosexual HIV epidemic while other parts of the continent, and poor people in wealthier nations, do not. Note that disease status in this argument has nothing to do with risky sexual practices, including early sexual debut, and many lifetime and multiple concurrent sexual partners, as knowledge-based rational action HIV prevention strategies would have us believe (as argued by John Nkonyana, Lesotho's Director of Disease Control, HIV/AIDS). Given the relationship between male circumcision and genital ulcer diseases, wherein circumcised men suffer fewer genital ulcer diseases, it was suggested that male circumcision might protect against HIV infection.

Biological evidence suggests that surgical removal of the foreskin from the head of the penis reduces likelihood of HIV infection (Morris and Wamai 2012). The exact mechanism of action is still unclear. However, it appears that removal of the foreskin may operate to protect against HIV infection in a number of interacting ways (Anderson, Politch, and Pudney 2011). HIV target cells are present in the foreskin epithelium, but they are also found in other areas of the penis, including the shaft. Sexually transmitted

Nicola Bulled, "Biomedical Shift: Medical Male Circumcision" in *Prescribing HIV Prevention: Bringing Culture into Global Health Communication*, pp. 175-191. © 2015 Left Coast Press, Inc. All rights reserved.

infections (STIs) can affect any of these sites and increase susceptibility to HIV acquisition by causing abrasions, minor trauma, and inflammation, eroding the protective epithelial layer, and attracting and activating HIV target cells. The foreskin also creates a moist cavity that encompasses the entire penile tip, trapping microbes causing STIs and HIV, increasing the risk of STI and HIV acquisition not only through the inner foreskin, but also through other sites covered by the foreskin (McCoombe and Short 2006; Patterson et al. 2002).

Ecological descriptions of areas in sub-Saharan Africa with low prevalence of male circumcision and high HIV prevalence have provided support for claims that complete removal of the foreskin could offer protection from HIV infection (Bongaarts et al. 1989; Halperin and Bailey 1999; Moses et al. 1990). An examination of the relationship between male circumcision and HIV prevalence across 118 developing countries offered additional support (Drain et al. 2006). Systematic reviews of observational studies comparing HIV risk between circumcised and uncircumcised men in the same population found that circumcised men were consistently at lower risk of HIV infection. These reviews include an assessment of 37 studies conducted across the globe (Siegfried et al. 2005) and an evaluation of 27 studies conducted in sub-Saharan Africa (Weiss, Quigley, and Hayes 2000). A meta-analysis of 15 studies, adjusting for potential confounding factors, showed the reduction in HIV risk to be large (58 percent) and statistically significant (adjusted risk ratio 0.42) (Weiss, Quigley, and Hayes 2000). Subsequent observational studies have found similar reductions in risk of HIV infection among circumcised men that are not related to differences in behavior patterns (see Baeten et al. 2005; Quinn et al. 2000; Reynolds et al. 2004).

Three randomized clinical control trials of circumcision among consenting healthy adult men in Uganda, Kenya, and South Africa were initiated in 2002-2003 to provide evidence of the causative link between circumcision status and HIV infection (Auvert et al. 2005; Bailey et al. 2007; Byakika-Tusiime 2008; Gray, Kigozi, et al. 2007). Interim analysis found a highly significant reduction in risk of HIV infection among the men randomly assigned to circumcision. This result compelled independent Data and Safety Monitoring Boards to stop each trial early. Collectively, 10,908 uncircumcised, HIV-negative men were randomly assigned to intervention or control groups and followed for up to two years. A random-effects meta-analysis of the combined study results found a protective effect of 58 percent, corresponding to that found in the observational studies (Weiss et al. 2008). Furthermore, in the Ugandan and Kenyan trials, circumcised men were at approximately half the risk of self-reported or clinically diagnosed genital ulcer disease during the trial. This finding offers additional evidence of the strong protective effect of circumcision against other STIs, especially genital ulcer disease (Weiss et al. 2006). Subsequent analysis of the roll-out of *voluntary* medical male circumcision within the population of Orange Valley, South Africa (the site of one of the randomized control trials), revealed significant reductions in HIV levels within the community, even though, given the non-trial situation, causality could not be established (Auvert et al. 2013).

Recognizing the relative cost effectiveness, limited interactions with a health facility, lowered reliance on individual negotiations of risk reduction, and projected long-lasting benefits, the world has rapidly accepted MMC as a highly valuable HIV prevention strategy. Many southern African countries have incorporated MMC into their national HIV prevention strategies. As recently stated by Wamai and colleagues (2012, 118), "There is no biomedical intervention currently being implemented that has been demonstrated scientifically to be more efficacious or cost-effective than male circumcision."

Despite international pressures for a nationwide scale-up of MMC services, the Lesotho government has delayed efforts. Two public clinics in the capital city of Maseru offer MMC services, though capacity within these clinics is not sufficient to meet population levels deemed necessary to effect a reduction in national HIV prevalence. No government-initiated communication initiatives have been developed to inform and educate the public about the scientific findings of the protective benefits of MMC against HIV infection in the region. As discussed in this book, communication is a vital (though not the only) component of successful disease-prevention interventions, informing, persuading and motivating laypersons to consider new strategies.

Communication is even more vital in this particular case. In Lesotho two forms of male circumcision exist: MMC, the surgical procedure conducted in a sterile clinic or surgery theatre, and the traditional circumcision conducted outside "in the mountains" during initiation *(lebollo)* rites. Many in Lesotho continue to regard these as synonymous practices, although important distinctions between the two procedures likely influence the level of protection (or risk) offered against HIV infection. In this chapter, I examine the circulation of knowledge regarding MMC as an HIV prevention strategy, from knowledge production through domestic dissemination and finally to acquisition and rational action by the man-on-the-street. First, I provide an overview of the development of global policies on MMC. Then, I examine the hesitance of Lesotho's national HIV policy makers to MMC scale-up as an indicator of resistance to the current global public health prevention approaches. Finally, I offer insights on the understanding by laypersons in Lesotho of MMC as an HIV prevention strategy, given the lack of consistent informational messaging from domestic knowledge disseminators. Although

MMC provides biological protection against HIV infection, the individual must still be convinced to undergo the surgical procedure, which like other behavioral risk reduction strategies requires the ability to process knowledge.

Establishing Global Directives on MMC

In response to the results of the clinical trials taking place in Kenya, Uganda, and South Africa, the WHO and UNAIDS convened the conference titled "Male Circumcision and HIV Prevention: Research Implications for Policy and Programming" in Montreux, Switzerland, 6–8 March 2007. According to Dr. Kim Dickson, coordinator of the joint WHO/UNAIDS working group on male circumcision and HIV prevention and the Inter-agency Task Team on male circumcision and HIV prevention, the meeting offered an opportunity to review the research results and consider what they meant for in-country HIV prevention policy and programming. As Dickson described in an interview prior to the meeting, the aim was "to bring around the table as many stakeholders as possible to look at and discuss many of the issues that male circumcision can raise, and, if possible, give guidance and recommendations for Member States and other stakeholders" (UNAIDS 2007).

A diverse group of participants attended the meeting, including academic researchers, members of international health organizations, gender relations specialists, representatives of UN funding agencies (World Bank, UNICEF, UN Population Fund) and of other public and private institutions (Global Fund, the French ANRS [National Agency for AIDS Research], Bill and Melinda Gates Foundation), association members, youth organization members, human rights activists, and the editor of a scientific journal. Sixteen representatives from Member States and 11 civil society representatives, including women's health advocates and a delegate from the Global Network of People Living with HIV, were invited to "present their own reading of the results and also to raise the issues that they face in their countries and in the context of their activities" (Dickson quoted in UNAIDS 2007). According to Dickson, particular attention had been paid to inviting people representing different positions, as this was the first time that such a wide range of stakeholders was able to exchange views and discuss the consequences of MMC as an additional prevention method in response to HIV.

A written statement on the Conclusions and Recommendations of the meeting was released on the 28 March 2007.[1] The WHO/UNAIDS statement read:

> The partial protective effect of male circumcision is remarkably consistent across the observational studies (ecological, cross-sectional and cohort) and the three randomized controlled trials conducted in diverse

settings.... The efficacy of male circumcision in reducing female to male transmission of HIV has been proven beyond reasonable doubt. This is an important landmark in the history of HIV prevention.

The heterogeneous collection of meeting participants gathering around a table, each to offer their voice, suggests the development of a multi-disciplinary, multi-occupational, and truly global policy. However, such formal platforms of communication do not necessarily provide opportunities for all stakeholders to offer their perspectives (Dutta 2011). The meeting was primarily attended by medical scientists (75% biomedical training), with very few social scientists and community members (Garenne, Giami, and Perrey 2013). No traditional healers or circumcisers were present. Traditional healers and circumcisers have a long standing stake in the discussion, yet as no representative was invited to what was meant to be a global collaborative meeting, they were effectively silenced from the conversation. Furthermore, with such a short time between study findings, the conference, and the release of official policy recommendations, there was no time to conduct additional research on contextual variations or concerns raised by meeting participants. Might the intentions of the Montreux conference, as an open-ended technical consultation among multiple stakeholders, be an overstatement?

What the timing of events, meeting content, and attendees reveal is a heavy emphasis on biomedical evidence for this new and potentially highly-effective prevention technology. The results of the randomized control trials were accepted with very little scrutiny as to their effectiveness beyond the highly controlled clinical trial setting. However, as has been argued, biological effectiveness does not always translate into effective public health interventions, given highly varied geographic and cultural context (Aggleton 2007; Black 1996; de Camargo et al. 2013; Dowsett and Couch 2007; Garenne, Giami, and Perrey 2013; Sanson-Fisher et al. 2007). Dowsett and Couch offer the example of a circumcised male, possibly experiencing a ritual cut or partial removal of foreskin during a traditional circumcision procedure, believing himself to be at lower risk because he is 'circumcised' and continuing his regular occasionally unprotected sexual behaviors as he moves between low and high HIV prevalence areas. The Montreux conference and the resulting WHO/UNAIDS statement provided no space for considering a situation like this and the role that other stakeholders (e.g., traditional circumcisers and healers) have in developing and shaping strategies.

Encouraging only MMC as an HIV prevention strategy, and failing to consider how domestic government officials and important community leaders interpret trial results and communicate these results to their constituents, limits the effectiveness of the strategy to adapt to highly mobile patterns of migration and social change, including integration of biomedical strategies, rapidly changing sexual cultures, and markers of identity (Dowsett and Couch 2007; Aggleton 2007).

Resisting MMC Policies

In Lesotho, nine hospitals have been assessed and equipment and consumables procured to support increased MMC, given global funding directives. MMCs are performed in government hospitals, filter clinics and private surgeries at a cost that varies from 50 to 600 LSL (6-74 USD). In 2007, a male clinic was established in Lesotho's capital city, Maseru, run by the Lesotho Planned Parenthood Association (LPPA). According to Program Officer Tefo Lephowa,[2] 240 men, of age 17 years and up, undergo circumcision at the clinic every month.[3] Demand has continued to increase to the point where men are placed on an ever-lengthening waiting list. An assessment of MMC estimated that between 4,000 and 6,000 MMC surgeries are performed each year (MoHSW 2008). The majority of clients seeking services are adult men in urban areas. Rural health facilities have neither the amenities nor the personnel to perform MMC surgeries, even if there were demand. Furthermore, the costs of MMC remain prohibitive for many individuals, especially those in rural areas who are not engaged in the formal economy and have the additional expense of traveling to an urban service facility.

Despite these efforts to scale-up and meet what appears to be a growing demand for service provision, the Lesotho government is unwilling to fully support MMC as an HIV prevention strategy. In this section, I trace the government's hesitance to respond to global directives to scale-up MMC services. I also examine why there may be a reluctance to put forward an educational health communication campaign that clearly distinguishes MMC (as an HIV risk reduction surgery) from initiation-embedded circumcision. By circulating knowledge of the potential benefits of MMC and/or developing local strategies to regulate *lebollo*-based circumcisions,[4] the government could endorse circumcision as a health promotion strategy while making use of existing cultural structures, attitudes, and practices. In so doing, current divisions between modern-traditional, rational-irrational, and uninfected-infected could be largely eliminated in an approach that satisfies and promotes both global health institution directions and domestic concerns.

The government cites three factors, namely, the apparent failings of circumcision as a protective measure against HIV at the population level, funding limitations, and infrastructural weaknesses, as reasons for their decision. First, the government claims that there is no evidence to suggest that male circumcision is protective against HIV infection in Lesotho. Drawing on domestic surveillance data (the Lesotho demographic and health survey), as established by global health bureaucracies, the government argues that the relationship between self-reported male circumcision and HIV "does not conform to the expected pattern of higher prevalence among uncircumcised men" (MoHSW 2009, 212). HIV prevalence is, in fact, higher in circumcised men than uncircumcised men (21 percent compared to 16 percent, respectively). Also, with 52 percent of men already circumcised, only slight reductions in national HIV prevalence will be obtained by increasing the proportion of men circumcised to 80 percent per model projections (Gray et al. 2003; Nagelkerke et al. 2007; Williams et al. 2006). However, the Lesotho Demographic and Health Survey (DHS) data does not account for distinctions in type of circumcision performed (i.e., traditional *lebollo* or MMC), nor does it confirm self-reported circumcision status through visual inspection. A study conducted among recent military recruits in Lesotho indicated that not all circumcisions are complete and the surgeries therefore do not provide the anticipated level of protection against HIV infection (Thomas et al. 2011).

The contradictory relationship between male circumcision and HIV observed in Lesotho may also relate to the age at which circumcision is performed. Traditional circumcision occurs for many after sexual debut. Hence men often have been exposed to HIV before circumcision. Should some initiation candidates be infected with HIV prior to circumcision, they risk transmitting infection to their fellow initiates, should traditional healers not use sterile instruments and procedures while performing the circumcision (see Brewer et al. 2007). This possibility was noted by Mathoriso Monaheng, former Director of Administration at the Lesotho AIDS Program Coordinating Agency, who was quoted in a local newspaper in 2003 as saying, "The problem [of initiation rites] is that they are using one knife to circumcise boys, that knife is used by everybody" (Staff reporter 2003, 10). However, warnings of the dangers of sharing cutting instruments have compelled many people to supply their own sterile razor blades when seeking health care from traditional healers. It is likely that initiation candidates now, over 10 years since the publication of Monaheng's statement, currently do the same.

Second, the Lesotho government has argued that cost and limitations in infrastructure have further halted a full scale-up of MMC initiatives. The Ministry of Health and Social Welfare has only been considering MMC surgeries performed by trained surgeons. The national guidelines stipulate that the 'sleeve/dorsal slit method' is the standard method for MMC in Lesotho. Of the three methods for MMC—forceps-guided, dorsal slit, and sleeve—sleeve is considered the most difficult, followed by dorsal slit. Forceps guided, considered the easiest method, can be performed by trained health professionals (nurses or even traditional healers) and need not be performed by surgeons. The decision to require the most complex surgical strategy suggests that the national government wants to restrict MMC to trained surgical experts, a position that places additional barriers to MMC and reduces overall access owing to high costs and limited staffing. The estimated cost of scaling-up MMC to achieve a level that would effectively reduce HIV prevalence is 125 million LSL (15 million USD), 17 percent of the 2011 national HIV/AIDS budget, with an annual cost of 10 million LSL (1.22 million USD) (MoHSW 2008). Scale-up of such a magnitude would, it is estimated, prevent one HIV infection for every 6.1 individuals circumcised. It would also save 2,136 LSL (262 USD) per individual infection averted in life-long anti-retroviral treatments and other prevention measures (USAID 2007). Yet, Lesotho currently does not have a sufficient number of surgeons to perform MMC, and few health care facilities have the capacity for performing sterile surgical procedures.

Third, the Ministry of Health and Social Welfare has argued that in addition to barriers offered by limited funding and infrastructure, culture has been an obstacle to developing a national male circumcision policy that would involve the support and implementation of MMC services. In 2009, the Director General of Health, Dr. Mpolai Moteetee was quoted in a newspaper article titled "Health Ministry has no intention of campaigning for circumcision" as saying that "circumcising young children [neonatal circumcision]…is against the Basotho culture" (Linake 2009, 8). The title of this article suggests that the government is against all circumcision practices regardless of age or venue. Moteetee's actual statement regarding neonatal circumcisions suggests that circumcision still serves as a marker of manhood, thus an important part of cultural and individual identity. Not only is neonatal circumcision considered irrelevant in the male circumcision conversation in Lesotho, but circumcision in general must be regarded as part of the larger conception of culture and identity, not just a medical procedure.

According to the Ministry of Health and Social Welfare, disagreements with traditional healers have further limited scale-up. While the national government neither regulates nor supports the circumcision procedures performed by traditional healers during initiation, it has suggested the implementation of standardized certification requirements for all traditional healers, perhaps in an effort to more closely monitor *lebollo* circumcision practices (Linake 2010). Traditional healers argue that they have been appointed by their forefathers and require no certification from the government.

Moreover, by supporting the most difficult method of MMC, any possibility that traditional healers could perform government-supported safe and effective circumcision surgeries as part of initiation rites is eliminated, even with government-sponsored training. The promotion of MMC may result in a significant reduction in clientele for traditional healers who perform circumcisions as a livelihood. Louise Vincent (2008b, 87), examining the male circumcision conversations in South Africa, argues that traditional healers, or other community leaders involved in the preservation of traditional culture, resist "the intrusion of state influence into a domain where some of the poorest and most marginalized in the society seek to maintain a limited hold on power." She suggests that such individuals have limited marketable skills and opportunities for the assertion of power or status. As the region becomes more integrated into global markets, these cultural leaders cannot readily covert their currency into the coinage of the modern liberal capitalist order (Vincent 2008b, 89). Consequently, 'tradition' is viewed as a limited currency with which to trade for power, and one that state regulations risk further devaluing.

Traditional healers have been involved in other HIV prevention and care services in Lesotho and the region. In Lesotho, traditional healers have been trained to provide community level support for long-term adherence to antiretroviral therapy alongside expert patients, community health workers, and police officers (NAC 2010c, 56). Traditional healers are also trained in the identification of the symptoms of tuberculosis, as well as providing HIV prevention information, conducting testing, and monitoring treatment (Furin 2011; The Global Fund 2008). In these programs, traditional healers are paid for referring their patients to biomedical facilities for medical treatment. This incentive suggests that, while biomedical initiatives recognize the importance of traditional healers in the community, the desire is to limit their direct involvement in HIV prevention and care efforts and their voices in directing future policy.

The limited involvement of traditional healers may relate to the state's desire (possibly pushed by larger global forces) to limit the value placed on local culture. As expressed by the LCE students and the domestic news media, 'culture' in Lesotho is connected to an historical base for social and political discrimination and oppression and is associated with traditional practices of uneducated, un-modern individuals residing in rural areas. As such, political leaders and, more generally, individuals who wish to be perceived as connected to the modern global enterprise, distance themselves from such traditions, identifying themselves and their country as modern, democratic, and capitalist. To collaborate with *lebollo* instructors and traditional healers might suggest that the government of Lesotho supports traditional cultural practices.

The concerns raised by the Lesotho government over developing national policies for MMC position the issue of male circumcision at the divide between modern and traditional. The international community supports new sanitary methods for male circumcision that are "safe and proper" and which take place in *modern* hospitals. This, by implication, is in opposition to the unsafe and improper circumcisions that take place at *traditional* initiation schools (Vincent 2008b, 81). By supporting MMC, the government might be seen as undermining long-practiced traditions. In contrast, by supporting traditional practices the government might be seen as at odds with the progressive, civilized, and sanitary practice of the modern. As a result, the national government has chosen to remain silent, resisting global directives to scale-up services using surveillance data as the language through which they are able to communicate with global health institutions and funding agencies. Such hesitance to develop and endorse a national MMC strategy suggests both a desire for change and greater equality within the established global health communication platforms and for greater independence and self-governance in domestic HIV prevention policy.

Domestic Interpretations of MMC

Generations of Bantu boys throughout sub-Saharan Africa have undergone initiation rites and the associated circumcision procedures, despite the risks associated with the unsterile conditions and the occasional loss of life as a result of bacterial infection (Magubane 1998; Marck 1997; Paige and Paige 1981; Richards 1982; Turner 1969; Wagner 1949). The circumcision procedure serves as an important marker of the elaborate ceremonies of passage to adulthood. Anthropologist Victor Turner (1957, 291) argued that rituals such as initiation rites act as a social glue, "compensat[ing] to some extent for the limited range of effective political control and for the instability of kinship... to which political value is attached." Furthermore, circumcision as a ritual symbol should be regarded as revealing "crucial values of the community" (Turner 1969, 2). The fraternal interest group theory suggests that male circumcision is performed as a way for fathers to demonstrate their allegiance to a family, clan, or village (Paige and Paige 1981) by submitting their sons to initiation, knowing the brutality of the acts their sons will have to undergo. According to this theory, the ceremony is not designed to impact the child; rather, it occurs at a time when the father's political and military potential becomes a source of concern to his lineage. The continuation of the practice in Lesotho suggests that initiation rites *(lebollo)* and associated circumcision still serve an important role in the maintenance of social structures and national identities among a significant portion of the Basotho society.

However, the practice has been in decline since the arrival of Christian missionaries in Lesotho in the 1800s. During this period, initiation rites were discouraged (particularly) among people in urban areas who were investing in higher education and engaging in the formal economy. The missionaries objected to initiation rites, citing them as a backwards and ungodly practice. The advent of the AIDS era offered further cause to abandon initiation ceremonies and associated circumcision practices, given concerns that the reuse of unsterilized cutting instruments contributed to HIV transmission. More recently, expectations of modernity have impacted the people of Lesotho, becoming a cultural factor in popular attitudes about *lebollo*-associated circumcision. As stated by a young, fashionably dressed Mosotho woman while we talked together with her German boyfriend in a chic café in the bordering South African town of Ladybrand, "You can't put 'From the Mountain' (local reference to geographic location of *lebollo* practices) on your resume."

Perhaps in response to reduced demand or interest in initiation practices, circumcision as an element of initiation rites in the region appears to have been modified in some cases, either replaced by ritualistic cuts or abandoned completely. A study conducted among a sample of young adult men undergoing physical examinations during the Lesotho Defense Force recruitment process found that of the individuals self-reporting circumcision by traditional initiation, almost half (42 percent) had no foreskin removed (Thomas et al. 2011). Some groups, communities, families, or individuals have completely abandoned the initiation process. The Zulus of South Africa abandoned the practice during the reign of King Shaka, as all boys of initiation age were needed for military service. It was believed that 10 years of military service was sufficient to prove loyalty to the chief. Other groups likely abandoned the practice of circumcision and initiation as a consequence of Western influences, including the intentional weakening of clan loyalties and the rise in cultural value placed on individual agency (Marck 1997; Wagner 1949).

In Lesotho, boys arriving back from initiation school, smeared with dirt and wrapped in blankets and driven through the capital city in open-back trucks, received a mixed response from onlookers. Some cheered and clapped their hands, others clucked their tongues, jeered, and shook their heads. Men who elected not to attend initiation school explained that in contemporary society one cannot afford to spend three to six months away from formal education or employment. Many explained that their fathers had not undergone circumcision, so consequently they had not and neither would their children. Families could not always afford to pay the initiator's fees or associated expenses such as food, a new blanket, and clothing for when a boy emerges as a man.[5] Others purported that initiation rites were contrary to their religious doctrine, or that initiation rites were the practices of people who were neither educated nor modern. Many admitted to being fearful of the procedure, particularly given its mystery and dangers. Individuals in Lesotho were not naïve to the risks associated with circumcisions. In recent years, increasing reports from neighboring South Africa have made apparent the significant dangers associated with traditional circumcision practices. During the 2006-2007 initiation season, 27 initiates reportedly died in the Eastern Cape province (on the southern border of Lesotho), 63 underwent penile amputations, and 562 were hospitalized (reported in Vincent 2008a; b). Men in Lesotho cited these risks as reasons for electing not to engage in *lebollo* practices.

According to the 2009 Lesotho surveillance data, 90 percent of the men who self-identified as circumcised (over 50 percent of the male populations) underwent the traditional initiation process of *lebollo* (MoHSW 2009). Attendance at initiation schools varied by dwelling area, education level, and socioeconomic status. Men living in rural areas were more likely to self-report being circumcised as compared to men living in urban areas (59 and 34 percent, respectively). Men who had never been to school were more likely to report being circumcised as compared to men who had completed primary or secondary school (79, 24, and 26 percent, respectively). Finally, men with a lower socioeconomic status were more likely to report circumcision, with 74 percent of men in the lowest wealth quintile reporting circumcision as compared to 29 percent of men in the highest wealth quintile.

Local youth perceptions of male circumcision offer insights into the complexity of implementing biomedical interventions and the importance of clear communication to inform and motivate individuals to engage with the approach. The lack of a clearly communicated policy on male circumcision has generated speculation and considerable confusion regarding MMC as an HIV prevention strategy. I asked students whether a circumcised man's chances of getting HIV from occasional exposure through unprotected sex were lower than those of a man who has never been circumcised.[6] One third (of 556 students) said that the likelihood of infection was no different. Students were not always aware that circumcision could be performed in a clinical setting, knowing only about *lebollo*-based circumcision. Some students clarified that if a man were circumcised in a clinic his chances of HIV infection declined, while if circumcised during initiation his risk of HIV increased. This perspective draws on the shared understanding that unsterile cutting instruments can transmit HIV. Some students noted that only if the clinic used a new sterile blade to perform the surgery would risk of HIV infection decrease as a result of circumcision. The confusion surrounding MMC is evident in the following statements from students:

> Student 1: No, I do not believe that [clinic-based circumcision reduces HIV infection]. Because if you are circumcised or if someone is not circumcised and you have sex with someone who is HIV positive both of them not using condoms, both of them are going to contract HIV. It does not matter whether you are circumcised or not. (female, Maseru campus, urban, 21 years)

> Student 2: I don't think it is 100% safe. I think that whether or not he is circumcised he will still get HIV. I saw them at my place, died because of HIV, even if they come from circumcision. I mean traditional, I don't know those from hospitals. (female, Maseru campus, rural, 26 years)

Student 3: I am not sure. Is it true that when a male is circumcised he has a less chance of being infected? That I am not quite sure of it. (male, Maseru campus, urban, 24 years)

Note that two of the three students are female.[7] The voice of women remains important in the MMC debate. Although women are not concerned with undergoing MMC themselves, and will never know of the particulars of the highly secretive traditional circumcision ceremony, they may have younger brothers and future sons for whom they will have to consider circumcision options, possibly even opting for neonatal circumcision. In the United States, the American Academy of Pediatrics (AAP 2012, e757) issued a positive, though not prescriptive, report of neonatal circumcision noting that current evidence indicates that the health benefits of neonatal male circumcision outweigh the risks. They further added, "Parents should weigh the health benefits and risks in light of their own religious, cultural, and personal preferences, as the medical benefits alone may not outweigh these other considerations for individual families." A review of the literature by Morris, Bailis and Wiswell, (2014, 1) concluded that "As with vaccination, circumcision of newborn boys should be part of public health policies."

Although few students knew of the particulars of *lebollo* or the associated circumcision ceremony, having not attended themselves (and none would reveal if they had), years of educational messaging warning of the risks of sharing of cutting instruments had convinced the students that male circumcision as performed by a traditional healer/initiator was risky and increased HIV risk. This perception is clear in the following statements of two female students[8]:

We don't know what is happening there [at the initiation schools]. We don't know if they are using different blades.

In the Basotho culture, where people go for initiation and they are circumcised. I don't really know what happens in the process of circumcision, if they use one blade or they use different blades. If they use only one blade that means there is transmission of AIDS there.

These statements further indicate that students separate themselves from the individuals who continue to engage in traditional practices such as initiation rites or from those who associate with "the Basotho culture." Such practices are seen as old-fashioned, outdated, and un-modern. The practice is stigmatized as something found among individuals who have limited education, given their location in rural areas and continued belief in witchcraft and sorcery, as noted by a male LCE-Maseru student, who commented, "My family used to believe in traditional doctors where we used to share one blade for cutting our skin. This was done for protection against lightning, witches and devil spirit."

Youths' confusion was further complicated by unclear statements from government officials, as well as the implementation of MMC services throughout the country without any strong support or promotional campaigns by voices of authority. For example, in 2011, Dr Limbamba, Lesotho's NAC strategic planner, was quoted in a local newspaper as having made the announcement, "Although many believe male circumcision to be one of the main contributors to the high [HIV] infection rate, research shows that it actually combats the spread of the virus" (Staff Reporter 2011). Dr Limbamba did not clarify which type of circumcision strategy, and whether one circumcision strategy remains risky (and why), while another is safe and protective (and why). Without complete and accurate knowledge, youth in Lesotho are unable to make informed decisions regarding their engagement in HIV prevention strategies, making evident the power dynamics inherent in the circulation of knowledge that contribute to the failures of current prescriptive HIV prevention strategies. In the case of MMC, knowledge disseminators have chosen to withhold information preventing the public from engaging as rational actors. Of course, we should not assume that knowledge alone is empowering. However, by not knowing of the potential benefits of MMC, at the level of the individual and potentially the population, and not being able to access MMC services, the public is disempowered, at risk, and infected.

Opposing Global Health Institution Directives

The resistance to scale-up MMC efforts in Lesotho, despite general acceptance of global HIV directives over the past 20 years, further offers an indication that the global hegemony of Western knowledge, including biomedicine and science, is and always has been vulnerable to challenges from political and religious leaders (Epstein 2007; Fassin 2007; Nattrass 2007).[9] Powerful national state actors have offered considerable resistance against global HIV programs and their local NGO and social movement mediators (Cassidy and Leach 2007). Consider, for example, former South African President Thabo Mbeki's well known dissident science position on AIDS. Mbeki aligned himself with unorthodox scientists including David Rasnick and Peter Doesberg, who challenged conventional biomedical approaches to HIV and AIDS. Mbeki's refusal to accept scientific orthodoxy, believing that science has been used as a vehicle for neo-imperialism, is evident in statements he made in a letter published in the South African newspaper, *Mail and Guardian*. Mbeki wrote, "They [scientists] proclaim that our continent [Africa] is doomed to an inevitable mortal end because of our devotion to the sin of lust" (Mbeki, *Mail and Guardian*, 26 October 2001, in Mbali 2004). For Mbeki, being forced to respond to the local HIV epidemic through the biomedical paradigm was unacceptable. His dissent placed an international spotlight on the political economy of biomedical research (Schneider 2002) and the power structures of global public health.

The increasing involvement of international health agencies in health programs in the global South has unleashed more periodic backlashes from governments claiming that these humanitarian interventions represent foreign interests and constitute Western threats to national sovereignty. In fact, the very processes of globalization with which global humanitarian efforts are intimately connected and that have perpetuated modes of oppression and control across the globe, have also created openings for challenging unequal, unjust, and powerful structures at the center through the creation of solidarity networks across global borders (Moghadam 2009). "Narratives of colonialism coexist with narratives of resistance that seek to rupture the dominant narratives of power and control through which the colonial forces created their systems of oppression," argues Mohan Dutta (2011, 52).

Acts of resistance suggest that nation states and individuals are attempting to redefine their positions in the global public health structures. As noted by Dutta (2011, 45), "The hegemony of Western ways of knowing was often accomplished through the languages of rationality, science and medicine, positioned as the antithesis of the irrationalities of the natives." Anna Tsing has suggested that resistance against dominant knowledge, ideologies, and structures is to be expected, as ideas and products increasingly flow and circulate around the globe. She used the metaphor of "friction," with both its positive and negative aspects, to describe the interactions that occur as the global and local interact. She argued that despite unequal and heterogeneous encounters between global and local entities, the friction that results can often lead to new arrangements of culture and power (Tsing 2004, 5). Nation states have served as a mechanism for multi- and transnational corporations (the colonizers of the twenty-first century), by ensuring the creation and maintenance of markets that serve the interests of the dominant social classes and the continued control of power by the global North (Dutta 2011; Harvey 2005). Resistance to global directives at the state level suggests desires for transformation of existing global power structures. Such resistance has been discussed under multiple frameworks including "globalization from below," "transnational activism," "transnational social movement," and "grassroots organizing" (Ganesh et. al 2005).

In Summary

The case of MMC in Lesotho offers a clear view of the circulation of knowledge for HIV prevention. Using this new HIV prevention strategy we can trace the flow of knowledge from the global South (observational, ecological, randomized controlled trial studies) to the global North (the conference at Montreux) and back to the global South (as policy). Directors of global public health institutions expect domestic agents to serve as knowledge disseminators, passively passing on 'globally established' knowledge to the layman. However in this case, the domestic knowledge disseminators (government officials and cultural leaders) have adjusted the UNAIDS message. Rather than scaling-up services and promoting MMC, the domestic government has delayed, listed rationale based on domestic surveillance (as implemented by global public health institutions), and not advocated for MMC publically. Consequently, the intended recipients of the message are unable to make a rational choice to undergo MMC, given the insufficient, incomplete, and contradictory knowledge.

In Lesotho, two circumcision practices exist side-by-side. Though it is waning as a practice, rural men continue to undergo circumcision through traditional *lebollo* ceremonies. Men in urban areas have either elected not to be circumcised or are circumcised in modern MMC facilities. Other than defining which type of MMC surgery can be performed in Lesotho, the government has resisted global health institution directives calling for the significant scale-up of MMC services and the establishment of a formulated message on its position on MMC as an HIV prevention strategy.

The government may not have wanted to support either traditional or modern circumcision practices for two primary reasons. First, collaborations with *lebollo* instructors and traditional healers could suggest the government of Lesotho supports traditional cultural practice. For years, the nation state of developing countries, acting as a tool in the colonial and now neoliberal enterprise, distanced themselves from local traditions in an attempt at identifying themselves and their countries as modern, democratic, and capitalist. Supporting traditional cultural practice would appear to counter the development advances made. Second, given the considerable objection raised in South Africa to government regulation of traditional circumcision practices, the Lesotho government's unwillingness to communicate publicly their decisions about circumcision may have been a political step to retain the support of rural constituents, given that national elections were held in early 2012. Presenting the debate as a modern value system clashing with a traditional system risks suggesting that cultural practices are pristine and static, yet increasingly contaminated by outside interference. With biomedical HIV directives largely produced by international agencies (though influenced by experts in the global South), which have the financial capacity to ensure their directives are implemented, HIV prevention strategies such as MMC can be viewed as the 'contaminating outside interference.' The 'contamination' might appear less forced if domestic agents, including cultural leaders and traditional healers were offered an opportunity to reassemble the MMC approach to fit with their current practices. Instead, they are silenced in the international discussion and forced to comply with directives that may not be socially appropriate or prove cost-effective in an already limited health and HIV budget.

Furthermore, calls for MMC place male circumcision within the restricted purview of the modern biomedical community. Biomedicine has justified its need to oversee and control life events, such as male circumcision, by grounding itself in science wherein knowledge about the body and disease is systematized and objective. As Foucault (1973, 54) argued, medicine "assumes a normative posture, which authorizes it not only to distribute advice as to a healthy life, but also to dictate the standards for physical and moral relations of the individual and of the society in which he lives." Observations and causative experimentation based on germ theory and employing gold standard randomized control trials provides the evidence needed to rationalize surgical removal of foreskin from every boy and man in the AIDS belt. By employing statistical surveys, biomedicine has defined 'healthy' and 'pathology' relative to an act, which continues to hold significant meaning. Notes Vincent (2008b, 81), "Doctors and hospitals are one of the primary mechanisms through which certain practices are authorized and rendered legitimate while others are marginalized and rendered illegitimate." Male circumcision may be yet another standardized biomedical response to threats of disease, with certain individuals procuring rights to 'appropriate' forms of circumcision/technology/knowledge. Poor and marginalized individuals, particularly those who are not integrated into the global system from which prescriptions on disease prevention come, may turn to traditions as a way of gaining or maintaining social standing in the local community.

As indicated by data gathered from youth, silence of, as well as contradictory statements made by, national leaders has resulted in considerable local confusion. Traditional and clinic-based circumcisions are viewed as one and the same, having no association with HIV other than increasing the risk of infection if unsterilized cutting instruments are used. Consequently, what could potentially be an effective public health intervention is mired in contestations over current global health communication frameworks and discourse that pit global-modern against local-traditional. The voice of the subaltern continues to be lost in such debates, and his beliefs, attitudes, values, and behaviors become even further marginalized by dominant global ideologies.

Bringing Culture to
Global Health Communication

In this book I have examined how the prescriptive nature of knowledge-based global HIV prevention strategies has affected the knowledge, explanatory accounts, and practices of youth in Lesotho. By focusing on the movement of HIV knowledge (how people know what they know) and the impact of this knowledge (how people interpret health education messages), rather than just the content of HIV education campaigns (what is being taught), this examination offers evidence that current knowledge-based HIV prevention strategies and general global health campaigns do not account for dynamic social systems and multiple knowledge domains. We must consider the fact that positionality relative to knowledge communication (producers, disseminators, receivers) is a significant component in debates about general health inequities. The web of knowledge producers, disseminators, receivers and their interactions that comprise what we know as HIV prevention science generates particular categories of knowledge, consciousness, and reality related to HIV prevention. To achieve their desired outcomes, global health campaigns cannot simply be scaled-up, universalized, and made 'culturally-sensitive.'

In exploring the ideological constructions of biomedical knowledge production, dissemination, and acquisition and the related reduction in risk behavior, it is evident that the information and practices necessary to become rational and self-regulating are unequally distributed. Examinations of recent health epidemics, including the HIV pandemic, reveal that competing narratives are often reduced to a dominant scientific account, backed by a vast scientific network and imposed globally through international health organizations, NGOs, and a system of expert knowledge that includes leading scholars, academic institutions, and journals (Epstein 1996; Eves 2012; Patton 1990; Pigg 1996; Treichler 1991). As a result, national responses to epidemics generally disregard local interpretations, local context,

Nicola Bulled, "Bringing Culture to Global Health Communication" in *Prescribing HIV Prevention: Bringing Culture into Global Health Communication*, pp. 193-205. © 2015 Left Coast Press, Inc. All rights reserved.

and local solutions (Leclerc-Madlala 2002; McNeill 2011; Pigg 2005; Sae-thre and Stadler 2009). The transnational social movement, for instance, continues to be largely represented by the global North and by participants from privileged, middle-class backgrounds (Basu and Dutta 2009; Basu 2004; 1995; Desai 2005).

The continued dominance of Western ideologies, devaluing alternatives, presents an additional barrier to equitable global health communication platforms. The West has taught individuals in developing nations that in en-acting certain health initiatives, engaging in certain behaviors, and buying certain products they will be able to overcome their inferiority. The growth of global consumer capitalism has developed a means by which hegemonic ideas, behaviors, and lifestyles can be marketed and demand created, al-though these ideas are frequently in conflict with one another. Youth in Le-sotho, with access to modern commodities and media, become oriented to a global culture that values the fulfillment of individual rights, sexual liberalization, and the authenticity of the individual through self-consti-tution, self-assertion, self-transformation, self-governance, self-reliance, and self-maintained wellbeing (echoing Foucault's (1998) 'technologies of self'). Desiring to live modern lifestyles (portrayed by local and global media as being economically successful and sexually liberated), youth are reconfiguring modern identity through their own localities. They engage with consumer culture and maintain multiple sexual partners as a way to acquire modern commodities and/or express sexual liberation. Rather than drawing on 'technologies of self' in the same way as discussed by Foucault (1998), by purposefully engaging in risk as a way to acquire self-governance and self-reliance, youth engage in what appears as 'normal' sexual activi-ties (as displayed through media) without realizing the potential hazardous consequences.

Charles Briggs and colleagues' examinations of disease outbreaks, includ-ing cholera and dengue fever in Venezuela and H1N1 in the United States, suggest that social divisions are created and perpetuated based upon relative positioning to knowledge sources, or spheres of biocommunicability, and the mostly one-way flow of information between these spheres (Briggs 2003, 2005; Briggs and Hallin 2010; Briggs and Hallin 2007; Briggs and Mantini-Briggs 2003; Briggs and Nichter 2009; Mantini-Briggs 2013). In this, much like other biomedical technologies, biomedical knowledge has generated social stratifi-cations based not only on access to knowledge, but also on the power-laden relationships involved in knowledge creation and transfer—those authorized to produce and disseminate knowledge (the expert and the well-informed citizen) versus those who actively or passively receive the message (the man-on-the-street).

The rules for knowledge production, including what constitutes knowledge, are largely determined by dominant social and cultural institutions across the globe that represent an implicit interest in the status quo. The basic requirements of civil society such as literacy, formal education, nuclear family units, and private property are considered necessary for involvement in knowledge-producing platforms. These requirements exclude significant sectors of the population. As explained by Mohan Dutta (2011, 184), marginalized individuals "exist in the interstices of modern civil societies, rendered invisible through the lack of access to the discursive spaces of the mainstream public spheres where issues are debated and policies are formulated." Given their inferior social positions, there is limited opportunity for individuals from the marginalized sectors of the globe to participate in knowledge-production at the domestic, international, or global levels, as discursive opportunities are not accessible. For instance, rural dwelling individuals in Lesotho are perceived as being socially inferior, given their lower levels of educational attainment. They are shut out of discussions of national HIV prevention policy, even if they are considered by their own society as being at greatest risk for HIV infection. As a result, HIV prevention strategies are produced for them and likely fail to address the structural factors that perpetuate risk behaviors.

The long-standing focus of global disease prevention strategies on Western-oriented biomedical knowledge development has further fostered inequities of power and resources. These power imbalances are less a consequence of the unfamiliarity of peoples around the globe or disagreement with biomedical perspectives and solutions, and more a result of inequitable distribution of biomedical knowledge. The dominant (funders, researchers, and global policy institutions largely positioned in the global North) are dictating who gets what knowledge and under what circumstances. They force compliance and provide access to knowledge solely to cement their own strong positions and deter challengers. Those who fail to participate in the system are further ostracized. Much as the colonial legacy has taught people in developing countries that they are backward, ignorant, and tainted, contemporary global health and development agencies have dominated the production and dissemination of health information, signaling to local actors that they neither appropriately conceptualize their disease situations nor have strategies in place to address the situation.

The vertical, local-global-local approach that pushes forward in the name of the efficiency mechanisms of free market economies, rather than trying to fully engage with the communities involved or develop bottom-up community-based strategies, has profound implications for global HIV prevention initiatives. Take, for instance, the most recent biomedical HIV prevention development—oral- and gel-based antiretroviral (ARV) pre-exposure prophylactics

(PrEP)—which global industry, philanthropists, and academia have endorsed as a "defining moment in the global AIDS response" (Karim and Karim 2011, e23). Planning for the deployment of PrEP globally has proceeded despite widely varying study results,[1] opposition to clinical trials,[2] and considerable indications that efficacy will depend on a great number of yet-to-be explored contextual factors (e.g., knowledge, adherence, drug resistance, tolerance, longer term effects, drug interactions, side-effects, real life context factors that differ from clinical trial control contexts, impacts of other diseases).

As the majority of Lesotho's HIV budget is provided by funds from global agencies, the Ministry of Health and Social Welfare will soon experience significant external pressures to consider how PrEP can be implemented as a core component of its prevention strategy. Given existing health system strains that are, in part, the result of previous vertical approaches to HIV program implementation, simply delivering a drug proven efficacious in clinical trial settings may not be adequate in a low-resource setting such as Lesotho (Kenworthy and Bulled 2013). Consequently, hard decisions will have to be made about which citizens are most deserving of life-saving (PrEP) or life-prolonging (ARV) interventions. These decisions, and the method by which these decisions are made, convey unmistakable messages about which citizens are most valuable and who is to be held responsible for their diseased or healthy bodies. Decisions will likely be made on the pragmatic grounds of efficacy and efficiency, and, if history offers any indication of the future, will not involve dialogue with individuals most impacted by such strategies. Consequently, this new biomedical technology has the potential to promote social and health inequities fostering stigma, blame, and discrimination through ill-devised, efficiency-driven deployment strategies.

As an alternative strategy to addressing health inequities, culture-centered projects of social change are constituted in the creation of dialogic spaces at local sites where communities can come together and articulate their views in order to develop locally appropriate and effective interventions (Basu and Dutta 2009). Dutta-Bergman (2004a, b, c) argued that one-way diffusion of predetermined solutions to health problems (e.g., MMC and ABC) perpetuates the existence of global inequities by not taking into account the agency of marginalized people. By not listening to their voices and securing the necessary mechanisms by which to promote risk-reduction behavior change, disease-prevention campaigns "stand the risk of stigmatizing and marginalizing members of target communities by not making available the means of achieving behavior change" (Dutta and Basnyat 2008, 263). In her exploration of Botswana's expanding HIV epidemic, despite years of concerted education campaigns, testing, and treatment programs, Georgia Rakelmann (2014) points to new forms of collaborative action and an expansion of 'expertise' that includes the voices of traditional healers, religious leaders, and health workers. Communication and knowledge creation through dialogue in common spaces of articulation are fundamental to the mobilizing of participants in processes of social change and structural transformations.

The struggle for the creation of such spaces, therefore, is a struggle for ensuring that new and dissenting voices can be heard, alternative rationalities be articulated, and new and creative ways of understanding, organizing, and mobilizing resources be considered. The legitimacy and existence of such open spaces for dialogue is always contingent upon the relationships of power and the continuous negotiations with dominant structures (Dutta 2011). The critical culture-centered approach to health communication positions health disparities as tied to these structural levels of inequalities. The approach calls for scholars and practitioners to move beyond the limited knowledge-risk behavior change model of health disparities to address structural or environmental factors that perpetuate engagement in risk, irrespective of knowledge.

The systematic erasure of the voices of marginalized individuals from dominant discursive spaces that manufacture knowledge and then utilize this knowledge to create policies and interventions, is increasingly being resisted. Globalization has offered new opportunities to articulate this resistance (Pal and Dutta 2008a, b). The increasing speed and volume of the flow of people, capital, ideas, goods, images, and services across national borders (Appadurai 1996, 2001; Keohane 2002; McMichael 2005, 2008) has simultaneously amplified fundamental problems of equity, suffering, social justice, and governance. Globalization scholar Arjun Appadurai (1996) argues that both disjuncture and flow are the markers of globalization. While goods, services, and people have flowed across borders, multiple points of interruptions, frictions, and possibilities of resistance within global systems have simultaneously been created (Appadurai 2001). The amalgamation of local and global in globalization processes offers occasions for locals to engage in globally-situated issues and for the continuous suffusion of the local within the global (Dutta 2011). For example, HIV activist groups (e.g., ACT UP, Treatment Action Commission) have shaped global HIV policies by mobilizing at both local and global levels.

Rather than follow the dictates of global health institutional authorities by enacting or complying with public health interventions and policies, governments, organizations, and individuals are offering up acts of defiance. Certain forms of HIV knowledge have been contested by select national groups (traditional healers, youth league members) and government representatives (President Thabo Mbeki of South Africa, President Yahya Jammeh of The Gambia, former South African Minister of Health Manto Tshabalala-Msimang), generating resistance as part of emergent regional modernities and nationalist politics within the globalized world. At the 2012 XIX International AIDS Conference, Teguest Guerma, leader of the African Medical and Research Fund, argued for a readjustment of African engagement in HIV policy. Guerma suggested that the international AIDS community dictates global prescriptions on HIV, making promises, and rapidly shifting priorities based on global health institution determinants and argued that "if we [Africans] don't know what we want to do, we don't want others to come and tell us what to do."[3] She challenged current notions of expert knowledge as being developed in and by elites in the global North, and she called for "country ownership, [for Africans] to take over responsibilities for the [HIV] epidemic and other health problems in Africa." Africans and other experts from the global South have participated in global health knowledge production for some time (Crane 2013; Feierman 2011; Fullwiley 2011; Iliffe 1998). However, the contributions made, or allowed to be made, by individuals from developing countries are not proportional to the experience of disease (Dutta 2008a; 2011). Moreover, merely having someone present at the discussion table does not afford him the ability to speak or to be heard. Instead the voice of expertise needs, as Guerma argued, to come from within, with local needs identified by locals, to gain the support of those involved and ensure that new initiatives are "owned by Africans."

The calls of African leaders to look inwards for solutions to their HIV epidemics suggest renegotiations of the African position within the global power structure, not a reassertion of local/indigenous knowledge. The challenge posed by Teguest Guerma, of the African Medical and Research Fund, of finding African solutions does not imply shutting out the international community completely. Rather, in calling for the establishment of "global solidarity," she proposes a new more equitable system, with greater involvement by domestic leadership, communities, and individuals in determining what, where and how prevention (and treatment) initiatives and policies are implemented. Anthropologist Merrill Singer (1994, 1323) noted that "the AIDS text is multivocal, and includes not only the voice of authority but also the voice of resistance." Arguments for the development of "local solutions to local problems" suggest that attempts to rework the arrangements of knowledge and power and of expert and lay person are being pushed forward from the bottom up. In challenging hegemonic structures there is recognition of their existence and the limitations that they impose upon those existing on the margins of society. Rather than 'international' agencies developing global health-related knowledge interventions and policies *for* local situations, comprehension of and solutions to disease epidemic(s) should be developed *with* or *by* locals in collective partnership-based 'global' health actions.[4]

As I have shown in this book, by exploring not just the content of the HIV knowledge construct but also the ideological constructions of the ever expanding global circuitry of knowledge distribution, it becomes evident that while access to the information and practices necessary to become rational and self-regulating is granted to some, it continues to be withheld from others. Furthermore, involvement in the production of knowledge has been limited to a few elites based in global organizations and academic institutions with Western-centric ideologies. Although biomedical knowledge is perceived to be empowering and emancipatory, claiming to be 'truth' in its connection with scientific objectivity, measurement, and replication, it has commanded global power and, through its inequitable distribution, maintained global inequities (Robbins 2009). The culture-centered approach recognizes that dialogic interactions create opportunities for marginalized communities to articulate their viewpoints in a context that has traditionally silenced them. With appropriate communication strategies, cultural work, and collaborations within specific cultural contexts, HIV prevention strategies that rely on behavior change, such as the 'abstain, be faithful and use condoms' approach and those that utilize new biomedical technologies including medical male circumcision, do not need to be positioned at a divide between the modern-traditional, global-local.

Reimaging Global Health Prevention

For dominant social institutions to become open to listening to the voices of marginalized individuals, communities, and even nations that have been historically erased, communicative procedures and practices need to be reconfigured. Participation in dialogic forums offers marginalized groups opportunities for constructing alternative narratives and knowledge that resist the status quo of geopolitical inequities. The United Nations Permanent Forum on Indigenous Issues (UNPFII) is one discussion platform that presents the issues, ideas, and interests of indigenous actors within global policy discussions. Debates involve local, national, as well as global policy-makers, opening up a space for dialogue with indigenous communities and creating opportunities for shaping policies on the basis of indigenous interests.

Although the United Nations has created an opportunity for marginalized sectors to engage with the dominant structures of knowledge production through dialogue, indigenous actors run the risk of being co-opted within these structures. For example, the agendas of marginalized indigenous communities are bounded by the framework of the United Nations. Thus, while dialogue becomes a tool for representing relevant issues and agendas of marginalized communities in dominant discursive spaces, it also becomes a hegemonic apparatus for erasing authentic opportunities for dialogue. The very requirements of certain skill sets and knowledge about dialogic procedures in dominant platforms such as the UNFPII, including specific rules, procedures, and processes, ensure these discursive platforms are inaccessible to the marginalized sectors. By consequence, these opportunities for discussions operate in a sphere of domination and control that parallels other components of global public health institutions. Dialogue simply becomes a way of dominating marginalized groups, serving as a hegemonic device that minimizes resistance. Representative members of marginalized communities present at the communication table become tokens, rather than members of an authentic dialogic engagement that brings about structural reform.

The politics of representation through dialogue is not one of attempting to be in the shoes of the marginalized, but rather one of working with the marginalized sectors to represent issues of importance to them in mainstream discursive spaces (Dutta 2011). Similarly, engagement does not merely involve occasional conversations with community figureheads by local representatives of global organizations. Nor does it entail hiring local staff and training them to conduct interventions by the standards of the global health organizations with little acknowledgment of their input or belief that their input represents the concerns of the larger community. To fully engage with marginalized communities, efforts should be made to build communicative platforms within communities, both materially and communicatively, in order to address the structural capacities that limit involvement. This approach could include developing skills training for participation in formal institutional dialogic spaces or bringing informal conversations into the community.

The Global Dialogues Project offers an example of creating a platform to allow the voice of people impacted by disease to be expressed. Through the generation of film based on the video contests, local narratives (and their knowledges) inform global health institution policies, and on the ground engagements stimulate social mobilization. In Lesotho, generating platforms for communication could and should occur at multiple levels. At the government level, employees involved in collaborations with international stakeholders, developing policies, and making funding decisions must have access to the latest academic and policy literature. Only by having access to the latest global conversations will local elites be able to engage in discussions with international collaborators as equals. Empowered with current information, they will be more able to engage in the conversation, and less compelled to engage in particular interventions simply because they can offer no sound evidence to counter the claims made by the global health institution experts.

Similarly, at the level of the individual, some competence in health literacy is required in order to participate in knowledge production. As noted earlier in this book, health literacy is positively correlated with improved health status of those living with HIV (Kalichman et al. 2000; Kalichman and Rompa

2000). Consequently, what we teach about HIV and our indicators of HIV knowledge cannot be limited to a 'template of facts' on routes of transmission and means of prevention. We must offer a deeper, contextually appropriate understanding of HIV to empower individuals to manage their lives despite disease posing a constant threat to health, family, and livelihoods. We can no longer rely on catchy phrases and moral impositions. If we expect people to utilize biomedical facilities to first 'know their status' and then, if infected, receive complicated treatments that require a lifetime of adherence despite significant side effects, we need to deliver accurate messages (e.g., not every sexual encounter is risky). What is important here is that individuals know that knowledge is never complete and constantly evolving.

The current vertical approach of health education campaigns that has predominated the global response to the HIV pandemic, in limiting access to information by simplifying messages of prevention, has denied marginalized individuals, those greatest at risk for HIV infection, their rights to participate in the creation of contextually appropriate and effective HIV prevention campaigns. Rather than being joint partners in the development of knowledge and understanding of this new threat to human existence, individuals most at risk for HIV infection have become dominated by and alienated from their own disease experience. To supersede their condition as objects requires people to act, as well as reflect, upon the reality that they would like to transform in order to gain critical consciousness (Freire 1972).

Structural factors must be addressed to ensure that individuals and communities are able to acquire knowledge and are afforded the ability to develop skills of critical thinking and communication. Greater national investments in education allowing for more and better trained teachers, smaller classroom sizes, and more engagement between students and teachers might help move education away from a banking style towards one that develops critical consciousness. Teguest Guerma, in her call for "local solutions to HIV" in Africa, pointed to the empowerment of communities through education and training. She called, specifically, for the training of health workers in Africa and the use of innovative health technologies and learning tools. Studies assessing implementation of Life Skills education suggest that educators teaching about HIV, sexuality, and life skills are not offered additional training to equip them with necessary pedagogical skills (Chendi 1999; Kolosoa and Makhakhane 2010). Consequently, both teachers and learners feel uncomfortable discussing sexual and reproductive health topics that specifically address HIV risk (Gachuhi 1999). Improvements in pedagogical training related to HIV and, as in Lesotho, constant reassessment of the applicability of the pedagogical tools used to address dynamic disease epidemics will ensure that teachers feel empowered to meet the needs of their students. Along these lines, greater access to the Internet appears to be expanding local perspectives, as people become more aware of the vast diversities in peoples, perspectives, and realities that exist in the world. An appreciation is developing in Lesotho for different world views, alternate perspectives, and diverse opinions and ways of living.

Youth in Lesotho are making strides to increasingly involving themselves in spaces of dialogue and knowledge creation, sometimes through rebellious actions. In late May of 2011, the Lesotho Ministry of Health and Social Welfare held a meeting to review the newly revitalized National HIV Behavior Change Communication strategy. Youth members of the major national political parties were invited to attend with the idea that they may easily influence behavior change among party followers. As reported in the national newspaper, the *Public Eye*, "the meeting did not go as smooth as was anticipated" (Matope 2011b, 4). Youth league representatives refused to cooperate with the meeting's agenda, reflecting their desire for bottom-up participatory approaches. The youth league argued that it was inappropriate not to allow them to participate in the development of the Behavior Change Communication strategy. They complained that they had been invited to this meeting primarily to be informed of their role as knowledge disseminators rather than being allowed to have a voice in the development of the Behavior Change Communication strategy. Mr. Molai Mosoaboli of the Basotho National Party argued that it was useless for the youth league members to be involved at this point in the process of strategy development, stating, "It is as good as arresting someone before investigations. What is it that they want from us after shutting-us-out in the beginning?" (Matope 2011b). Youth league members noted that funding continued to be used for ineffective prevention strategies, including behavior change communication interventions that were never fully implemented. Furthermore, they suggested that behavior change communication programs were not addressing the underlying factors that pushed youth into HIV risk behaviors. Mosoaboli voiced his concern, noting, "It is useless to fund strategies like these because they don't directly help uplift the lives of the youths…promoting behavior-change without economic empowerment is like trying to move a mountain from Thaba-Tseka to plant it here in Maseru" (Matope 2011b, 4).

The dissenting voices of the youth representatives presented at this meeting were viewed by many as "savaging," destructive, and an example of the growing differences between generations. Freire (1972) argued that young people in their rebellion are denouncing and condemning the unjust model of a society of domination. In documenting the relationship between the gay rights movement and HIV activism in the United States, Steven Epstein (2003) wrote:

> In the field of biomedicine, for example, certainly the patient who 'does her homework' and confronts her doctor with alternative perspectives

about her own conditions is making a foray of sorts into the domain of lay participation [what I term 'well-informed citizen']. But when groups of patients suffering from the same disease establish new organizations, elaborate a collective sense of self, and then act in concert to challenge the medical conceptualization of their condition and its treatment, then the intervention is potentially both more radical in character and more transformative in its consequences.

Youth in Lesotho, and all marginalized sectors of society, should be encouraged to continue to voice their concerns by attending collaborative or informative political meetings, and be sought out for their unique perspectives to ensure that they are represented in the knowledge production process.

Local community collaborations that have placed greater attention on empowering all community members, rather than privileging the voices of elected representatives, local elites (frequently one in the same) or international experts, have been considered exemplars of HIV prevention success. These efforts target the structural inequalities of societies in order to reduce risk and limit the responsibilities placed upon individuals to alter engagement in high risk behaviors. Uganda's community-based efforts, for example, have served as a model of success. Journalist and epidemiologist Helen Epstein argued in her book *Invisible Cure* (2007) that community cohesion is the reason for the reduction in Uganda's HIV prevalence by two-thirds from 1992 to 2003. Epstein draws on sociologist Felton Earls' term "collective efficacy"—the ability of people to join together to help each other in a sense of deeply rooted compassion on common humanity (Sampson, Raudenbush, and Earls 1997). Open dialogue about HIV risk behaviors and prevention strategies, as well as sharing the burden of taking care of the sick and orphaned in hundreds of small community initiatives in "spirit of collective action and mutual aid," argued Epstein (2007, 160), is Uganda's "invisible cure" for HIV.

These efforts seem simplistic when placed in contrast to Lesotho's HIV prevention programs, which offer a very direct, heavily Westernized, and less successful approach. The distinction in responses to the two epidemics is notably in the placement of marginalized sectors of society in the dialogic spaces of HIV prevention. In Uganda, communities engaged openly in HIV discourse, being empowered to practice what were locally considered appropriate prevention strategies. By contrast, communities in Lesotho have only been further marginalized by Western dictates, with regards to both direct HIV prevention strategies and structures of representation. In being more involved in discursive spaces, not simply through elite representatives, marginalized individuals and communities most gravely impacted have the potential to identify, manipulate, and reduce disease burdens.

Role of Culture-Centered
Critical Health Communication

While methodologies utilized by practitioners and academics at the center of knowledge production need to be continually interrogated for the values they represent and the assumptions they carry out (Dutta 2011; Sangaramoorthy 2014), practitioners and academics also play an important role in ensuring the involvement of marginalized sectors in dialogic spaces. Through accurate representations in published journal articles and policy documents, practitioners and scholars relay the voices of the marginalized sector to the broader global community. However, we must be cautious here as privileged academics can never truly "represent" the lived experiences of marginalized populations (Beverly 2004; Dutta and Basu 2013). Anthropologists, and the deep ethnographic methods we employ, serve as one avenue to uncover and understand the experiences of marginalized populations. Long-term engagements with communities, living within communities, conscious reflection of one's own geopolitical position, and direct involvement of community members in the process of representation, including obtaining feedback on interpretations, analyses, and even writings, all help to minimize the obscuring of perspectives and voices by academics in their attempts to represent a world that is not their own. With concerted conscious effort, "The location of dialogic spaces within broader structures [can] connect dialogic politics with the politics of structural transformations, working toward bringing about fundamental shifts in…inequalities and injustices" (Dutta 2011, 182).

In this vein, critical culture-centered communication processes and strategies for social change question representation of voice. Whose agendas are represented in dominant discursive spaces? Whose voices are privileged within such spaces, and whose voices are erased? How can we continually seek out opportunities that engage the marginalized in knowledge producing communication? In the culture-centered approach, voice is a key theoretical construct, as it offers an opening for the possibilities of change. "The very voices that have been systematically pathologized, scripted, and erased from the ontological and epistemiological bases of knowledge production and praxis return to the discursive spaces of global politics through dialogue" (Dutta 2011, 169). Knowledge-production through dialogue offers a way for meanings to be co-created by the involved actors (Dutta 2007, 2008a, c; Dutta-Bergman 2004b, c). Dialogic interactions allow for the development of relationships of authenticity where the interactions between the participants open up space for mutual learning (Dutta 2011; Freire 1972). Dialogue leads us to consider alternative worldviews, highlighting the taken-for-granted assumptions of the mainstream (e.g., Western ideologies, biomedicine, and neoliberalism) and its conventions. Articulated through dialogue, alternative rationalities interrogate the dominant narratives of development and modernity and draw our attention to the spaces of structural violence (Dutta 2011).

For the 'expert' engaging in social change research and praxis, a dialogic engagement with the margins begins with humility, reflexivity, and openness to learning through engagement, thus shifting the traditional role of the expert from a producer of knowledge situated at the centers of power to a listener who works in solidarity with the marginalized sectors (the man-on-the-street). Dialogue offers a moment in which the critical gaze can be turned inwards, questioning the assumptions and privileges that constitute the 'expert,' and interrogating the foundations of the Western knowledge structures that freeze the other as passive subjects of studies (Ellis and Bochner 2000; Jones 2005; Tomaselli, Dyll, and Francis 2008). In this sense, dialogue becomes an epistemological tool for the politics of social change and structural transformation by creating spaces for alternative ideas, understandings, and solutions. (Dutta 2011).

By articulating issues from the viewpoint of marginalized individuals, the configuration of problems and the development of solutions are shifted into the realm of those individuals and communities, offering them empowerment and agency. Rather than depicting the marginalized as bodies to be targeted in large-scale universal campaigns that focus on top-down logics of knowledge-based individual behavior change, effective strategies for HIV prevention can be developed using the dialogic approach, which centers itself on the role of purposefully listening to marginalized voices, making note of problem configurations as seen through their perspectives and creating spaces of change through their agendas. By so doing, cultural identities and traditions, frequently considered barriers to effective and efficient disease prevention strategies, become dynamic as the 'old' can be deconstructed and reconstructed in 'new' forms. In renegotiating how knowledge is produced and circulated, people disempowered by the prescriptions of biomedical and neoliberal hegemony can become reclassified as global citizens.

HIV Knowledge Questions (in English)

This appendix presents results of the factor analysis of the HIV-knowledge component of the survey conducted on 496 first and third year Lesotho College of Education students. The factor analysis aimed to identify the psychometric characteristics and patterns of relationships among the questions, including in the HIV-knowledge scale. The initial Eigenvalues showed that the first factor explained 10 percent of the variance, the second factor 7 percent, and the third factor 6 percent. Upon examination of the screeplot, using the elbow criterion, I forced a three factor solution. The loadings were examined using the varimax rotations of the factor loading matrix. The three-factor solution resulted in a factor structure with items 7, 16, 21, 24, 25 and 26 loading on one factor; items 12, 15, 17, 18 and 23 on a second; and items 10, 11 and 19 loading on the third. Criteria for inclusion in a factor were 0.4 or higher on the home factor and <0.40 on the other factor.

Factor 1

7. People can get HIV from witchcraft.
16. You can get infected by tongue kissing with someone who has HIV.
21. People admitted to hospital can get infected with HIV because the hospital is dirty.
24. The symptoms of HIV are the same as the symptoms of sugar diabetes.
25. HIV is a punishment from God.
26. Traditional healers can cure HIV/AIDS.

Factor 2

12. You can get the HIV from having sex with someone, even if you know everyone they have slept with.
15. If the HIV test is negative, it means the person is not infected.

17. A person with a sexually transmitted disease (STD), such as gonorrhea or syphilis is more likely to get the HIV than a person who doesn't have a STD.
18. A circumcised man's chances of getting HIV from occasional exposure through unprotected sex are lower than those of a man who has never been circumcised.
23. A person should retest 3 months after having an HIV test to confirm the result.

Factor 3

10. Sharing a toothbrush can transmit HIV.
11. It is ok for youth to have more partners. If one disappears they will still be left with someone to be close to.
19. HIV was produced in a laboratory.

Other Factors

1. There is the same amount of HIV in blood as there is in saliva.
2. It is possible for a person to be cured of HIV and AIDS.
3. Almost all babies born to mothers with HIV get HIV/AIDS.
4. If you feel healthy, you can be sure that you don't have HIV.
5. A person can get HIV from a mosquito bite.
6. You can get HIV by caring for someone who is HIV infected without gloves.
8. A mother who has HIV cannot pass the virus to her child by breast-feeding.
9. There are special medications available to treat someone with HIV.
13. The chance of transmitting HIV sexually is very high during the first 3 weeks of infection.
14. Condoms are an effective way to prevent HIV infection.
20. Scientists have discovered a cure for HIV, but they won't give it to infected people.
22. If you marry a person who is infected with HIV, you will be infected with HIV.

Preface

1. Whoopi Goldberg convinced the executives at Disney to make *Sarafina!* by agreeing to reprise her hit role as the singing nun in *Sister Act 2: Back In The Habit.*

2. I attended English speaking schools. Afrikaans was taught as the compulsory second language. An African language (either isiZulu or isiXhosa, depending on geographic location) was taught as a third language for the years Standard 3, 4, and 5, or what is now Grade 5, 6, and 7. I was very proud to be awarded the prize for isiZulu in my last year of primary school, though I had no option to continue my study of the language in high school and was not encouraged to do so.

3. These images of the violence of the apartheid state were creatively portrayed in the 2009 independent South African science-fiction film *District 9.*

4. Here I refer to the South African descriptor of my skin tone.

5. The Lesotho College of Education's (LCE) main campus, located in Maseru, opened its doors to students in 1975. Formally known as the National Teacher's Training College, LCE united three denominational teachers colleges connected to the Roman Catholic Church, the Lesotho Evangelical Church, and the Anglican Church of Lesotho, becoming the single national teacher's training college. In 2002, it began to operate autonomously, breaking connections with the religious institutions and the National University of Lesotho. By 2010, 4,190 students were enrolled at LCE-Maseru. Residential space is available for 900 first- and third-year students. Second-year students are deployed to primary and secondary schools throughout Lesotho for a year of teaching practice. In 2006, a satellite campus opened in the rural town of Thaba-Tseka, 70 miles east of the capital in the Maluti Mountain range. The majority (89 percent) of students still attend classes on the LCE-Maseru campus. The median age of LCE students is 23 years. Females comprised 66 percent of the student population.

Chapter 1

1. I use the term "biomedicine" to refer to the body of knowledge and associated clinical and experimental practices grounded in the medical sciences that were gradually consolidated in Europe and North America from the 19th century on. I do not limit this conception of medicine to one that is only focused on human biology; rather, I am referencing the term employed historically to distinguish one form of medicine from the practices of allopathic and what is termed in Lesotho "traditional" medicine.

2. Andrew Natsios' testimony before US House of Representatives Committee on International Relations. 2001. "Hearing: The United States' War on AIDS." Accessed August 10, 2012. www.commdocs.house.gov/committees/intlrel/hfa72978.000/hfa72978_0.htm

3. According to the UNAIDS Global Report on AIDS (2012), 8 million people received highly active anti-retroviral therapy (HAART) in 2011. HAART was first announced at the 11th International Conference on HIV/AIDS held in Vancouver in 1996, where researchers revealed viral dynamics and the effectiveness of different anti-viral drugs to inhibit the virus lifecycle. A typical HIV treatment regime combines three drugs, two nucleoside/nucleotide reverse transcriptase inhibitors and a protease inhibitor, or two nucleoside/nucleotide reverse transcriptase inhibitors and a non-nucleoside/nucleotide reverse transcriptase inhibitor. The US Food and Drug Administration approved the first protease inhibitor in December, 1995, with two additional protease inhibitors approved early the following year, ushering in the era of HAART. Brazil became the first country to begin a national antiretroviral distribution program in 1996. HAART was first introduced in Lesotho in 2004 with the opening of the GlaxoSmithKline (makers of Emtriva [FTC], Epivir [3TC], Epzicom [abacavir], and Retrovir [AZT]) HIV/AIDS clinic, Senkantana. At present, the cost of HAART is about 10,000-12,000 USD/patient/year in the US. This cost is likely to increase with new agents and more aggressive treatment. See John G. Bartlett's (2006) *Ten Years of HAART: Foundation for the Future* for a review of the history of HAART.

4. See the special issue "Anti-retrovirals for treatment and prevention–new ethical challenges" in *Developing World Bioethics*, August 2013, Volume 13, Issue 2, for a full discussion of this complex topic.

5. Illness is the subjective experience of disease, sickness, or simply feeling that something is not right whether or not there is a diagnosis of disease (Eisenberg 1977; Hahn 1983; Kleinman 1980; Young and Garro 1982).

6. Disease is the medically defined, objective pathology afflicting the patient (e.g., malaria, cancer, PTSD). Sickness is the social manifestation of the body's physical reaction to a disease (e.g., fever, pain, rashes) that entitles the person to take on the socially defined sick role (Parsons 1951).

7. Stated in the DHS as "Limiting sexual intercourse to one uninfected partner."

Chapter 2

1. See World Health Organization webpage on 'Public Health Surveillance.' www.who.int/topics/public_health_surveillance/en/

2. Following an extensive study of the development industry in Lesotho, anthropologist James Ferguson (1994) blamed Lesotho's current development situation on colonial rule, geographic and economic dependence, South African political and economic dominance (particularly during the apartheid era), and internal instability.

3. Though advancing the view of HIV by including more of the general population, like any national survey of this kind, interpretations of the data should be regarded with some caution. For example, the DHS employed a household sampling strategy, but data is reported at the individual level. Given employment migration patterns, men of reproductive age are under-represented; men comprise only 27 percent of the sample though they make up 49 percent of the Lesotho population. Furthermore, while 90 percent of surveyed individuals were eligible for HIV testing, the test results for only two-thirds of the sample are included in the report.

4. Conversation with Tefo Lephowa, Program Officer for Information, Education and Communication at the Lesotho Planned Parenthood Association (LPPA) on September 15, 2011.

5. Personal Communication with John Nkonyana, Director of Disease Control at the Ministry of Health and Social Welfare, Lesotho, on October 18, 2011.

6. Funding for KYS-plus is being provided by the UN and PEPFAR. Operational assistance will be provided by Population Services International, Christian Health Association of Lesotho, and Lesotho Network of AIDS Service Organizations.

7. 2004 was the year that South Africa initiated universal antiretroviral treatment distribution in five major hospitals in Gauteng province, following significant local and international efforts to fight the denialist stance of then President Thabo Mbeki. For more on this topic see Fassin 2007; Kalichman 2009; Mbali 2004; McNeill 2011; Robins 2010.

Chapter 3

1. Established in 1994, the Bill and Melinda Gates Foundation has become the largest private funder of global health research and implementation, disbursing over $15 billion for global health (Bill and Melinda Gates Foundation 2009).

2. Giles Bolton (2008) and William Easterly and Tobias Pfutze (2008) offer a substantial discussion on the inefficiencies in the administration of development aid.

3. The Inspector General found that, in Mauritania, 70 percent of funds (6.7 million USD) were unsupported; in Mali, 39 percent of funds (4.3 million USD) were unsupported; in Djibouti, 30 percent (5.2 million) were unsupported; in Zambia, 6.7 million USD were unsupported (six percent of the funds examined by the Inspector General); in Haiti, 1.26 million USD were spent on ineligible expenses (three percent of the funds examined) (The Global Fund 2010). Despite what these findings suggest and Western media's emphasis on corruption in Africa, economist Jeffrey Sachs (2005) points out that, according to the Freedom House index, the level of corruption in African states is no different on average than that for other low-income countries globally.

4. In a government report updated in 2005 it was estimated that at least 60 percent of U.S. foreign-aid funding never leaves the United States (Tarnoff and Nowels 2005). The 2011 version of this report offers no estimation, but suggests that as much as 90 percent of U.S. foreign-aid is spent on U.S. manufactured weapons, pharmaceuticals, vehicles, computers and other equipment, overhead, travel, and salary-and-benefit packages for the highly trained experts deployed to manage programs abroad (Tarnoff and Lawson 2011).

5. Many of the programs that received funding were modeled on U.S. programs (e.g., True Love Waits) that strictly promote 'abstinence-only until marriage.' The U.S. government has spent hundreds of millions of dollars on such programs in American schools since 1996. Under these programs, teachers are barred from mentioning condoms and other birth control options (except to highlight their failure rates). They stress that heterosexual intercourse within marriage is the only safe and acceptable form of sexual behavior. To date, evaluations of abstinence-only programs suggest that they fail to reduce rates of teen pregnancy or sexually transmitted diseases (Hauser 2004; Center for Health and Gender Equity 2004).

6. Initial examinations of Uganda's 'Kinsey' data were conducted by Michel Carael (based at the United Nations). Re-analysis was conducted by Daniel Halperin (based with the U.S. government).

7. There are many such international organizations currently operating in Lesotho, including Partners in Health, Save the Children, and the Lesotho-Boston Health Alliance, to name only a few. See the Letsema website (www .letsema.org) for a more complete list of NGOs conducting HIV focused work in Lesotho. The AIDS epidemic in Lesotho has established a booming aid-economy in Lesotho's capital, which has only in recent years, as a consequence of the global economy downturn, begun to slow. My own indicator of the impact of aid agencies and their expatriate employees is the availability of

ground coffee and coffee presses within the local markets. Locals continue to prefer instant coffee made with chicory, sold under the local brand—Ricoffy.

8. The brand name "Trust" was not selected to convince consumers that these condoms are effective in preventing disease transmission or pregnancy, as this would imply that other condoms brands are not trust-worthy.

9. A "luscious lips" sticker accompanying the Silkee promotional campaign remains stuck on my international cell phone. It always stimulates much conversation.

10. When I enquired why this pack of condoms was so expensive, the student did not know. I pointed out that it was flavored and we decided that that must be why. Discretely and rather nervously, the student (and his male friend) asked me what flavored meant and the purpose of the flavoring. I explained, hoping that my internal flustering was not externally evident. We all giggled. I thanked them and handed the condoms back, hoping they would get used one way or another.

11. Newsprint was a major distributor of HIV information among youth in Lesotho. While there were no daily newspapers in Lesotho, over 65 publications were available. Two weekly circulating local papers, the privately owned *Public Eye* and the *Lesotho Times,* were the most popular, and were read by most individuals who had regular access either through their employers or in libraries. Both papers sold at around 5 LSL each, the equivalent of a loaf of bread. Though no circulation data exists, editors estimated that on average 20,000 papers were printed each week, depending on how popular the print issue was likely to be. The newsprint audience was mostly limited to individuals in urban areas, as major local newspapers did not have distribution networks in the rural mountainous zones of the country. South African papers such as *The Sowetan* and *The Times* were also available to students at both the LCE campus libraries. Staff at LCE enjoyed a free local newspaper, *The Informative*, which was delivered directly to administrative offices every Tuesday. The paper was owned and operated by a local pair of sisters, who in recent years had expanded their media enterprise to include the first locally produced fashion magazine, *Finite*. All other local papers were owned and managed by Zimbabweans, a point of considerable contention among locals. All major newspapers available in Lesotho were predominantly in English. Both the *Public Eye* and *Lesotho Times* printed a small section in Sesotho, mostly translating the news stories from English.

12. Libuseng Nyaka wrote many HIV feature pieces for the *Public Eye*, becoming the domestic voice of HIV knowledge dissemination for a period of time.

13. Though there is the presumption that modernity is quintessentially Western, Stacy Leigh Pigg has noted that "there are 'other' and 'many' modernities" (1996, 164).

Chapter 4

1. Proverbs 5:15-18 (New International Version): Drink water from your own cistern, running water from your own well. Should your springs overflow in the streets, your streams of water in the public squares? Let them be yours alone, never to be shared with strangers. May your fountain be blessed, and may you rejoice in the wife of your youth.

2. Personal communication with Mpjo Maketela, Life Skills, the National Curriculum Development Center of the Ministry of Education, on February 16, 2012.

3. Kick4Life is an HIV-related initiative founded in 2005 delivering a range of sports-based projects including health education, voluntary testing, and life-skills development.

4. Phela Health and Development Communications (www.phela.org.ls/) is an NGO based in Lesotho, distributing HIV and associated health literature and media messages, including the One Love campaign.

5. Personal communication with Mokete Hlaelae, Executive Director, Lesotho Inter-religious AIDS Consortium (LIRAC), on October 11, 2011.

6. Personal Communication with M. Mabafokeng, resident HIV tester and counselor at Lesotho College of Education, on February 6, 2012.

7. Singhal and Rogers (1999, 101) argued that the Indian entertainment-education TV drama *Hum Log* "launched the era of commercially sponsored programs" on state-sponsored television. The authors argue that the introduction of commercial products (in this case Maggi noodle soup) demonstrated the combined power of strategic marketing, program planning, and television diffusion.

8. According to the World Bank (2010), only 13 percent of households in Lesotho own a television. The *Kheto ea ka!* audience was by default restricted to individuals who owned or had access to televisions, electricity, and satellite provider contracts. The message was thus limited to the middle- and upper-class population, likely perpetuating existing local social divisions related to HIV-risk.

Chapter 5

1. For examples in Lesotho, see Akeke, Mokgatle, and Oguntibeju 2007; ALAFA 2010; Colvin and Sharp 2000; CRS/WVI/USAID/PEPFAR 2009; NAC 2008, 2010b.

2. Chikovore and colleagues (2009) used this strategy to assess HIV knowledge among primary school students in rural areas of Zimbabwe. Students were asked to write their questions while seated in the classroom. While the close quarters of the classroom resulted in a bit of chatting and some concern over the effect of the teacher's presence, the authors determined that the questions were significantly varied and personal, eliminating concerns of bias.

3. Of the 791 questions recovered, 71.5 percent were from females, whose median age was 22 years, consistent with the demographic distribution of the entire LCE student population. All texts were translated if necessary, transcribed verbatim, and coded.

4. Questions were assigned only a single code rather than multiple codes. If a question related to multiple concepts, I determined the theme that seemed most relevant. I elected to use single rather than multiple codes, as a second component of the knowledge-assessment strategy involved the students themselves sorting questions into piles based on relatedness. Students were asked to place each question into a single pile. Thus to compare my own coding of the questions with how students sorted questions into piles, I and the students had to limit each question to a single defining category.

5. Similar gaps in knowledge were discovered more recently by Merrill Singer (2011) and colleagues among injection drug users not in treatment in Rio de Janeiro, Brazil, who subsequently failed to engage with prevention measures.

6. I purposefully selected a stratified random sample of 76 students representing the different groups (urban-Maseru, rural-Maseru, urban-Thaba-Tseka, rural-Thaba-Tseka), enrollment years (first and third), and gender (male and female). The intent was to obtain a sample whereby relationships between factors such as urban-rural home environment, campus location, and gender could be examined. Each pile sort activity took place in a private setting such as a vacant classroom, conference room, or office and lasted approximately one hour.

7. Scientific examinations of archival blood and lymph samples maintained for years in clinic and laboratory freezers have pieced together an understanding of where HIV came from. From a scientific perspective it is commonly accepted that HIV emerged zoonotically in central Africa as a mutated form of a simian virus. However, not until Jacques Pepin published his book, *The Origins of AIDS* (2011) had anyone traced HIV from its first appearance in central Africa to the Americas, Europe, Asia, and beyond. Pepin (2011) theorized that public health workers in the French territories of central Africa spread HIV between rural villagers and ultimately to urban areas by reusing syringes and needles for the treatment of tropical diseases. First initiated by French colonial doctor Eugene Jamot in 1917 to control sleeping sickness in Oubangui-Chari, disease-specific mobile control teams roamed through villages in the region on campaigns to treat and control other tropical diseases including leprosy, yaws, syphilis, and malaria. Until antibiotics became more readily available in the mid-1900s, drugs against infectious diseases were not very effective and had to be administered by injections, often intravenously, so as to maximize the drug concentration in the blood and other tissues. Given that transmission of HIV is ten times more effective through the sharing of needles and syringes than via sexual intercourse, and co-infec-

tion with tropical disease further increases the chance of HIV infection, this is the most probable theory of amplification (Pepin 2011). From rural areas, HIV moved into the nascent cities of central Africa and continued on its next phase of transmission, which involved sexual dissemination following travel, migration, and trading routes throughout the world and the rest of Africa (Timberg and Halperin 2012).

Local perceptions of the origin(s) of HIV throughout Africa include various conspiracy theories such as the use of the virus in a CIA-backed germ-warfare campaign against blacks, poison in food, and witchcraft or magic (Posel 2004; Rödlach 2006; 2011; Stadler 2003a). In 1986, allegations were made in newspapers throughout Africa that HIV had been developed at a US military laboratory and introduced into Africa by American and British doctors (Mzala 1988). The authors of the newspaper article, presumed to be Soviet propagandists, inserted the names of local white physicians wherever the story appeared. Continuing along these lines, Namibian President Sam Nujoma declared that HIV was invented by an American biological development program during the Vietnam War (Rompel 2001). The epidemic has even been attributed to condoms (McNeill 2009). A young man in Mozambique explained to anthropologist James Pfeiffer, "that if one hangs a JeitO condom (local condom brand) up to dry in the sunlight for a day, one can eventually see the HIV virus squirming inside" (2004, 94). International HIV researchers have recently made claims that the significant burden of HIV in African countries is the direct result of high levels of iatrogenic infections (Gisselquist et al. 2002; Gisselquist et al. 2003). These claims have not been backed by evidence collected by global organizations.

Conspiracy theorists in South Africa have claimed that the virus was originally sprayed in police tear gas (McLean 1990). They have also suggested that the disease was deliberately spread to black prostitutes by infected ex-African National Congress guerrillas working for the police (*New Nation News* 1991 June 28-July 4). A file on Chemical and Biological Warfare opened by the South African Truth and Reconciliation Commission (1998) revealed that during the last years of the apartheid government, laboratories were developing chemical and biological weapons, including anthrax, with the intent to eliminate black leaders (De Lange 2000; Fassin 2003; Gould and Folb 2000; Hogan 2000; Sapa 2000). According to Dr. Wouter Basson, the chemical and biological weapons program's scientific director, HIV was among the infectious agents considered (Niehaus and Jonsson 2005). During the regime of South Africa's apartheid government, the AIDS acronym was commonly known to stand for the "Afrikaner Invention to Discourage Sex" (Stadler 2003a; b; Van der Vliet 2001).

In Lesotho, as in many other countries heavily afflicted by HIV, church leaders regarded the mystery of HIV (i.e., that some people were infected while others were not) as a consequence of the sinful behaviors of the entirety of humanity (De Waal 2003; Smith 2003; Wardlow 2008). Sometimes the behaviors of certain individuals identified with HIV were considered retribution for sinful actions. HIV was linked with what are locally considered 'immoral' and 'disrespectful' behaviors including sex before or outside of marriage.

8. Classes of students were randomly selected from the LCE weekly timetable to complete the self-administered survey. A total of 570 surveys was collected from LCE-Maseru and LCE-Thaba-Tseka students. A larger proportion of the students from LCE-Thaba-Tseka were included to ensure statistical representation. Due to the age criteria (age 18-26), 74 were excluded, leaving 496 eligible surveys. Overall the student survey sample was similar to the demographic distribution of the LCE student population. More females completed surveys than males, given the uneven distribution of students by gender, which was further increased by disproportionate attendance in classes.

9. As the reliability measure for the knowledge scale was low, I conducted factor analysis to tease out the relationships among the questions included in the knowledge scale (see Appendix). Based on the results, I forced a three factor solution. Statements included in Factor One specifically referenced misconceptions of HIV, including the belief that HIV is a result of witchcraft or God, that symptoms of HIV are similar to those of diabetes, that HIV can be transmitted via kissing, and that traditional healers can cure HIV. These misconceptions are not common, but appear to be shared by a select group of students. Statements loading heavily on Factor Three included misconceptions of HIV that are more commonly held, such as the statements that HIV can be transmitted by sharing toothbrushes, that it is acceptable to have multiple sexual partners, and that HIV was originally produced in a laboratory. Items loading on Factor Two are those that students were particularly unsure of, as the ideas they address are not clearly right or wrong, for example, the risk of getting HIV even if you know all your sexual partners prior sexual partners, the certainty of HIV screening results, and the impact of STIs and male circumcision on risk of HIV infection.

10. When evaluated as separate scales, the standardized Cronbach alpha of items in Factor One was 0.515, for items that loaded on Factor Two alpha was 0.434, and for items loading on Factor Three alpha was 0.341.

11. This question did not distinguish between medical (clinic-based) and traditional (*lebollo*-based) circumcisions. If performed correctly, and using sanitary practices, either method should provide protection from HIV infection. Differential rates of STIs were, after all, first noticed among communities of men who engaged in initiation based traditional circumcisions and were not limited to those who had been circumcised in biomedical facilities.

12. The wording of the statement—"It is ok for youth to have more partners. If one disappears they will still be left with someone to be close to."—reflects how local discourse constructs multiple concurrent sexual partnerships. Al-

though partnerships do not always involve sex, that level of specification is not offered in local educational campaigns, as discussing sex openly is taboo.

13. International standards define MCP as more than one sexual partner in a 12-month period. I limited the time period to 6 months, as I wanted to identify more closely the overlap of relationships. The less time between relationships, the greater the risk.

14. As the question was not raised by students, my knowledge scale did not include questions about the risk of transmitting HIV by sharing food with an infected individual.

15. This variable for HIV knowledge is normally distributed with Skewness= -0.86 and Kurtosis=1.16 (between -1 and +1 required for measuring normal distribution).

Chapter 6

1. Students' perceptions of rural space and individuals from rural areas are reminiscent of Mayer and Mayer's (1961) 'Red' people. Though most students from LCE are from rural areas themselves, they fall into Mayer and Mayer's category of 'School.' More recently, James Ferguson (1999, 109) described urban/rural distinctions of migrant laborers in Zambia, not as dichotomous, or categorized, but rather as placed on a non-linear continuum based on familiarity with cosmopolitan or local stylistic repertoires.

2. My students in the United States find this approach frustrating as well. Despite the extensive access to information, the university culture in the United States still seems largely focused on the passive provision of information, rather than the development of critical thought directing where to seek out information and how to utilize it.

3. I will be forever grateful to Professor Fiona Vernal at the University of Connecticut, for carefully showing me the other perspective, without judgment or criticism of my ignorance.

4. Research in southern Africa indicates that individuals engage with multiple concurrent sexual partners (MCP) for many diverse and complex reasons (Shelton et al. 2004). Both genders prominently report dissatisfaction with their primary partner including lack of communication and romance, monotony, domestic discord, partner's lack of skill in lovemaking, and desire for variety of sexual practices (Leclerc-Madlala 2004; One Love 2008; Parker et al. 2007; PSI 2008; Swidler and Watkins 2007; Tawfik and Watkins 2007; Watkins 2004). Women are more likely to engage in MCP with older men, for economic and social support, less based on transactional fee-for-service and more related to social norms of economic support from men as part of sexual relationships, expectation of gifts, desire for luxury goods, and social status (NAC 2009a ; One Love 2008; Romero-Daza 1994b; Tawfik and Wat-

kins 2007). Other reasons include insurance against the loss of one's main partner (One Love 2008; PSI 2008; Swidler and Watkins 2007), a strategy to find the "right" life partner (One Love 2008), peer pressure (One Love 2008; PSI 2008), geographic separation (One Love 2008; Parker et al. 2007; PSI 2008), and revenge in response to a partner's infidelity (One Love 2008; Swidler and Watkins 2007). Women perceive that modern lifestyles afford them the freedom to behave more like men by having multiple sexual partners (Tawfik and Watkins 2007). The backdrop of polygamy contributes to this perception (One Love 2008; Tawfik and Watkins 2007), as does the belief that men's desires are uncontrollable and reflect prowess (One Love 2008; PSI 2008; Leclerc-Madlala 2004), while women serve a traditional passive role in sex (One Love 2008).

Chapter 7

1. The full text of the recommendations can be found at: www.who.int/hiv/mediacentre/MCrecommendations_en.pdf.

2. Conversation with Tefo Lephowa, Program Officer for Information, Education and Communication at the Lesotho Planned Parenthood Association (LPPA) on September 15, 2011.

3. Despite images posted on the Internet and in local newspapers of men lining up outside supposed MMC clinics, in my observations of the male clinic in Maseru I never saw a single individual enter or exit the clinic, and certainly no orderly lines of men waiting their turn.

4. The neighboring government of South Africa released the Application of Health Standards in Traditional Circumcision Act No. 6 of 2001 in an effort to monitor traditional circumcision ceremonies.

5. A local traditional healer and President of a Traditional Healers Association in Lesotho, Malefetsane Liau, contradicted this point, telling me in personal conversations that there were no set fees established. Rather, individuals and families donated to a central fund.

6. This question did not distinguish between MMC and *lebollo*-associated circumcision. As long as the foreskin is completely removed using sterile instruments, either practice should theoretically afford the individual the same level of protection from HIV.

7. Male students were less willing to comment on MMC, highlighting the importance of researcher subjectivities influencing data collection.

8. It is perhaps expected that females would know less of the details of male-specific ceremonies. Nevertheless, these women may at some point need to decide whether or not to circumcise their sons, either as neonates or adolescents. In addition, one would expect that all members of society would have some idea of what takes place at an important and central cultural rite.

9. This pattern is not peculiar to Africa. Although AIDS was first reported in the medical and popular press in 1981, it was only in October of 1987 that US President Ronald Reagan publically spoke about the epidemic. By the end of that year 59,572 AIDS cases had been reported and 27,909 of those individuals had died. Regan sided with conservatives who said the government should not provide sex education information stating, "How that information is used must be up to schools and parents, not government. But let's be honest with ourselves, AIDS information cannot be what some call 'value neutral.'" (see ACT UP 2012; Bronski 2004; Shilts 1987).

Chapter 8

1. The iPREX trial demonstrated a reduction in infections among men-who-have-sex-with-men who took a daily dosage of *Truvada* to prevent infections: 44% overall and 92% among those with biological evidence of regimen adherence (Grant et al. 2010). In subsequent trials, proven efficacies of ARV-based PrEP have varied greatly, from no effect to 73%. Two trials among high-risk women were discontinued in full or in part due to an inability to show any difference in HIV infection between treatment and placebo groups (FHI360 2011; Van Damme et al. 2012; VOICE [MTN-003] 2011).

2. PrEP trials planned in Cambodia, Cameroon, Nigeria, Thailand, and Malawi have been halted by community groups or terminated (see Ahmad 2004; Singh and Mills 2005; Ukpong and Peterson 2009).

3. Teguest Guerma was interviewed on National Public Radio by Michel Martin on July 26, 2012. www.npr.org/2012/07/26/157424209/finding-africas-solutions-to-hiv-aids

4. In the definitions of international and global health offered by Global Health Education Consortium, 'International Health' relates to health practices, policies, and systems in other countries, stressing differences rather than commonalities. The concept focuses more on bilateral foreign aid activities to control disease in resource poor countries and less on medical mission work. 'Global Health' relates to health issues and concerns that transcend national borders, class, race, ethnicity, and culture. The term stresses the commonality of health issues, which require a collective (partnership-based) action. (globalhealtheducation.org/Pages/GlobalvsInt.aspx)

AAP, American Academy of Pediatrics Task Force on Circumcision. 2012. "Circumcision policy statement." *Pediatrics* 130 (3):e756-e785.

Abdool Karim, Q., S. S. Abdool Karim, J. A. Frohlich, A. C. Grobler, C. Baxter, L. E. Mansoor, A. B. Kharsany, S. Sibeko, K. P. Mlisana, Z. Omar, T. N. Gengiah, S. Maarschalk, N. Arulappan, M. Mlotshwa, L. Morris, and D. Taylor. 2010. "Effectiveness and safety of tenofovir gel, an antiretroviral microbicide, for the prevention of HIV infection in women." *Science* 329 (5996):1168-1174.

ACT UP. 2012. "Reagan's AIDSGATE." AIDS Coalition to Unleash Power. Accessed 2 May, 2012. www.actupny.org/reports/reagan.html

Adams, Vincanne, and Stacy Leigh Pigg. 2005. "Introduction: The moral object of sex." In *Sex in development: Science, sexuality, and morality in global perspective*, edited by Vincanne Adams and Stacy Leigh Pigg, 1-38. Durham, NC: Duke University Press.

Afrobarometer. 2004. "Public opinion and HIV/AIDS: Facing up to the future?" Accessed 1 February, 2008. www.afrobarometer.org/papers/AfrobriefNo14.pdf

Aggleton, Peter. 2007. "'Just a snip'?: A social history of male circumcision." *Reproductive Health Matters* 15 (29):15-21.

Ahlberg, Beth Maina. 1994. "Is there a distinct African sexuality? A critical response to Caldwell." *Journal of International African Institute* 64 (2):220-242.

Ahmad, Khabir. 2004. "Trial of antiretroviral for HIV prevention on hold." *Lancet Infectious Diseases* 4 (10):597.

Ahmed, Nazeema, Alan J. Flisher, Catherine Mathews, Wanjiru Mukoma, and Shahieda Jansen. 2009. "HIV education in South Africa schools: The dilemma and conflicts of educators." *Scandinavian Journal of Public Health* 32 (Suppl 2):48-54.

AIDS.gov. 2012. "A timeline of AIDS." U.S. Department of Health & Human Services. Accessed 1 June, 2013. www.aids.gov/hiv-aids-basics/hiv-aids-101/aids-timeline/

Airhihenbuwa, C. O., R. J. DiClemente, G. M. Wingood, and A. Lowe. 1992. "HIV/AIDS education and prevention among African-Americans: A focus on culture." *AIDS Education and Prevention* 4 (3):267-276.

Airhihenbuwa, Collins O., Bunmi Makinwa, and Rafael Obregon. 2000. "Toward a new communication framework for HIV/AIDS." *Journal of Health Communication* 5 (Suppl 1):101-111.

Airhihenbuwa, Collins O. 1990-1991. "A conceptual model for culturally appropriate health education programs in developing countries." *International Quarterly of Community Health Education* 11:53-62.

Airhihenbuwa, Collins O. 1993. "Health promotion for child survival in Africa: Implications for cultural appropriateness." *International Journal for Health Education* 12 (3):10-15.

Airhihenbuwa, Collins O. 1995. *Health and culture: Beyond the Western paradigm.* Thousand Oaks, CA: Sage.

Airhihenbuwa, Collins O., and Michael J. Ludwig. 1997. "Remembering Paolo Freire's legacy of hope and possibility as it relates to health education/ promotion." *Journal of Health Education* 28:317-319.

Airhihenbuwa, Collins O. 1989. "Perspectives on AIDS in Africa: Strategies for prevention and control." *AIDS Education and Prevention* 1 (1):57-69.

Airhihenbuwa, Collins, and Rafael Obregon. 2000. "A critical assessment of theories/models used in health communication for HIV/AIDS." *Journal of Health Communication* 5 (Suppl 1):5-15.

Akeke, V. A., M. Mokgatle, and O. O. Oguntibeju. 2007. "Assessment of knowledge and attitudes about HIV/AIDS among inmates of Quthing prison, Lesotho." *West Indian Medical Journal* 56 (1):48-54.

ALAFA. 2010. *Peer education and behavior change: KAP 2009 qualitative study.* Maseru, Lesotho: Apparel Lesotho Alliance to Fight AIDS.

Albarracin, D., J. C. Gillette, A. N. Earl, L. R. Glasman, M. R. Durantini, and M. H. Ho. 2005. "A test of major assumptions about behavior change: A comprehensive look at the effects of passive and active HIV-prevention interventions since the beginning of the epidemic." *Psychological Bulletin* 131 (6):856-897.

Albert, E. 1989. "AIDS and the press: The creation and transformation of a social problem." In *Images of issues: Typifying contemporary social problems,* edited by Joel Best, 39-54. Hawthorne, NY: Aldine de Gruyter.

Alcena, Valiere. 1986. "AIDS in third world countries." *New York State Journal of Medicine* 86:446.

Amazigo, Uche, Nancy Silva, Joan Kaufman, and Daniel Obikeze. 1997. "Sexual activity and contraceptive knowledge and use among in-school adolescents in Nigeria." *International Family Planning Perspectives* 23 (1):28-33.

Ambrose, David. 1976. *The guide to Lesotho.* Johannesburg, South Africa: Winchester Press.

American Medical Association. 1999. "Health literacy: Report of the Council of Scientific Affairs." *Journal of American Medical Association* 281:552-557.

Amuyunzu-Nyamongo, Mary K., and Monica A. Magadi. 2006. "Sexual privacy and early sexual debut in Nairobi informal settlements." *Community, Work and Family* 9 (2):143-158.

Anderson, Deborah, Joseph A. Politch, and Jeffrey Pudney. 2011. "HIV infection and immune defense of the penis." *American Journal of Reproductive Immunology* 65 (3):220-229.

Anderson, Elizabeth S. 1995. "The democratic university: The role of justice in the production of knowledge." *Social and Political Philosophy* 12 (2):189-219.

Anderson, Kermyt G. 2010. "Life expectancy and the timing of life history events in developing countries." *Human Nature* 21 (2):103-123.

Andreasen, Alan R. 1995. *Marketing social change: Changing behavior to promote health, social development, and the environment.* San Francisco, CA: Jossey-Bass.

Ankrah, E. Maxine. 1991. "AIDS and the social side of health." *Social Science & Medicine* 32 (9):967-980.

Ankrah, E. Maxine. 1989. "AIDS: Methodological problems in studying its prevention and spread." *Social Science & Medicine* 29 (3):265-276.

Appadurai, Arjun. 1996. *Modernity at large: Cultural dimensions of globalization.* Minneapolis, MN: University of Minnesota Press.

Appadurai, Arjun. 2001. *Globalization.* Durham, NC: Duke University Press.

Arowujolu, A. O., A. O. Ilesanmi, O. A. Roberts, and M. A. Okunola. 2002. "Sexuality, contraceptive choice and AIDS awareness among Nigerian undergraduates." *African Journal of Reproductive Health* 6 (2):60-70.

Ashforth, Adam. 2005. *Witchcraft, violence and democracy in South Africa.* Chicago, IL: University of Chicago Press.

Asiimwe-Okiror, Godwil, Alex A. Opio, Joshua Musinguzi, Elizabeth Madraa, George Tembo, and Michel Carael. 1997. "Change in sexual behaviour and decline in HIV infection among young pregnant women in urban Uganda." *AIDS* 11 (14):1757-1763.

Auvert, Bertran, Dirk Taljaard, Emmanuel Lagarde, Joelle Sobngwi-Tambekou, Remi Sitta, and Adrian Puren. 2005. "Randomized, controlled intervention trial of male circumcision for reduction of HIV infection risk: The ANRS 1265 Trial." *PLoS Medicine* 2 (11):e298.

Auvert, Bertran, Dirk Taljaard, Dino Rech, Pascale Lissouba, Beverley Singh, Julie Bouscaillou, Gilles Peytavin, Séverin Guy Mahiane, Rémi Sitta, Adrian Puren, and David Lewis. 2013. "Association of the ANRS-12126 male circumcision project with HIV levels among men in a South African township: Evaluation of effectiveness using cross-sectional surveys." *PLoS Medicine* 10 (9):e1001509.

Baeten, Jared M., Barbra A. Richardson, Ludo Lavreys, Joel P. Rakwar, Kishorchandra Madaliya, Job J. Bwayo, and Joan K. Kreiss. 2005. "Female-to-male infectivity of HIV-1 among circumcised and uncircumcised Kenyan men." *Journal of Infectious Diseases* 191 (4):546-553.

Bailey, Robert C., Stephen Moses, Corette B. Parker, Kawango Agot, Ian Maclean, John N. Krieger, Carolyn F. Williams, Richard T. Campbell, and Jechoniah O. Ndinya-Achola. 2007. "Male circumcision for HIV prevention in young men in Kisumu, Kenya: A randomised controlled trial." *Lancet* 369 (9562):643-656.

Baker, David W. 1995. "Reading between the lines: Deciphering the connections between literacy and health." *Journal of General Internal Medicine* 14:315-317.

Ballard, Danny J., David M. White, and Mary A. Glascoff. 1990. "AIDS/HIV education for preservice elementary teachers." *Journal of School Health* 60 (6):262-265.

Bandura, Albert. 1977. *Social learning theory*. Englewood Cliffs, NJ: Prentice-Hall.

Bandura, Albert. 1986. *Social foundations of thought and action: A social cognitive theory*. Englewood Cliffs, NJ: Prentice-Hall.

Bandura, Albert. 2001. "Social cognitive theory of mass communication." *Media Psychology* (3):265-299.

Bardhan, Nilanjana R. 2001. "Transnational AIDS/HIV news narratives: A critical exploration of overarching frames." *Mass Communication & Society* 4:283-310.

Bardhan, Nilanjana R. 2002. "Accounts from the field: A public relations perspective on global AIDS/HIV." *Journal of Health Communication* 7 (3):221-244.

Barry, Andrew. 2001. *Political machines: Governing a technological society*. London: Athlone.

Barth, Fredrik. 2002. "An anthropology of knowledge." *Current Anthropology* 43 (1):1-11.

Bartlett, John G. 2006. Ten years of HAART: Foundation for the future. *Medscape Education*. Accessed 20 August, 2013. www.medscape.org/ viewarticle/523119

Basu, Amrita. 1995. *The challenge of local feminisms: Women's movements in global perspectives*. Boulder, CO: Westview.

Basu, Amrita. 2004. "Women's movements and the challenge of transnationalism." *Curricular Crossings: Women's Studies and Area Studies*. Amherst University, MA. www.amherst.edu/~mrhunt/womencrossing/basu.html

Basu, Ambar. 2010. "Communicating health as an impossibility: Sex work, HIV/ AIDS, and the dance of hope and hopelessness." *Southern Communication Journal* 75 (4):413-432.

Basu, Ambar, and Mohan J. Dutta. 2009. "Sex workers and HIV/AIDS: Analyzing participatory culture-centered health communication strategies." *Human Communication Research* 35:86-114.

Bearman, Peter S., and Hannah Bruckner. 2001. "Promising the future: Virginity pledges and the transition to first intercourse." *American Journal of Sociology* 106 (4):859-912.

Beltran, Luis Ramiro. 1975. "Research ideologies in conflict." *Journal of Communication* 25:187-193.

Beltran, Luis Ramiro. 1980. "A farewell to Aristotle: 'Horizontal' communication." *Communication* 5:5-41.

Bernard, H. Russell, Gery W. Ryan, and Stephen P. Borgatti. 2009. "Green cognition and behavior: A cultural domain analysis." In *Networks, resources, and economic action*, edited by Clemens Greiner and Waltraud Kokot, 189-215. Cologne, Germany: Dietrich Reimer Verlag.

Bertrand, Jane, Kevin O'Reilly, Julie Denison, Rebecca Anhang, and Michael Sweat. 2006. "Systematic review of the effectiveness of mass communication programs to change HIV/AIDS-related behaviors in developing countries." *Health Education Research, Theory and Practice* 21 (4):567-597.

Beverly, John. 2004. *Subalternity and representation: Arguments in cultural theory.* Durham, NC: Duke University Press.

Biehl, Joao. 2007. *Will to live: AIDS therapies and the politics of survival.* Princeton, NJ: Princeton University Press.

Bill and Melinda Gates Foundation. 2009. Global health program fact sheet. Accessed 15 February, 2013. docs.gatesfoundation.org/global-health/documents/global-health-fact-sheet-english-version.pdf

Billingsley, Andrew, and Barbara Morrison-Rodriguez. 1998. "The black family in the 21st century and the church as an action system: A macro perspective." In *Human behavior in the social environment from an African American perspective,* edited by Letha A. (Lee) See, 31-47. Binghamton, NY: Haworth Press.

Black, Nick. 1996. "Why we need more observational studies to evaluate the effectiveness of health care." *British Medical Journal* 312 (7040):1215-1218.

Blanc, Ann Klimas, and Brent Wolff. 2001. "Gender and decision-making over condom use in two districts in Uganda." *African Journal of Reproductive Health* 5 (3):15-28.

Blumenreich, Megan, and Marjorie Siegel. 2006. "Innocent victims, fighter cells, and white uncles: A discourse analysis of children's books about AIDS." *Children's Literature in Education* 37 (1):81-110.

Bogart, Laura M., Frank H. Galvan, Glenn J. Wagner, and David J. Klein. 2010. "Longitudinal association of HIV conspiracy beliefs with sexual risk among black males living with HIV." *AIDS and Behavior* 2011 (15):6.

Bogart, Laura M., Seth C. Kalichman, and Leickness C. Simbayi. 2008. "Endorsement of a genocidal HIV conspiracy as a barrier to HIV testing in South Africa." *Journal of Acquired Immune Deficiency Syndromes* 49 (1):115-116.

Bogart, Laura M., and Sheryl Thornburn. 2003. "Exploring the relationship of conspiracy beliefs about HIV/AIDS to sexual behaviors and attitudes among African American adults." *Journal of the National Medical Association* 95 (11):1057-1065.

Bogart, Laura M., and Sheryl Thornburn. 2005. "Are HIV/AIDS conspiracy beliefs a barrier to HIV prevention among African Americans?" *Journal of Acquired Immune Deficiency Syndromes* 38 (2):213-218.

Bogart, Laura M., Glenn Wagner, Frank H. Galvan, and Denedria Banks. 2010. "Conspiracy beliefs about HIV are related to antiretroviral treatment nonadherence among African American men with HIV." *Journal of Acquired Immune Deficiency Syndromes* 53 (5):648-655.

Bohnert, Amy S., and Carl A. Latkin. 2009. "HIV testing and conspiracy beliefs regarding the origins of HIV among African Americans." *AIDS Patient Care STDS* 23 (9):759-763.

Bolton, Giles. 2008. *Africa doesn't matter: How the West has failed the poorest continent and what we can do about it*. New York: Arcade.

Bonacci, Mark A. 1992. *Senseless casualties: The AIDS crisis in Asia*. Washington, DC: Asia Resource Center.

Bongaarts, John, Priscilla Reining, Peter Way, and Francis Conant. 1989. "The relationship between male circumcision and HIV infection in African population." *AIDS* 3 (6):373-377.

Borawski, F., L. Lovegreen, C. Demko, D. Guwatudde, K. Abbott, and S. Stewart. 2001. *Evaluation of the teen pregnancy prevention programs funded through the wellness block grant (1999-2000)*. Cleveland, OH: Center for Health Promotion and Research, Department of Epidemiology and Biostatistics, Case Western Reserve University.

Boscarino, J. A., and R. J. DiClemente. 1996. "AIDS knowledge, teaching comfort, and support for AIDS education among school teachers: A statewide survey." *AIDS Education and Prevention* 8 (3):267-277.

Bourdieu, Pierre. 1991. *Language and symbolic power*. Translated by C. Raymond and M. Adamson. Cambridge, MA: Harvard University Press.

Bowker, Geoffrey C., and Susan Leigh Starr. 1999. *Sorting things out: Classification and its consequences*. Cambridge, MA: MIT Press.

Brandt, Allan M., and Paul Rozin, eds. 1997. *Morality and health*. New York, NY: Routledge.

Brewer, Devon D., John J. Potterat, John M. Roberts, Jr., and Stuart Brody. 2007. "Male and female circumcision associated with prevalent HIV infection in virgins and adolescents in Kenya, Lesotho, and Tanzania." *Annals of Epidemiology* 17 (3):217-226.

Briggs, Charles L., and Daniel Hallin. 2010. "Health reporting as political reporting: Biocommunicability and the public sphere." *Journalism* 11 (2):149-165.

Briggs, Charles L. 2003. "Why nation-states and journalists can't teach people to be healthy: Power and pragmatic miscalculation in public discourses on health." *Medical Anthropology Quarterly* 17 (3):287-321.

Briggs, Charles L. 2005. "Communicability, racial discourse, and disease." *Annual Review of Anthropology* 34:269-291.

Briggs, Charles L., and Daniel C. Hallin. 2007. "Biocommunicability: The neoliberal subject and its contradictions in news coverage of health issues." *Social Text* 25 (4):43-66.

Briggs, Charles L., and Clara Mantini-Briggs. 2003. *Stories in the time of cholera: Racial profiling in a medical nightmare*. Berkeley, CA: University California Press.

Briggs, Charles L., and Mark Nichter. 2009. "Biocommunicability and the biopolitics of pandemic threats." *Medical Anthropology* 28 (3):189-198.

Brislin, Richard W., and Tomoko Yoshida, eds. 1994. *Improving intercultural interactions: Modules for cross-cultural training programs*. Thousand Oaks, CA: Sage.

Bronski, Michael. 2004. The truth about Reagan and AIDS. *Z Magazine* January. Accessed 26 October, 2012. www.zcommunications.org/the-truth-about-reagan-and-aids-by-michael-bronski

Brown, Darigg C., Rhonda BeLue, and Collins O. Airhihenbuwa. 2011. "HIV and AIDS-related stigma in the context of family support and race in South Africa." *Ethnicity & Health* 21 (3):441-458.

Browning, Christopher R. 2005. "Sexual initiation in early adolescence: The nexus of parental and community control." *American Sociological Review* 70:758-778.

Bryman, Alan. 2006. "Integrating quantitative and qualitative research: How is it done?" *Qualitative Research* 6 (1):97-113.

Bukali de Graca, F. L. 2004. *HIV/AIDS prevention and care in Mozambique, a socio-cultural approach: Literature and institutional assessment, and case studies on Manga, Sofala Province and Morrumbala District, Zambezia Province, Maputo.* Maputo, Mozambique: UNESCO.

Bulled, Nicola. 2011. "'You can find anything online': Biocommunicability of cyber-health information and its impact on how the NET generation accesses health care." *Human Organization* 70 (2):153-163.

Bulled, Nicola, and Richard Sosis. 2010. "Examining the influence of life expectancy of reproductive timing, total fertility, and education attainment." *Human Nature* 21 (3):269-289.

Burgard, Sarah A., and Susan M. Lee-Rife. 2009. "Community characteristics, sexual initiation, and condom use among young black South Africans." *Journal of Health and Social Behavior* 50:293-309.

Bureau of Democracy, and Human Rights and Labor. 2011. *2010 human rights report: Lesotho.* Washington, DC: U.S. Department of State.

Caldwell, John C. 1995. "Lack of male circumcision and AIDS in sub-Saharan Africa: Resolving the conflict." *Health Transition Review* 5 (1):113-117.

Caldwell, John C., and Pat Caldwell. 1993. "The nature and limits of the sub-Saharan African AIDS epidemic: Evidence from geographical and other patterns." *Population and Development Review* 19 (4):817-848.

Caldwell, John C., and Pat Caldwell. 1994. "The neglect of an epidemiological explanation for the distribution of HIV/AIDS in sub-Saharan Africa: Exploring the male circumcision hypothesis." *Health Transition Review* 4 (Suppl):23-46.

Caldwell, John C., and Pat Caldwell. 1996. "The African AIDS epidemic." *Scientific American* 274 (3):62-63, 66-68.

Camacho, Ariana Ochoa, Gust A. Yep, Prado Y. Gomez, and Elissa Velez. 2008. "El poder y la fuerza de la pasion: Toward a model of HIV/AIDS education and service delivery from the 'bottom-up.'" In *Emerging perspectives in health communication: Meaning, culture and power,* edited by Heather M. Zoller and Mohan J. Dutta, 224-246. New York, NY: Taylor & Francis.

Cameron, D. William, Lourdes J. D'Costa, Gregory M. Maitha, Mary Cheang, Peter Piot, J. Neil Simonsen, Allan R. Ronald, Michael N. Gakinya, J. O. Ndinya-Achola, Robert C. Brunham, and Francis A. Plummer. 1989. "Female to male transmission of human immunodeficiency virus type 1: Risk factors for seroconversion in men." *Lancet* 2 (8660):403-407.

Campbell, Catherine. 2000. "Selling sex in the time of AIDS: The psycho-social context of condom use by sex workers on a southern African mine." *Social Science & Medicine* 50 (4):479-494.

Carter, Erica, and Simon Watney. 1989. *Taking liberties: AIDS and cultural politics*. London, UK: Serpent's Tail.

Cassidy, Rebecca, and Melissa Leach. 2007. "Citizenship, global funding and AIDS treatment controversy: A Gambian case study." Citizen Engagement in a Globalizing World, Brighton, 10-11 October 2007.

Castells, Manuel. 2010. *The power of identity: The information age: Economy, society and culture*. 2nd ed. Sussex, UK: Wiley-Blackwell.

CDC. 1981. "Kaposi's sarcoma and *Pneumocystis* pneumonia among homosexual men—New York City and California." *Morbidity and Mortality Weekly Report (MMWR)* 30 (25):305-308.

CDC. 2011. *CDC fact sheet: Estimates of new HIV infections in the United States, 2006-2009*. Atlanta, GA: Centers for Disease Control.

Ceci, C. 2004. "Nursing, knowledge and power: A case analysis." *Social Science & Medicine* 59:1879-1889.

Center for Health and Gender Equity. 2004. *Debunking the myths in the US global AIDS strategy: An evidence-based analysis*. Washington, DC: Center for Health and Gender Equity.

Central Bank and Bureau of Statistics. 1995. *Survey of Basotho migrant mineworkers. Maseru, Lesotho*: Central Bank and Bureau of Statistics.

Chakanza, J. C. 1998. "Unfinished agenda: Puberty rites and the response of the Roman Catholic Church in southern Malawi 1901-1904." In *Rites of passage in contemporary Africa*, edited by James Leland Cox, 168-175. Cardiff, UK: Cardiff Academic Press.

Chandrasekaran, C. 1966. "Recent trends in family planning research in India." In *Family planning and population programs*, edited by Bernard Berelson. Chicago, IL: University of Chicago Press.

Check, Erika. 2006. "New methods suggest AIDS toll lower than estimated." *Nature Medicine* 12 (11):1224-1224.

Chendi, Helen. 1999. *HIV/AIDS life skills programmes in southern Africa: The case of the Kingdom of Lesotho*. Geneva, Switzerland: UNICEF.

Chikovore, Jeremiah, Lennarth Nystron, Gunilla Lindmark, and Beth Maina Ahlberg. 2009. "HIV/AIDS and sexuality: Concerns of youths in rural Zimbabwe." *African Journal of AIDS Research* 8 (4):503-513.

Christakis, Nicholas. 1989. "Responding to a pandemic: International interests in AIDS control." *Daedalus* 118 (2):113-134.

Church, Cathleen A., and Judith Geller. 1989. Lights! Camera! Action! Promoting family planning with TV, video, and film. In *Population Reports*. Baltimore, MD: Johns Hopkins University, Population Information Program.

CIA. 2010. *The World Factbook: Africa, Lesotho*. McLean, VA: Central Intelligence Agency.

Clarke, Adele, Janet K. Shim, Laura Mamo, and Jennifer R. Fosket. 2003. "Biomedicalization: Technoscientific transformations of health, illness, and US biomedicine." *American Sociological Review* 68 (2):161-194.

Clarke, Juanne N. 1992. "Cancer, heart disease, and AIDS: What do the media tell us about these diseases?" *Health Communication* 4 (2):105-120.

Colvin, M., and B. Sharp. 2000. "Sexually transmitted infections and HIV in a rural community in the Lesotho highlands." *Sexually Transmitted Infections* 76 (1):39-42.

Conrad, Charles, and Denise Jodlowski. 2008. "Dealing drugs on the border: Power and policy in pharmaceutical reimportation debates." In *Emerging perspectives in health communication: Meaning, culture and power*, edited by Heather M. Zoller and Mohan J. Dutta, 365-389. New York, NY: Routledge.

Conrad, Peter. 1994. "Wellness as a virtue: Morality and the pursuit of health." *Culture, Medicine & Psychiatry* 18 (3):385-401.

Cowan, Frances M., Lisa F. Langhaug, George P. Mashungupa, Tellington Nyamurera, John Hargrove, Shabbar Jaffar, Rosanna W. Peeling, David W. Brown, Robert Power, Anne M. Johnson, Judith M. Stephenson, Mary T. Bassett, Richard J. Hayes, and Regai Dzive Shiri Project. 2002. "School-based HIV prevention in Zimbabwe: Feasibility and acceptability of evaluation trials using biological outcomes." *AIDS* 16 (12):167-168.

Crane, Johanna Tayloe. 2013. *Scrambling for Africa: AIDS, expertise, and the rise of American global health science*. Ithaca, NY: Cornell University Press.

Crosby, Ricard, Stephanie Sanders, William L. Yarber, and Cynthia A. Graham. 2003. "Condom-use errors and problems: A neglected aspect of studies assessing condom effectiveness." *American Journal of Preventive Medicine* 24:367-370.

CRS/WVI/USAID/PEPFAR. 2009. Lesotho faith-based HIV prevention campaign: Baseline survey report. Maseru, Lesotho: Catholic Relief Services.

Curran, James W., and Harold W. Jaffe. 2011. AIDS: The early years and CDC's response. *Morbidity and Mortality Weekly Report* (MMWR) 60 (4):64-69.

Curtis, Tom. 1992. "The origin of AIDS. A startling new theory attempts to answer the question: Was it an act of God or an act of man?" *Rolling Stone*, March 19, 54-61, 106-108.

Das, Veena. 2007. *Life and words: Violence and the descent into the ordinary*. Berkeley, CA: University of California Press.

Das, Veena, and Ranendra K. Das. 2005. "Urban health and pharmaceutical consumption in Delhi, India." *Journal of Biosocial Science* 38:69-82.

Dawson, Lori J., Michelle L. Chunis, Danielle M. Smith, and Anthony A. Carboni. 2001. "The role of academic discipline and gender in high school teachers' AIDS-related knowledge and attitudes." *Journal of School Health* 71 (1):3-8.

de Bruin, Wändi Bruine, Julie S. Downs, Baruch Fischhoff, and Claire Palmgren. 2007. "Development and evaluation of an HIV/AIDS knowledge measure for adolescents focusing on misconceptions." *Journal of HIV/AIDS Prevention in Children & Youth* 8 (1):35-57.

de Camargo, Kenneth Rochel, André Luiz de Oliveira Mendonça, Christophe Perrey, and Alain Giami. 2013. "Male circumcision and HIV: A controversy study on facts and values." *Global Public Health* 8 (7):769-783.

De Lange, I. 2000. "HIV blood 'was stored for war.'" *The Citizen*, May 25.

De Waal, Alex. 2003. "A disaster with no name: The HIV/AIDS pandemic and the limits of governance." In *Learning from HIV and AIDS*, edited by G. Ellison, M. Parker and C. Campbell, 238-267. Cambridge, UK: Cambridge University Press.

Dearing, James W., and Everett Rogers. 1996. *Agenda-setting*. Thousand Oaks, CA: Sage.

Deetz, Stanley A. 1991. *Democracy in an age of corporate colonization*. Albany, NY: SUNY Press.

Delamont, Sara. 1992. *Fieldwork in educational settings: Methods, pitfalls, and perspectives*. London, UK: Falmer Press.

Denison, Julie, Kevin O'Reilly, George Schmid, Caitlin Kennedy, and Michael Sweat. 2008. "HIV voluntary counseling and testing and behavioral risk reduction in developing countries: A meta-analysis, 1990–2005." *AIDS and Behavior* 12 (3):363-373.

Dennis, Ruth E., and Michael F. Giangreco. 1996. "Creating conversation: Reflections of cultural sensitivity in family interviewing." *Exceptional Children* 63:103-116.

Desai, Manisha. 2005. "Transnationalism: The face of feminist politics post-Beijing." *International Social Science Journal* 184:319-330.

DFID. 2006. Helping Lesotho's factory workers to stitch up HIV and AIDS. Maseru, Lesotho: Department for International Development.

Dietrich, John W. 2007. "The politics of PEPFAR: The President's emergency plan for AIDS relief." *Ethics & International Affairs* 21 (3):277-292.

Dilger, Hansjörg. 2003. "Sexuality, AIDS and the lures of modernity: Reflexivity and morality among young people in rural Tanzania." *Medical Anthropology* 22 (1):23-52.

Doniger, Andrew S., Edgar Adams, Cheryl A. Utter, and John S. Riley. 2001. "Impact evaluation of the 'Not Me, Not Now' abstinence-oriented, adolescent pregnancy prevention communications program, Monroe County, NY." *Journal of Health Communication* 6 (1):45-60.

Dowsett, Gary W., and Murray Couch. 2007. "Male circumcision and HIV prevention: Is there really enough of the right kind of evidence?" *Reproductive Health Matters* 15 (29):33-44.

Drain, Paul K., Daniel T. Halperin, James P. Hughes, Jeffrey D. Klausner, and Robert C. Bailey. 2006. "Male circumcision, religion, and infectious diseases: An ecologic analysis of 118 developing countries." *BMC Infectious Diseases* 6:172.

Dutta-Bergman, Mohan J. 2004a. "An alternative approach to social capital: Exploring the linkage between health consciousness and community participation." *Health Communication* 16:393-409.

Dutta-Bergman, Mohan J. 2004b. "Poverty, structural barriers, and health: A Santali narrative of health communication." *Qualitative Health Research* 14 (8):1107-1122.

Dutta-Bergman, Mohan J. 2004c. "The unheard voice of Santalis: Communicating about health from the margins of India." *Communication Theory* 14 (3):237-263.

Dutta-Bergman, Mohan J. 2005. "Theory and practice in health communication campaigns: A critical interrogation." *Health Communication* 182:103-122.

Dutta, Mohan J. 2009. "On Spivak: Theorizing resistance—Applying Gayatri Chakravorty Spivak in public relations." In *Social theory on public relations*, edited by Oyvind Ihlen, Betteke van Ruler and Magnus Fredriksson, 278-300. London, UK: Routledge.

Dutta, Mohan J., and Mahuya Pal. 2010. "Public relations and marginalization in a global context: A postcolonial critique." In *Public relations in global cultural contexts*, edited by Nilanjana Bardhan and C. Kay Weaver, 195-225. London, UK: Routledge.

Dutta, Mohan J. 2007. "Communicating about culture and health: Theorizing culture-centered and cultural-sensitivity approaches." *Communication Theory* 17:304-328.

Dutta, Mohan J. 2008a. *Communicating health: A culture-centered approach*. Cambridge, UK: Polity.

Dutta, Mohan J. 2008b. "A critical response to Storey and Jacobson: The co-optive possibilities of participatory discourse." *Communication for Development and Social Change: A Global Journal* 2:81-90.

Dutta, Mohan J. 2008c. "Participatory communication in entertainment education: A critical analysis." *Communication for Development and Social Change: A Global Journal* 2:53-72.

Dutta, Mohan J. 2011. *Communicating social change: Structure, culture, and agency*. New York, NY: Taylor & Francis.

Dutta, Mohan J, and Iccha Basnyat. 2008. "Interrogating the radio communication project in Nepal: The participatory framing of colonization." In *Emerging perspectives in health communication: Meaning, culture and power*, edited by Heather M. Zoller and Mohan J. Dutta, 247-265. New York, NY: Taylor & Francis.

Dutta, Mohan J., and Ambar Basu. 2001. "Culture, communication and health: A guiding framework." In *Routledge handbook of health communication. (2nd ed)*, edited by Teresa L. Thompson, Roxanne Parrott and Jon F. Nussbaum, 320-334. New York, NY: Routledge.

Dutta, Mohan J., and Ambar Basu. 2013. "Negotiating our postcolonial selves: From the ground to the ivory tower." In *Handbook of autoethnography*, edited by Stacy Holman Jones, Tony E. Adams and Carolyn Ellis, 143-161. Walnut Creek, CA: Left Coast Press, Inc.

Easterly, William. 2006. *The white man's burden: Why the West's effort to aid the rest have done so much ill and so little good*. New York, NY: Penguin.

Easterly, William, and Tobias Pfutze. 2008. "Where does the money go? Best and worst practices in foreign aid." *Brookings Global Economy and Development Working Paper* 21.

Eisenberg, Leon. 1977. "Disease and illness: Distinctions between professional and popular ideas of sickness." *Medicine & Psychiatry* 1:9-23.

Ellis, Carolyn, and Arthur P. Bochner. 2000. "Autoethnography, personal narrative, reflexivity." In *The Sage handbook of qualitative research*, edited by Norma K. Denzin and Yvonna S. Lincoln, 733-768. Thousand Oaks, CA: Sage.

Epstein, Helen. 2007. *The invisible cure: Why we are losing the fight against AIDS in Africa*. New York, NY: Farrar, Straus & Giroux.

Epstein, Steven. 1996. *Impure science: AIDS, activism, and the politics of knowledge*. Berkeley, CA: University of California Press.

Epstein, Steven. 2003. "Inclusion, diversity, and biomedical knowledge-making: The multiple politics of representation." In *How users matter: The co-construction of users and technologies*, edited by Nelly Oudshoorn and Trevor Pinch, 173-190. Cambridge, MA: MIT Press.

Escobar, Arturo. 1995. *Encountering development: The making and unmaking of the third world*. Princeton, NJ: Princeton University Press.

Eves, Richard. 2012. "Resisting global AIDS knowledges: Born-again Christian narratives of the epidemic from Papua New Guinea." *Medical Anthropology* 31 (1):1-16.

Eves, Richard, and Leslie Butt. 2008. "Introduction." In *Making sense of AIDS: Culture, sexuality, and power in Melanesia*, edited by Leslie Butt and Richard Eves, 1-23. Honolulu, HI: University of Hawai'i Press.

Fassin, Didier. 2003. "The embodiment of inequality: AIDS as a social condition and the historical experience in South Africa." *EMBO Reports* 4 (Spec No):S4-9.

Fassin, Didier. 2007. *When bodies remember: Experiences and politics of AIDS in South Africa*. Berkeley, CA: University of California Press.

Fauci, Anthony S. 1983. "Acquired immune deficiency syndrome: The ever broadening clinical spectrum." *Journal of the American Medical Association* 250:2375-2376.

Feierman, Steven. 2011. "When physicians meet: Local medical knowledge and global public goods." In *Evidence, ethos and experiment: The anthropology and history of medical research in Africa*, edited by Wenzel Geissler and Catherine Molyneux, 171-196. New York, NY: Berghahn Books.

Feldman, Douglas A. 2003a. "Problems with the Uganda model for HIV/AIDS prevention." *Anthropology News* 44 (7):6.

Feldman, Douglas A. 2003b. "Reassessing AIDS priorities and strategies for Africa: ABC vs. ACCDGLMT." *AIDS and Anthropology Bulletin* 15 (2):5-9.

Ferguson, James. 1994. *The anti-politics machine: Development depolitization and bureaucratic power in Lesotho*. Chicago, IL: University of Chicago Press.

Ferguson, James. 1999. *Expectations of modernity: Myths and meanings of urban life on the Zambian copperbelt*. Berkeley, CA: University of California Press.

FHI360. 2011. "FEM-PrEP Project." Accessed 28 November, 2011. www.fhi.org/en/Research/Projects/FEM-PrEP.htm

Fink, Aaron J. 1986. "A possible explanation for heterosexual male infection with AIDS." *New England Journal of Medicine* 315:1167.

Ford, L. A., and G. A. Yep. 2003. "Working along the margins: Developing community-based strategies for communicating about health with marginalized groups." In *Handbook of health communication*, edited by Teresa L. Thompson, Alicia M. Dorsey, Katherine I. Miller and Roxanne Parrott, 241-261. Mahwah, NJ: Lawrence Erlbaum Associates.

Fordyce, Lauren. 2008. *A new look at Thai AIDS: Perspectives from the margin*. New York, NY: Berghahn.

Foster, George M. 1976. "Disease etiologies in non-Western medical systems." *American Anthropologist* 78 (4):773-782.

Foucault, Michel. 1973. *The birth of the clinic: An archeaology of medical perception*. Translated by A. M. Sheridan Smith. New York, NY: Vintage.

Foucault, Michel. 1977. *Discipline and punish: The birth of the prison*. Translated by Alan Sheridan. New York, NY: Vintage.

Foucault, Michel. 1978. *The History of Sexuality, vol. 1: The will to knowledge*. Translated by Robert Hurley. New York, NY: Pantheon.

Foucault, Michel. 1979. "On Governmentality." *Ideology and Consciousness* 6 (Autumn):5-22.

Foucault, Michel. 1991. "Governmentality." In *The Foucault effect: Studies in governmentality*, edited by Graham Burchell, Colin Gordon and Peter Miller, 87-104. Chicago, IL: University of Chicago Press.

Foucault, Michel. 1998. "Technologies of the self." In *Technologies of the self*, edited by Luther Martin, Huck Gutman and Patrick H. Hutton, 16-49. Amherst, MA: University of Massachusetts Press.

Foucault, Michel, and Colin Gordon. 1980. *Power/knowledge: Selected interviews and other writings, 1972-1977*. New York, NY: Pantheon.

Fowke, Keith, O. Anzala, J. Neil Simonsen, Nico J. Nagelkerke, E. N. Ngugi, and Francis A. Plummer. 1992. "Heterogeneity in susceptibility to HIV-1 in continuously exposed prostitutes" (Abstract for Poster PoC 4026). VIII International Conference on AIDS/III STD World Congress, Amsterdam, July.

Fowke, Keith R., Rupert Kaul, Kenneth L. Rosenthal, Julius Oyugi, Joshua Kimani, W. John Rutherford, Nico J. D. Nagelkerke, T. Blake Ball, Job J. Bwayo, J. Neil Simonsen, Gene M. Shearer, and Francis A. Plummer. 2000. "HIV-1-specific cellular immune responses among HIV-1-resistant sex workers." *Immunology and Cellular Biology* 78 (6):586-595.

Fox, Ashley. 2009. "The HIV poverty thesis re-examined: Poverty or inequality as an underlying cause of HIV in sub-Saharan Africa?" Doctoral dissertation, Graduate School of Arts and Sciences, Columbia University (3388441).

Frank, Lauren B., Joyee S. Chatterjee, Sonal T. Chaudhuri, Charlotte Lapsansky, Anurudra Bhanot, and Sheila T. Murphy. 2012. "Conversation and compliance: Role of interpersonal discussion and social norms in public communcation campaigns." *Journal of Health Communication* 17 (9):1050-1067.

Freire, Paulo. 1972. *Pedagogy of the oppressed*. New York, NY: Penguin Books.

Freire, Paulo. 1993. *Education for critical consciousness*. New York, NY: Continuum.

Fullwiley, Duana. 2011. *The enculturated gene: Sickle cell health politics and biological difference in West Africa*. Princeton, NJ: Princeton University Press.

Furin, Jennifer. 2011. "The role of traditional healers in community-based HIV care in rural Lesotho." *Journal of Community Health* 36 (5):849-856.

Gachuhi, Debbie. 1999. The impact of HIV/AIDS on education systems in the eastern and southern African region and the response of education systems to HIV/AIDS: Life skills programmes. Geneva, Switzerland: UNICEF.

Ganesh, Shiv, Heather Zoller, and George Cheney. 2005. "Transforming resistance, broadening our boundaries: Critical organizational communication meets globalization from below." *Communication Monographs* 72:169-191.

Gans, Herbert J. 1979. *Deciding what's news*. New York, NY: Pantheon.

Garenne, Michel, Alain Giami, and Christophe Perrey. 2013. "Male circumcision and HIV control in Africa: Questioning scientific evidence and the decision-making process." In *Global health in Africa: Historical perspectives on disease control*, edited by Tamara Giles-Vernick and James L. Webb Jr., 185-210. Athens, OH: Ohio University Press.

Garner, Robert C. 2000. "Safe sects? Dynamic religion and AIDS in South Africa." *Journal of Modern African Studies* 38 (1):41-69.

Geary, Cynthia W., Holly M. Burke, Laure Castelnau, Shailes Neupane, Yacine B. Sall, Emily Wong, and Heidi T. Tucker. 2007. "MTV 'Staying Alive' global campaign promoted interpersonal communication about HIV and positive beliefs about HIV prevention." *AIDS Education and Prevention* 19 (1):89-101.

Giorgianni, S. J., editor. 1998. *Responding to the challenge of health literacy, The Pfizer journal*. New York, NY: Impact Communications.

Gisselquist, David, John J. Potterat, Richard Rothenberg, Ernest M. Drucker, Stuart Brody, Devon D. Brewer, and Steven Minkin. 2003. "Examining the hypothesis that sexual transmission drives Africa's HIV epidemic." *AIDScience* 3 (10).

Gisselquist, David, Richard Rothenberg, James M. Potter, and Ernest M. Drucker. 2002. "HIV infections in sub-Saharan Africa not explained by sexual or vertical transmission." *International Journal of STD & AIDS* 13 (10):657-666.

Goffman, Erving. 1974. *Frame analysis: An essay on the organization of experience*. New York, NY: Harper & Row.

Gold, R. S., A. Karmiloff-Smith, M. J. Skinner, and J. Morton. 1992. "Situational factors and thought processes associated with unprotected intercourse in heterosexual students." *AIDS Care* 4 (3):305-323.

Goldenberg, Robert L. 2003. "The plausibility of micronutrient deficiency in relationship to perinatal infection." *Journal of Nutrition* 133:1645-1648.

Goldstein, Susan, Shereen Usdin, Esca Scheepers, and Garth Japhet. 2005. "Communicating HIV and AIDS, what works? A report on the impact evaluation of Soul City's fourth series." *Journal of Health Communication* 10:465-483.

Gortmaker, Steven L., and Jose Antonio Izazola. 1992. "The role of quantitative behavioral research in AIDS prevention." In *AIDS prevention through education: A world view*, edited by Jaime Sepulveda, Harvey Fineberg and Jonathan Mann, 37-56. Oxford, UK: Oxford University Press.

Gottlieb, Jerry B., and Dan Sarel. 1991. "Comparative advertising effectivness: The role of involvement and source credibility." *Journal of Advertising* 20 (1):38-45.

Gottlieb, M. S., H. M. Schanker, P. T. Ran, A. Saxon, J. D. Weisman, and I. Pozalski. 1981. "Pneumocystis pneumonia—Los Angeles." *Morbidity and Mortality Weekly Report (MMWR)* 30:250-252.

Gould, Chandré, and Peter Folb. 2000. "Perverted science and twisted loyalty." *The Sunday Independent,* October 8, 7.

Granich, Reuben M., Charles F. Gilks, Christopher Dye, Kevin M. De Cock, and Brian G. Williams. 2009. "Universal voluntary HIV testing with immediate antiretroviral therapy as a strategy for elimination of HIV transmission: A mathematical model." *Lancet* 373 (9657):48-57.

Grant, Robert M., Javier R. Lama, Peter L. Anderson, Vanessa McMahan, Albert Y. Liu, Lorena Vargas, Pedro Goicochea, Martin Casapia, Juan V. Guanira-Carranza, Maria E. Ramirez-Cardich, Orlando Montoya-Herrera, Telmo Fernandez, Valdilea G. Veloso, Susan P. Buchbinder, Suwat Chariyalertsak, Mauro Schechter, Linda-Gail Bekker, Kenneth H. Mayer, Esper G. Kallas, K. Rivet Amico, Kathleen Mulligan, Lane R. Bushman, Robert J. Hance, Carmela Ganoza, Patricia Defechereux, Brian Postle, Furong Wang, J. Jeff McConnell, Jia-Hua Zheng, Jeanny Lee, James F. Rooney, Howard S. Jaffe, Ana I. Martinez, David N. Burns, and David V. Glidden for the iPrEx Study Team. 2010. "Preexposure chemoprophylaxis for HIV prevention in men who have sex with men." *New England Journal of Medicine* 363 (27):2587-99.

Gray, Ronald H., Xianbin Li, Godfrey Kigozi, David Serwadda, Fred Nalugoda, Stephen Watya, Steven J. Reynolds, and Maria Wawer. 2007. "The impact of male circumcision on HIV incidence and cost per infection prevented: a stochastic simulation model from Rakai, Uganda." *AIDS* 21 (7):845-50.

Gray, Ronald H., Godfrey Kigozi, David Serwadda, Frederick Makumbi, Stephen Watya, Fred Nalugoda, Noah Kiwanuka, Lawrence H. Moulton, Mohammad A. Chaudhary, Michael Z. Chen, Nelson K. Sewankambo, Fred Wabwire-Mangen, Melanie C. Bacon, Carolyn F. Williams, Pius Opendi, Steven J. Reynolds, Oliver Laeyendecker, Thomas C. Quinn, and Maria J. Wawer. 2007. "Male circumcision for HIV prevention in men in Rakai, Uganda: A randomised trial." *Lancet* 369 (9562):657-666.

Gray, R. H., X. Li, M. J. Wawer, S. J. Gange, D. Serwadda, N. K. Sewankambo, R. Moore, F. Wabwire-Mangen, T. Lutalo, T. C. Quinn, and The Rakai Project Group. 2003. "Stochastic simulation of the impact of antiretroviral therapy and HIV vaccines on HIV transmission: Rakai, Uganda." *AIDS* 17 (13):1941-1951.

Grebe, Eduard, and Nicoli Nattrass. 2012. "AIDS conspiracy beliefs and unsafe sex in Cape Town." *AIDS and Behavior.* 16 (3):761-773

Green, Edward C. 1992. "Sexually transmitted disease, ethnomedicine and AIDS in Africa." *Social Science & Medicine* 35 (2):121-130.

Green, Edward C. 1999. "The involvement of African traditional healers in the prevention of AIDS and STDS." In *Anthropology in public health: Bridging differences in culture and society,* edited by R. A. Hahn. Oxford, UK: Oxford University Press.

Green, Edward C. 2003a. "New challenges to the AIDS prevention paradigm." *Anthropology News* 44 (6):5-6.

Green, Edward C. 2003b. *Rethinking AIDS Prevention.* Westport, CT: Praeger.

Green, Edward C., and Allison Herling Ruark. 2011. *AIDS, Behavior, and Culture: Understanding Evidence-Based Prevention.* Walnut Creek, CA: Left Coast Press, Inc.

Greene, Jennifer C., Valerie J. Caracelli, and Wendy F. Graham. 1989. "Towards a conceptual framework for mixed-method evaluation designs." *Educational Evaluation and Policy Analysis* 11 (3):255-274.

Grmek, Mirko D. 1989. *History of AIDS: Emergence and origin of a modern pandemic.* Translated by R. C. Maultiz and J. Duffin. Princeton, NJ: Princeton University Press.

Grube, A., and K. Boehme-Deurr. 1989. "AIDS in international magazines." *Journalism Quarterly* 66:686-689.

Guha, Ranajit. 1982. "On some aspects of the historiography of colonial India." In *Subaltern studies I,* edited by Ranajit Guha, 1-6. New Delhi, India: Oxford University Press.

Hahn, Robert A. 1983. "Biomedical practice and anthropological theory: Frameworks and directions." *Annual Review of Anthropology* 12:305-333.

Haignere, C. S., J. F. Culhane, C. M. Balsley, and P. Legos. 1996. "Teachers' receptiveness and comfort teaching sexuality education and using non-traditional teaching strategies." *Journal of School Health* 66 (5):140-144.

Halperin, Daniel, and Robert C. Bailey. 1999. "Male circumcision and HIV infection: Ten years and counting." *Lancet* 354 (9192):1813-1815.

Harris, Richard. 2001. *Morning edition.* Washington, DC: National Public Radio.

Harvey, David. 2005. *A brief history of neoliberalism.* Oxford, UK: Oxford University Press.

Hassan, Fareed, and Oladeji Ojo. 2002. *Lesotho: Development in a challenging environment. A joint World Bank-African Development Bank evaluation.* Geneva, Switzerland: World Bank Publications.

Hauser, Debra. 2004. *Five years of abstinence-only-until-marriage education: Assessing the impact.* Washington, DC: Advocates for Youth.

Hauser, Philip M. 2001. "The limitations of KAP surveys." In *Social research in developing countries: Surveys and censuses in the third world*, edited by Martin Bulmer and Donald P. Warwick, 65-69. London, UK: Routledge.

Hausman, Alice J., and Sheryl B. Ruzek. 1995. "Implementation of comprehensive school health education in elementary schools: Focus on teacher concerns." *Journal of School Health* 65 (3):81-85.

Helleve, Arnfinn, Alan J. Flisher, Hans Onya, Sylvia Kaaya, Wanjiru Mukoma, Caroline Swai, and Knut-Inge Klepp. 2009. "Teachers' confidence in teaching HIV/AIDS and sexuality in South African and Tanzanian schools." *Scandinavian Journal of Public Health* 32 (S2):55-64.

Helleve, Arnfin, Alan J. Flisher, Hans Onya, Wanjiru Mukoma, and Knut-Inge Klepp. 2009. "South African Life Orientation teachers' reflections on the impact of culture on their teaching in sexuality and HIV/AIDS." *Culture, Health and Sexuality* 11 (2):189-204.

Helleve, Arnfinn, Alan J. Flisher, Hans Onya, Wanjiru Mukoma, and Knut-Inge Klepp. 2011. "Can any teacher teach sexuality and HIV/AIDS? Perspectives of South African Life Orientation teachers." *Sex Education* 11 (1):13-26.

Himmelgreen, David A., Nancy Romero-Daza, David Turkon, Sharon Watson, Ipolto Okello-Uma, and Daniel Sellen. 2009. "Addressing the HIV/AIDS–food insecurity syndemic in sub-Saharan Africa." *African Journal of AIDS Research* 8 (4):401-412.

Hodgetts, Darrin, and Kerry Chamberlain. 2006. "Developing a critical media research agenda for health psychology." *Journal of Health Psychology* 11 (2):317-327.

Hogan, Heather. 2000. "Apartheid atrocities unravel in Basson trial." *Mail & Guardian*, 26 May.

Hogel, Janice. 2002. *What happened in Uganda? Declining HIV prevalence, behavior change and the national response.* Washington, DC: USAID.

Holborn, Lucy. 2010. *South Africa Survey 2009/2010.* Johannesburg, South Africa: South African Institute of Race Relations.

Hope, Ronald Kempe. 2003. "Promoting behavior change in Botswana: An assessment of the peer education HIV/AIDS prevention program at the workplace." *Journal of Health Communication* 8 (3):267-281.

Hornik, Robert, and Emile McAnany. 2001. "Theories and evidence: Mass media effects and fertility change." *Communication Theory* 11 (4):454-471.

Howard, Marion, and Judith Blarney McCabe. 1990. "Helping teenagers postpone sexual involvement." *Family Planning Perspectives* 22 (January/February):21-26.

Human Rights Watch & AIDS and Rights Alliance for Southern Africa. 2008. *A testing challenge: The experience of Lesotho's universal HIV counseling and testing campaign.* New York, NY: Human Rights Watch.

Iliffe, John. 1998. *East African doctors: A history of the modern profession.* Cambridge, UK: Cambridge University Press.

Islamic Medical Association of Uganda. 1998. AIDS education through Imams: A spiritually motivated community effort in Uganda. In *Best practice collection.* Kampala, Uganda: UNAIDS.

Izazola-Licea, J. A., J. L. Valdespino-Gomez, S. L. Gortmaker, J. Townsend, J. Becker, M. Palacios-Martinez, N. E. Mueller, and J. Sepulveda Amor. 1991. "HIV-1 seropositivity and behavioral and sociological risks among homosexual and bisexual men in six Mexican cities." *Journal of Acquired Immune Deficiency Syndromes* 4 (6):614-622.

James, Shamagonam, Priscilla Reddy, Robert A. C. Ruiter, Ann McCauley, and Bart van den Borne. 2006. "The impact of an HIV and AIDS life skills program on secondary school students in Kwazulu-Natal, South Africa." *AIDS Education and Prevention* 18 (4):281-294.

Janzen, John M. 1981. "The need for a taxonomy of health in the study of African therapeutics." *Social Science & Medicine* 15B:185-194.

Jill, Joseph G., Susanne B. Montgomery, Carol-Ann Emmons, Ronald C. Kessler, David G. Ostrow, Camille B. Wortman, Kerth O'Brien, Michael Eller, and Suzann Eshleman. 1987. "Magnitude and determinants of behavioral risk reduction: Longitudinal analysis of a cohort at risk for AIDS." *Psychology & Health* 1 (1):73-95.

Johansson, Kjell A., Bjarne Robberstad, and Ole F. Norheim. 2010. "Further benefits by early start of HIV treatment in low income countries: Survival estimates of early versus deferred antiretroviral therapy." *AIDS Research & Therapy* 7 (1):3.

Johnson, Blair T., Lori A. Scott-Sheldon, and Michael P. Carey. 2010. "Meta-synthesis of health behavior change meta-analyses." *American Journal of Public Health* 100 (11):2193-2198.

Johnson, Blair T., Colleen A. Redding, Ralph J. DiClemente, Brian S. Mustanski, Brian Dodge, Paschal Sheeran, Michelle R. Warren, Rick S. Zimmerman, William A. Fisher, Mark T. Conner, Michael P. Carey, Jeffrey D. Fisher, Ronald D. Stall, and Martin Fishbein. 2010. "A network-individual-resource model for HIV prevention." *AIDS and Behavior* 14:204-221.

Johnson, Deborah, June A. Flora, and Rajiv Nath Rimal. 1997. "HIV/AIDS public service announcements around the world: A descriptive analysis." *Journal of Health Communication: International Perspectives* 2 (4):223-234.

Jones, Chaunetta. 2011. "'If I take my pills I'll go hungry': The choice between economic security and HIV/AIDS treatment in Grahamstown, South Africa." *Annals of Anthropological Practice* 35 (1):67-80.

Jones, Stacy Holman. 2005. "Autoethnography: Making the personal political." In *The Sage handbook of qualitative research*, edited by Norma K. Denzin and Yvonna S. Lincoln, 763-791. Thousand Oaks, CA: Sage.

Jorgensen, Stephen R., Vicki Potts, and Brian Camp. 1993. "Project taking charge: Six-month follow-up of a pregnancy prevention program for early adolescents." *Family Relations* 42:401-406.

Jules-Rosette, Bennetta. 1980. "Changing aspects of women's initiation in southern Africa: An exploratory study." *Canadian Journal of African Studies* 13 (3):389-405.

Kaaya, Sylvia, Wanjiru Mukoma, Alan J. Flisher, and Knut-Inge Klepp. 2002. "School-based sexual health interventions in sub-Saharan Africa: A review." *Social Dynamics* 28 (1):64-88.

Kahn, James G., Elliot Marseille, and Bertran Auvert. 2006. "Cost-effectiveness of male circumcision for HIV prevention in a South African setting." *PLoS Med* 3 (12):e517.

(The Henry J.) Kaiser Family Foundation. 2011. "Kaiser Daily Global Health Policy Report: Global Fund Cancels Round 11 Grants, Approves New Strategy and Organization Plan." Accessed 8 January, 2013. globalhealth.kff.org/Daily-Reports/2011/November/29/GH-112911-Global-Fund-Round-11.aspx

Kalichman, Seth C. 2009. *Denying AIDS: Conspiracy theories, pseudoscience and human tragedy*. New York, NY: Copernicus Books.

Kalichman, Seth C., Eric Benotsch, Troy Suarez, Sheryl Catz, Jeff Miller, and David Rompa. 2000. "Health literacy and health related knowledge among persons living with HIV/AIDS." *American Journal of Preventive Medicine* 18 (4):325-331.

Kalichman, Seth C., and David Rompa. 2000. "Functional health literacy is associated with health status and health-related knowledge in people living with HIV/AIDS." *Journal of Acquired Immune Deficiency Syndromes* 25 (4):337-344.

Kalofonos, Ippolytos Andreas. 2010. "'All I Eat is ARVs': The paradox of AIDS treatment interventions in central Mozambique." *Medical Anthropology Quarterly* 24 (3):363-380.

Kapiga, Saidi H., and Joe L. P. Lugalla. 2002. "Sexual behavior and condom use in Tanzania: Results from the 1996 Demographic and Health Survey." *AIDS Care* 14 (4):455-469.

Karim, Salim Abdool, and Quarraisha Abdool Karim. 2011. "Antiretroviral prophylaxis: A defining moment in HIV control." *Lancet* 378 (9809):e23-5.

Kates, Jennifer, Adam Wexler, Eric Lief, Carlos Avila, and Benjamin Gobet. 2012. Financing the response to AIDS in low- and middle-income countries: International assistance from donor governments in 2011. *UNAIDS and Kaiser Family Foundation*. Accessed 25 November, 2012. www.kff.org/hivaids/upload/7347-08.pdf

Kathuria, R., P. Chirenda, R. Sabatier, and N. Dube. 1998. "Peer education to reduce STI/HIV transmission in Lusaka, Zambia." 12th International Conference on AIDS, Geneva.

Katzenstein, D., W. McFarland, M. Mbizvo, A. Latif, R. Machekano, J. Parsonnet, and M. Bassett. 1998. "Peer education among factory workers in Zimbabwe: Providing a sustainable HIV prevention intervention." 12th International Conference on AIDS, Geneva.

Kelly, Kevin, Warren Parker, and Graeme Lewis. 2001. "Reconceptualising behaviour change in the context of HIV/AIDS." In *Socio-political and psychological perspectives of South Africa*, edited by Christopher R. Stones. London, UK: Nova Science.

Kenworthy, Nora. 2011. "To eat and be eaten: Hunger struggles and the politics of HIV in Lesotho." Anthropology Southern Africa Annual Conference, Stellenbosch University, Stellenbosch, 5 September.

Kenworthy, Nora, and Nicola Bulled. 2013. "From modeling to morals: Imagining the future of HIV PrEP in Lesotho." *Developing World Bioethics* 13 (2):70-78.

Keohane, Robert O. 2002. *After hegemony: Cooperation and discord in the world political economy*. Princeton, NJ: Princeton University Press.

Kerr, Dianne L., Diane D. Allensworth, and Jacob A. Gayle. 1989. "The ASHA national HIV education needs assessment of health and education professionals." *Journal of School Health* 59 (7):301-307.

Ki-moon, Ban. 2011. *The Secretary General: Message on World AIDS day, 1 December 2011*. Geneva, Switzerland: United Nations.

Kim, Y. M., C. Marangwanda, and A. Kols. 1997. "Quality of counselling of young clients in Zimbabwe." *East African Medical Journal* 74 (9):514-518.

Kirby, Douglas B. 2001. *Emerging answers: Research findings on programs to reduce teen pregnancy*. Washington, DC: National Campaing to Prevent Teen Pregnancy.

Kirby, Douglas B. 2002. *Do Abstincence-only programs delay the intiation of sex among young people and reduce teen pregnancy?* Washington, DC: National Campaign to Prevent Teen Pregnancy.

Kirby, Douglas B., B. A. Laris, and Lori A. Rolleri. 2007. "Sex and HIV education programs: Their impact on sexual behaviors of young people throughout the world." *Journal of Adolescent Health* 40 (3):206-217.

Kleinman, Arthur. 1980. *Patients and healers in the context of culture*. Berkeley, CA: University of California Press.

Knight, Lindsay. 2008. *UNAIDS: The first 10 years*. Geneva, Switzerland: Joint United Nations Programme on HIV/AIDS.

Kolosoa, Lineo Clementina, and Bothephana Makhakhane. 2010. *Life skills for national development in Lesotho: Can ODL do it?* Maseru, Lesotho: Insitutute for Development Management and National University of Lesotho.

Kotanyi, Sophie, and Brigitte Krings-Ney. 2009. "Introduction of a culturally sensitive HIV/AIDS prevention in female initiation rites: An applied anthropological approach in Mozambique." *African Journal of AIDS Research* 8 (4):491-502.

Kraft, S. 1994. "42 nations vow to protect AIDS patients." *San Francisco Chronicle*, December 2, D3.

Latkin, Carl, Margaret R. Weeks, Laura Glasman, Carol Galletly, and Dolores Albarracín. 2010. "A dynamic social systems model for considering structural factors in HIV prevention and detection." *AIDS and Behavior* 14 (Suppl 2):222-238.

Latour, Bruno. 1987. *Science in action*. Cambridge, MA: Harvard University Press.

Leclerc-Madlala, Suzanne. 1997. "Infect one, infect all: Zulu youth response to the AIDS epidemic in South Africa." *Medical Anthropology* 17:363-380.

Leclerc-Madlala, Suzanne. 2001. "Virginity testing: Managing sexuality in a maturing HIV/AIDS epidemic." *Medical Anthropology Quarterly* 15 (4):533-552.

Leclerc-Madlala, Suzanne. 2002. "On the virgin cleansing myth: Gendered bodies, AIDS and ethnomedicine." *African Journal of AIDS Research* 1:87-95.

Leclerc-Madlala, Suzanne. 2004. "Transactional sex and the pursuit of modernity." *Social Dynamics* 29:1-21.

Leclerc-Madlala, Suzanne. 2005. "Popular responses to HIV/AIDS and policy." *Journal of Southern African Studies* 31 (4):845-856.

Lee, Benjamin, and Edward LiPuma. 2002. "Cultures of circulation: The imaginations of modernity." *Public Culture* 14 (1):191-213.

Lee, Renée Gravois, and Theresa Garvin. 2003. "Moving from information transfer to information exchange in health and health care." *Social Science & Medicine* 56 (3):449-464.

Lerner, Barron H. 1997. "From careless consumptives to recalcitrant patients: The historical construction of noncompliance." *Social Science & Medicine* 45 (9):1423-1431.

Lesotho Food Security Monitoring System. 2011. Quarterly Bulletin, March. Maseru, Lesotho.

Lester, Elli. 1992. "The AIDS story and moral panic: How the Euro-African press constructs AIDS." *Howard Journal of Communication* 7 (1):1-10.

Levenson Gingiss, P., and K. Basen-Engquist. 1994. "HIV education practices and training needs of middle school and high school teachers." *Journal of School Health* 64 (7):290-295.

Levenson Gingiss, P., and R. Hamilton. 1989a. "Evaluation of training effects on teacher attitutdes and concerns prior to implementing a human sexuality education program." *Journal of School Health* 59 (4):156-160.

Levenson Gingiss, P., and R. Hamilton. 1989b. "Teacher perspectives after implementing a human sexuality education program." *Journal of School Health* 59 (10):427-431.

Levi-Strauss, Claude. 1963. "The sorcerer and his magic." In *Structural anthropology*. New York, NY: Basic Books.

Lim, Khor. 1995. "Reporting AIDS: News representations in the Malaysian newspapers." *Journal of Development Communication* 7 (1):79-86.

Linake, 'Makuena. 2009. "Health ministry has no intentions of campaigning for circumcision." *Informative*, 13 July, 8.

Linake, 'Makuena. 2010. "Male circumcision crucial in reducing chances of HIV infection." *Informative*, 26 October. Accessed 2 February 2011. www .informativenews.co.ls/index.php/archives/2420-male-circumcision-crucial-in-reducing-chances-of-hiv-infections

Lock, Margaret. 2000. "Accounting for disease and distress: Morals of the normal and abnormal." In *The handbook of social studies in health and medicine*, edited by Gary L. Albrecht, Ray Fitzpatrick and Susan C. Scrimshaw, 259-276. Thousand Oaks, CA: Sage.

Lorway, Robert, Sushena Reza-Paul, and Akram Pasha. 2009. "On becoming a male sex worker in Mysore: Sexual subjectivity, 'empowerment', and community-based HIV prevention research." *Medical Anthropology Quarterly* 23 (2):142-160.

Lupton, Deborah. 1993. "AIDS risk and heterosexuality in the Australian press." *Discourse and Society* 4:307-328.

Lupton, Deborah. 1994a. *Moral threats and dangerous desires: AIDS in the news medias*. London, UK: Taylor & Francis.

Lupton, Deborah. 1994b. "Toward the development of critical health communication praxis." *Health Communication* 6:55-67.

Lupton, Deborah. 1995. *The imperative of health: Public health and the regulated body*. Thousand Oaks, CA: Sage.

Machel, Jozina A. 2001. "Unsafe sexual behaviour among schoolgirls in Mozambique: A matter of gender and class." *Reproductive Health Matters* 9 (17):82-90.

MacPhail, Catherine, and Catherine Campbell. 2001. "'I think condoms are good but, aai, I hate those things': Condom use among adolescents and young people in a Southern African township." *Social Science & Medicine* 52 (11):1613-27.

Magubane, Peter. 1998. *Vanishing cultures of South Africa: Changing customs in a changing world*. New York, NY: Rizzoli International Publications.

Maharaj, Pranitha. 2001. "Obstacles to negotiating dual protection: Perspectives of men and women." *African Journal of Reproductive Health* 5 (3):150-161.

Mahdavi, Pardis. 2008. *Passionate uprisings: Iran's sexual revolution*. Standford, CA: Stanford University Press.

Mahe, Tinadale, and Kim Travers. 1997-1998. "Evaluation of a peer health education project in The Gambia, West Africa." *International Quarterly of Community Health Education* 17 (1):43-56.

Maluleke, Thelmah X. 2003a. "Improving the health status of women through puberty rites for girls." *Health South African Gesondheid* 8 (3).

Maluleke, Thelmah X. 2003b. "Sexuality education, gender and health issues related to puberty rites for girls." *Health South African Gesondheid* 8 (3).

Maluleke, Thelmah X., and R. Troskie. 2003. "The views of women in the Limpopo province of South Africa concerning girls' puberty rites." *Health South African Gesondheid* 8 (3).

Mann, Jonathan M., Daniel Tarantola, and Global AIDS Policy Coalition. 1996. *AIDS in the world II: Global dimensions, social roots, and responses*. New York, NY: Oxford University Press.

Mann, Jonathan, Daniel Tarantola, and Thomas Netter. 1992. *AIDS in the world*. Cambridge, MA: Harvard University Press.

Manoff, Richard K. 1985. *Social marketing: New imperative for public health*. Westport, CT: Praeger.

Mantini-Briggs, Clara. 2013. "From revolutionary citizen to biocommunicable subject: Knowledge production and circulation in discource about Dengue Fever." American Anthropological Association, Chicago, November 24, 2013.

Marck, Jeff. 1997. "Aspects of male circumcision in sub-equatorial African cultural history." *Health Transition Review* 7 (Suppl):337-359.

Margolis, Howard. 1996. *Dealing with risk*. Chicago, IL: University of Chicago Press.

Matope, Tsitsi. 2011a. "AIDS battle: Lesotho on the back foot." *Public Eye*, 15 March, 2.

Matope, Tsitsi. 2011b. "Youths Savage AIDS Response." *Public Eye*, 27 May, 1.

Mattson, Marifran. 2000. "Empowerment through agency-promoting dialogue: An explicit application of harm reduction theory to reframe HIV test counseling." *Journal of Health Communication* 5 (4):333-347.

Mauldin, W. Parker. 1965. "Fertility studies: Knowledge, attitudes and practice." *Studies in Family Planning* 7 (1):1-10.

Mavhu, Webster, Lisa Langhaug, Bothwell Manyonga, Robert Power, and Frances Cowan. 2008. "What is 'sex' exactly? Using cognitive interviewing to improve the validity of sexual behavior reporting among young people in rural Zimbabwe." *Culture, Health & Sexuality* 10 (6):563-572.

Mavhu, Webster, Lisa Langhaug, Sophie Pascoe, Jeffrey Dirawo, Graham Hart, and Frances Cowan. 2011. "A novel tool to assess community norms and attitudes to multiple and concurrent sexual partnering in rural Zimbabwe: Participatory attitudinal ranking." *AIDS Care* 23 (1):52-59.

May, Todd. 1993. *Between genealogy and epistemology: Psychology, politics and knowledge in the thought of Michel Foucault*. University Park, PA: Pennsylvania State University.

Mayer, Philip, and Iona Mayer. 1961. *Townsmen or tribesmen: Conservatism and the process of urbanization in a South African city*. London, UK: Oxford University Press.

Mbali, Mandisa. 2004. "AIDS discourses and the South African state: Government denialism and post-apartheid policy-making." *Transformation* 54:104-122.

McAllister, Matthew P. 1992. "AIDS, medicalization, and the news media." In *AIDS: A communication perspective*, edited by T. Edgar, M. A. Fitzpatrick and V. S. Freimuth, 195-221. Hillsdale, NJ: Lawrence Erlbaum Associates.

McCombs, Maxwell. 1993. "The evolution of agenda-setting research: Twenty-five years in the marketplace in ideas." *Journal of Communication* 43:58-67.

McCombs, Maxwell. 2004. *Setting the agenda: The mass media and public opinion*. Cambridge, UK: Polity.

McCoombe, Scott G., and Roger V. Short. 2006. "Potential HIV-1 target cells in the human penis." *AIDS* 20:1491-1495.

Mckee, Neill, Jane Bertrand, and Antje Becker-Benton. 2004. *Strategic communication in HIV/AIDS epidemic.* New Delhi, India: Sage.

McLean, Diarmuid. 1990. "Communication report on the concerns of women in Khayelitsha." *AIDScan* 2 (4):9.

McLeod, Douglas, and Elisabeth M. Perse. 1994. "Direct and indirect effects of socioeconimc status on public affairs knowledge." *Journalism Quarterly* 71 (2):433-442.

McMichael, Phillip. 2005. "Globalization." In *The handbook of political sociology: States, civil societies and globalization,* edited by T. Janoski, R. Alford, A. Hicks, and M. Schwartz, 587-606. Cambridge, UK: Cambridge University Press.

McMichael, Phillip. 2008. *Development and social change. A global perspective.* Thousand Oaks, CA: Pine Forge Press.

McNeill, Fraser G. 2009. "'Condoms cause AIDS': Poison, prevention and denial in Venda, South Africa." *African Affairs* 108 (432):353-370.

McNeill, Fraser G. 2011. *AIDS, politics, and music in South Africa.* Cambridge, UK: Cambridge University Press.

Meekers, Dominique, and Megan Klein. 2001. *Determinants of condom use among unmarried youth in Yaounde and Douala, Cameroon. Working Paper No. 47.* Washington, DC: Population Services International.

Mertens, Donna M. 2005. *Research and evaluation in education and psychology: Integrating diversity with quantitative, qualitative, and mixed methods.* 2nd ed. Thousand Oaks, CA: Sage.

Mgomezulu, Victor Y., and A. G. Kruger. 2011. "Enhancing school HIV and AIDS strategic plan through expanded stakeholder involvement." *Africa Education Review* 8 (2):247-266.

Miller, Ann Neville, Mike Mutungi, Elena Facchini, Benard Barasa, Wycliffe Ondieki, and Charles Warria. 2008. "An outcome assessment of an ABC-based HIV peer education intervention among Kenyan university students." *Journal of Health Communication* 13 (4):345-356.

Mitchell, Claudia, and Ann Smith. 2003. "'Sick of AIDS': Life, literacy and South African youth." *Culture, Health and Sexuality* 5 (6):513-522.

Modo, I. V. O. 2001. "Migrant culture and changing face of family structure in Lesotho." *Journal of Comparative Family Studies* 32 (3):443-452.

Moghadam, Valentine. 2009. *Globalization and social movements.* Lanham, MD: Rowman & Littlefield.

MoHSW. 2005a. *'Know your status' campaign operational plan 2006-7: Gateway to comprehensive HIV prevention, treatment, care and support.* Maseru, Lesotho: Ministry of Health and Social Welfare.

MoHSW. 2005b. *Lesotho Demographic and Health Survey 2004.* Maseru, Lesotho: Ministry of Health and Social Welfare, Bureau of Statistics, ORC Macro.

MoHSW. 2006. *'Know your status' communication strategy.* Maseru, Lesotho: Ministry of Health and Social Welfare

MoHSW. 2008. *Situation analysis report: Male Circumcision in Lesotho.* Maseru, Lesotho: Ministry of Health and Social Welfare.

MoHSW. 2009. *Lesotho Demographic and Health Survey 2009.* Maseru, Lesotho: Ministry of Health and Social Welfare, Bureau of Statistics, ORC Macro.

MoHSW. 2011a. *Concept note on energized prevention of HIV transmission in Lesotho.* April 1. Maseru, Lesotho: Ministry of Health and Social Welfare.

MoHSW. 2011b. *Lesotho HIV prevention revitalization: Operational plan 2011*, released October 10, 2011. Maseru, Lesotho: Ministry of Health and Social Welfare.

Mollel, O., R. Olomi, J. Mwanga, and B. Mongi. 1995. "Peer education in Mererani mining settlement." In *Young people at risk: Fighting AIDS in northern Tanzania*, edited by Knut-Inge Klepp, Paul Biswalo and Aud Talle, 196-203. Oslo, Sweden: Scandinavian University Press.

Morokos, Hartmut B., and Stanley Deetz. 1996. "What counts as real? A constitutive view of communication and the disenfranchised in the context of health." In *Communication and disenfranchisement: Social health issues and implications*, edited by Eileen B. Ray, 29-44. Mahwah, NJ: Lawrence Erlbaum Associates.

Morris, Brian J., and Richard G. Wamai. 2012. "Biological basis for the protective effect conferred by male circumcision against HIV infection." *International Journal of STD & AIDS* 23 (3):153-9.

Morris, Brian J., Stefan A. Bailis, and Thomas E. Wiswell. 2014. "Circumcision rates in the United States: Rising or falling? What effect might the new affirmative pediatric policy statement have?" *Mayo Clinic Proceedings*:1-10.

Morse, Janice M., and Peggy A. Field. 1995. *Qualitative research methods for health professionals.* 2nd ed. Thousand Oaks, CA: Sage.

Moses, Stephen, Janet E. Bradley, Nico J. Nagelkerke, Allan R. Ronald, J. O. Ndinya-Achola, and Francis A. Plummer. 1990. "Geographical patterns of male circumcision practices in Africa: Association with HIV seroprevalence." *Internationl Journal of Epidemiology* 19 (3):693-697.

Moughutou, P. 1998. "Education of road haulers and taxi-drivers of Kumba Town on STD/AIDS prevention: Pilot project." 12th International Conference on AIDS, Geneva.

Mukoma, Wanjiru, Alan J. Flisher, Nazeema Ahmed, Shahieda Jansen, Catherine Mathews, Knut-Inge Klepp, and Herman Schaalma. 2009. "Process evaluation of school-based HIV/AIDS intervention in South Africa." *Scandinavian Journal of Public Health* 32 (Suppl 2):37-47.

Mupemba, Karen. 1999. "The Zimbabwe HIV prevention program for truck drivers and commercial sex workers: A behavior change intervention." In *Resistances to behavioural change to reduce HIV/AIDS infection in predominantly heterosexual epidemics in third world countries*, edited by John Caldwell, Pat Caldwell, John Anarfi, Kofi Awusabo-Asare, James Ntozi, I. O. Orubuloye, Jeff Marck, Wendy Cosford, Rachel Colombo and Elaine Hollings, 133-137. Canberra, Australia: Health Transition Centre, Australian National University.

Murphy, Alexandra G., Eric M. Eisenberg, Robert Wears, and Shawna J. Perry. 2008. "Contested streams of action: Power and deference in emergency medicine." In *Emerging perspectives in health communication*, edited by Heather M. Zoller and Mohan J. Dutta, 275-292. New York, NY: Routledge.

Muturia, Nancy, and An Soontae. 2010. "HIV/AIDS stigma and religiosity among African American women." *Journal of Health Communication* 15 (4):388-401.

Muyinda, Herbert, Jane Kengeya-Kayondo, Robert Pool and James Whitworth. 2001. "Traditional sex counseling and STI/HIV prevention among young women in rural Uganda." *Culture, Health and Sexuality* 3 (3):353-361.

Mzala, Comrade. 1988. "AIDS and the imperialist connection." *Sechaba* 22 (11):28.

Nabel, Gary J. 2001. "Challenges and opportunities for development of an AIDS vaccine." *Nature* 410 (April 19):1002-1007.

NAC. 2008. *Survey of HIV and AIDS related knowledge, attitudes and practices. Lesotho 2007.* Maseru, Lesotho: National AIDS Commission.

NAC. 2009a. *Behavior change communication in Lesotho: National behavior change communication strategy, 2008-2013.* Maseru, Lesotho: National AIDS Commission.

NAC. 2009b. *Lesotho HIV prevention response and modes of transmission analysis.* Maseru, Lesotho: National AIDS Commission.

NAC. 2009c. *Quarterly report on the national response to HIV/AIDS: Reporting period July through September 2009.* Maseru, Lesotho: National AIDS Commission.

NAC. 2010a. *The history of HIV and AIDS in Lesotho.* Maseru, Lesotho: National AIDS Commission.

NAC. 2010b. *UNGASS country report: Lesotho. January 2008-December 2009.* Maseru, Lesotho: National AIDS Commission.

NAC. 2010c. *UNGASS country report: Lesotho. Status of the national response to the 2001 declaration of commitment on HIV and AIDS.* January 2008-December 2009. Maseru, Lesotho: National AIDS Commission.

NAC. 2011. *Report on the national response to HIV and AIDS, reporting period 2006-2010.* Maseru, Lesotho: National AIDS Commission.

NAC. 2012. *Country progress report: Lesotho January 2010-December 2011.* Maseru, Lesotho: National AIDS Commission.

Nagelkerke, Nico J., Stephen Moses, Sake J. de Vlas, and Robert C. Bailey. 2007. "Modelling the public health impact of male circumcision for HIV prevention in high prevalence areas in Africa." *BMC Infectious Diseases* 7:16.

Nastasi, Bonnie K., and Marlene Berg, J. 1999. "Using ethnography to strengthen and evaluate intervention programs." In *Using ethnographic data: Interventions, public programming, and public policy*, edited by Jean J. Schensul, Margaret D. LeCompte, G. Alfred Hess, Bonnie K. Nastasi, Marlene J. Berg, Lynne Williamson, Jeremy Breecher and Ruth Glasser, 1-56. Walnut Creek, CA: AltaMira.

Nattrass, Nicoli. 2007. *Mortal combat: AIDS denialsim and the struggle for antiretrovirals in South Africa*. Scottsville, South Africa: University of KwaZulu-Natal Press.

Nelkin, Dorothy. 1991. "AIDS and the news media." *The Milbank Quarterly* 69 (2):293-307.

Netter, Thomas W. 1992. "The media and AIDS: A global perspective." In *AIDS prevention through education: A world view*, edited by Jamie Sepulveda, Harvey Fineberg and Jonathan Mann, 241-253. New York, NY: Oxford University Press.

New Nation News. 1991 June 28-July 4. Johannesburg, South Africa.

Ngugi, Elizabeth N., David Wilson, Jennifer Sebstad, Francis A. Plummer, and Stephen Moses. 1996. "Focused peer-mediated educational programs among female sex workers to reduce sexually transmitted disease and Human Immunodeficiency Virus transmission in Kenya and Zimbabwe." *Journal of Infectious Diseases* 174 (Suppl 2):S240-S247.

Nichter, Mark, and Mimi Nichter. 1996. "Modern methods of fertility regulation: When and for whom are they appropriate?" In *Anthropology and international health*, edited by Mark Nichter and Mimi Nichter. Amsterdam, The Netherlands: Gordon and Breach.

Niehaus, Isak, and G. Jonsson. 2005. "Dr. Wouter Basson, Americans, and wild beasts: Men's conspiracy theories of HIV/AIDS in South African lowveld." *Medical Anthropology Quarterly* 24 (2):179-208.

Njeuhmeli, Emmanuel, Steven Forsythe, Jason Reed, Marjorie Opuni, Lori Bollinger, Nathan Heard, Delivette Castor, John Stover, Timothy Farley, Veena Menon, and Catherine Hankins. 2011. "Voluntary medical male circumcision: Modeling the impact and cost of expanding male circumcision for HIV prevention in eastern and southern Africa." *PLoS Medicine* 8 (e1001132).

Noar, Seth M. 2008. "Behavioral interventions to reduce HIV-related sexual risk behavior: Review and synthesis of meta-analytic evidence." *AIDS and Behavior* 12 (3):335-353.

Noar, Seth M. 2006. "A 10-year retrospective of research in health mass media campaigns: Where do we go from here?" *Journal of Health Communication* 11 (1):21-42.

Nolen, Stephanie. 2008. *28: Stories of AIDS in Africa*. Toronto, Canada: Random House Digital.

Nunnally, Jum C., and Ira H. Bernstein. 1978. *Psychometric theory*. 2nd ed. New York, NY: McGraw-Hill.

Nutbeam, Don. 2000. "Health literacy as a public health goal: A challenge for contemporary health education and communication strategies into the 21st century." *Health Promotion International* 15 (3):259-267.

Nyaka, Libuseng. 2009b. "Youth join the fight against HIV/AIDS." *Public Eye*, 20 February, 2.

Nyaka, Libuseng. 2009a. "Gender and HIV." *Public Eye*, 6 March, 3-4.

Nyanzi, S. R. Pool, and J. Kinsman. 2001. "The negotiation of sexual relationships among school pupils in south-western Uganda." *AIDS Care* 13 (1):83-98.

Obidoa, Chinekwu Azuka. 2010. "The impact of social change on adolescent sexual behavior in Nigeria." PhD, Public Health, University of Connecticut.

O'Connor, A. 1991. "Lifting quarantine/Cuba relaxes policy of strict segregation of AIDS carriers." *Houston Chronicle*, August 18, 16.

Ogundare, D. 1998. "Evaluation of a workplace pilot behavioral intervention project among dock workers in the two sea ports in Lagos, Nigeria." 12th International Conference on AIDS, Geneva.

Olayinka, B. A., L. Alexander, M. T. Mbizvo, and L. Gibney. 2000. "Generational differences in male sexuality that may affect Zimbabwean women's risk for sexually transmitted disease and HIV/AIDS." *East African Medical Journal* 77 (2):93-97.

OneLove. 2008. *Multiple and concurrent sexual partnerships in southern Africa: A ten country research report*. Pretoria, South Africa: OneLove.

Packard, Randall M., and Paul Epstein. 1991. "Epidemiologists, social scientists, and the structure of medical research on AIDS in Africa." *Social Science & Medicine* 33 (7):771-794.

Paige, Karen Ericksen, and Jeffery M. Paige. 1981. *The politics of reproductive ritual*. Berkeley, CA: University of California Press.

Pal, Mahuya, and Mohan J. Dutta. 2008a. "Public relations in a global context: The relevance of critical modernism as a theoretical lens." *Journal of Public Relations Research* 20:159-179.

Pal, Mahuya, and Mohan J. Dutta. 2008b. "Theorizing resistance in a global context: Processes, strategies and tactics in communication scholarship." *Communication Yearbook* 32:41-87.

Papa, Michael J., Arvind Singhal, Sweety Law, Saumya Pant, Suruchi Sood, Everett M. Rogers, and Corinne Shefner-Rogers. 2000. "Entertainment-education and social change: An analysis of parasocial interaction, social learning, collective efficacy, and paradoxical communication." *Journal of Communication* 50 (4):31-55.

Parker, Richard. 2001. "Sexuality, culture and power in HIV/AIDS research." *Annual Review of Anthropology* 30:163-179.

Parker, Ruth M., David W. Baker, Mark V. Williams, and Joanne R. Nurss. 1995. "The test of functional health literacy in adults: A new instrument for measuring patients' literacy skills." *Journal of General Internal Medicine* 10 (10):537-541.

Parker, Warren, Benjamin Makhubele, Pumla Ntlabati, and Cathy Connolly. 2007. *Concurrent sexual partnerships amongst young adults in South Africa: Challenges for HIV prevention*. Glencoe, IL: Free Press.

Parsons, Talcott. 1951. *The social system*. New York: Free Press.

Passmore, John. 1972. *The perfectibility of man*. London, UK: Gerald Duckworth and Co.

Patterson, Bruce K., Alan Landay, Joan N. Siegel, Zareefa Flener, Dennis Pessis, Antonio Chaviano, and Robert C. Bailey. 2002. "Susceptibility to human immunodeficiency virus -1 infection of human foreskin and cervical tissue in explant culture." *American Journal of Pathology* 16:867-873.

Patton, Cindy. 1990. *Inventing AIDS*. New York, NY: Routledge.

Patton, Cindy. 1996. *Fatal advice: How safe-sex education went wrong*. Durham, NC: Duke University Press.

Paul, Benjamin D., ed. 1955. *Health, culture and community: Case studies of public reactions to health programs*. New York, NY: Russel Sage Foundations.

Pearce, Lisa. 2002. "Integrating survey and ethnographic methods for systematic anomalous case analysis." *Sociological Methodology* 32:103-132.

Pearsons, David N. 1990. *Teaching them unto your children: Contextualization of Basanga puberty rites in the United Methodist Church*. Ann Arbor, MI: University of Michigan Press.

Pelto, Pertti J., and Gretel H. Pelto. 1997. "Studying knowledge, culture, and behavior in applied medical anthropology." *Medical Anthropology Quarterly* 11 (2):147-163.

PEPFAR. 2010. *Fiscal Year 2009: PEPFAR Operational Plan*. Washington, D.C.: The U.S. President's Emergency Plan for AIDS Relief. Available at www.pepfar.gov/documents/organization/124050.pdf

Pepin, Jacques. 2011. *The origins of AIDS*. Cambridge, UK: Cambridge University Press.

Peters, Pauline E., Daimon Kambewa, and Peter A. Walker. 2010. "Contestations over 'tradition' and 'culture' in a time of AIDS." *Medical Anthropology* 29 (3):278-302.

Peterson, Robert A. 2001. "On the use of college students in social science research: Insights from a second-order meta-analysis." *Journal of Consumer Research* 28:450-461.

Petros, George, Collins O. Airhihenbuwa, and Leickness Simbayi. 2006. "HIV/AIDS and 'othering' in South Africa: The blame goes on." *Culture, Health & Sexuality* 8 (1):67-77.

Petryna, Adriana. 2002. *Life exposed: Biological citizens after chernobyl*. Princeton, NJ: Princeton University Press.

Pfeiffer, James. 2004. "Condom social marketing, pentecostalism, and structural adjustment in Mozambique: A clash of AIDS prevention messages." *Medical Anthropology Quarterly* 18 (1):77-103.

Phiri, Isabel A. 1998. "The initiation of Chewa women in Malawi. A Presbyterian women's perspective." In *Rites of passage in contemporary Africa*, edited by J. L. Cox, 129-146. Cardiff, UK: Cardiff Academic Press.

Pigg, Stacy Leigh. 1996. "The credible and the credulous: The question of 'villagers' beliefs' in Nepal." *Cultural Anthropology* 11 (2):160-201.

Pigg, Stacy Leigh. 2001. "Languages of sex and AIDS in Nepal: Notes on the social production of commensurability." *Cultural Anthropology* 16 (4):481-541.

Pigg, Stacy Leigh. 2005. "Globalizing the facts of life." In *Sex in development: Science, sexuality and morality in global perspective*, edited by Vincanne Adams and Stacy Pigg. Durham, NC: Duke University Press.

Pinto, Alvaro Vieira. 1960. *Consciencia e Realidade Nacional*. Vol. 2. Rio de Janeiro, Brazil: Textos Brasileiros de Filosofia.

Piotrow, Phyllis T., D. Lawrence Kincaid, Jose G. Rimen II, and Ward Rinehart. 1997. *Health communication: Lessons from family planning and reproductive health*. Westport, CT: Praeger.

Plummer, Francis A., Stephen Moses, and Jackoniah O. Ndinya-Achola. 1991. "Factors affecting female-to-male transmission of HIV-1: Implications of transmission dynamics for prevention." In *AIDS and women's reproductive health*, edited by Lincoln C. Chen, Jaime Sepulveda Amor and Sheldon Jerome Segal. New York, NY: Plenum.

PlusNews. 2011. HIV/AIDS: Clinton sets out new US focus. 14 November.

Poku, Nana K., and Alan Whiteside, eds. 2004. *The political economy of AIDS in Africa*. Burlington, VT: Ashgate.

Polgar, Steven. 1963. *Health action in cross-cultural perspective*. In *Handbook of medical sociolog*, edited by H. Freeman, S. Levine and L. Reeder, Englewood Cliffs, NJ: Prentice Hall.

Porter, Theodore. 1995. *Trust in numbers: The pursuit of objectivity in science and public life*. Princeton, NJ: Princeton University Press.

Posel, Deborah. 2004. "Sex, death and embodiment: Reflections on the stigma of AIDS in Agincourt, South Africa." Life and death in a time of AIDS: The southern African experience, Witwatersrand Institute for Social and Economic Research, Johannesburg, October 14-16.

Posel, Deborah. 2005. "Sex, death and the fate of the nation: Reflections on the politicisation of sexuality in post-apartheid South Africa." *Africa* 75 (2):125-153.

Power, J. Gerard. 1996. "Evaluating health knowledge: An alternative approach." *Journal of Health Communication* 1 (3):285-300.

Prater, Mary Anne, and Loretta A. Serna. 1993. "Teaching about HIV/AIDS and abuse: Special educators' perspectives." *Teacher Education and Practice* 8 (2):65-73.

Prejean, Jospeh, Ruiguang Song, Angela Hernandez, Rebecca Ziebell, Timothy Green, Frances Walker, Lillian S. Lin, Qian An, Jonathan Mermin, Amy Lansky, and H. Irene Hall. 2011. "Estimated HIV incidence in the United States, 2006-2009." *PLoS One* 6 (8):e17502.

Princeton Survey Research Associates. 1996. "Covering the epidemic: AIDS in the news media, 1985-1996." *Columbia Journalism Review* 35 (Special supplement):1-12.

PSI. 2008. *Research report: Concurrent heterosexual partnerships, HIV risk, and related determinants among the general population of Zimbabwe*. Washington, DC: Population Services International.

PSI Research & Metrics. 2010. *HIV/AIDS TRaC study examining consistent condom use and VCT uptake among men and women age 15-35 in Lesotho.* Washington, DC: Population Services International. Available at: www.psi.org/resources/publications

Quinn, Thomas C., Maria J. Wawer, Nelson Sewankambo, David Serwadda, Chaunjun Li, Fred Wabwire-Mangen, Mary O. Meehan, Thomas Lutalo, and Ronald H. Gray. 2000. "Viral load and heterosexual transmission of human immunodeficiency virus type 1: Rakai Project Study Group." *New England Journal of Medicine* 342:921-929.

Rabinow, Paul. 1992. "Articificiality and enlightenment: From sociobiology to biosociality." In *Incorporations*, Vol. 6, edited by Jonathan Crary and Sanford Kwinter, 234-252. New York: Zone Books.

Rakelmann, Georgia A. 2001. "'We sat there half the day asking questions, but they were unable to tell where AIDS comes from...': Local interpretations of AIDS in Botswana." *Afrika Spectrum* 36 (1):35-52.

Rakelmann, Georgia A. 2014. *Grabbed and buried: Social and cultural figures of the HIV/AIDS epidemic in Botswana.* Berlin, Germany: LIT Verlag.

Ramjee, Gita, Roshini Govinden, Neetha S. Morar, and Anthony Mbewu. 2007. "South Africa's experience of the closure of the cellulosc sulphate microbicide trial." *PLoS Medicine* 4 (7):e235.

Rasing, Thera. 1995. *Passing on the rites of passage: Girls' initiation rites in the context of an urban Roman Catholic Community.* London, UK: Avebury & Africa Studies Centre.

Rasing, Thera. 1999. "Globalization and the making of consumers: Zambian kitchen parties." In *Modernity on a shoestring: Dimensions of globalization, consumption and development in Africa and beyond*, edited by Ricard Fardon, Wim M. J. van Binsbergen and Rijk van Dijk, 227-247. Leiden, The Netherlands: EIDOS.

Rasing, Thera. 2001. *The bush burnt, the stones remain: Female initiation rites in urban Zambia.* African Studies Center, Leiden, The Netherlands: LIT Verlag.

Ray, Elieen Berlin, ed. 1996. *Communication and disenfranchisement: Social health issues and implications.* Mahwah, NJ: Lawrence Erlbaum Associates.

Rector, Robert. 2002. *The effectiveness of abstinence education programs in reducing sexual activity among youth.* Washington, DC: Heritage Foundation.

Reid, Allecia E., John F. Dovidio, Estrellita Ballester, and Blair T. Johnson. 2014. "HIV prevention interventions to reduce sexual risk for African Americans: The influence of community-level stigma and psychological processes." *Social Science & Medicine* 103:118-125.

Reid, Roddey. 1997. "Healthy families, healthy citizens: The politics of speech and knowledge in the California anti-secondhand smoke media campaign." *Science as Culture* 6 (4):541-581.

Reid, Roddey. 2004. "Tensions within California tobacco control in the 1990s: Health movements, state initiatives, and community mobilization." *Science as Culture* 29:541-581.

Remafedi, Gary. 1993. "The impact of training on school professionals' knowledge, beliefs, and behaviors regarding HIV/AIDS and adolescent homosexuality." *Journal of School Health* 63 (3):153-157.

Resnick, Michael D., Peter S. Bearman, Robert W. Blum, Karl E. Bauman, Kathleen M. Harris, Jo Jones, Joyce Tabor, Trish Beuhring, Renee E. Sieving, Marcia Shew, Marjorie Ireland, Linda H. Bearinger, and J. Ricard Udry. 1997. "Protecting adolescents from harm: Findings from the national longitudinal study on adolescent health." *Journal of American Medical Association* 278 (10):823-832.

Resnicow, K., R. L. Braithwaite, C. Dilorio, and K. Glanz. 2002. "Applying theory to culturally diverse and unique populations." In *Health behavior and health education: Theory, research, and practice (3rd Ed)*, edited by Karen Glanz, Barbara K. Rimer and Frances M. Lewis, 485-509. San Francisco, CA: Jossy-Bass.

Reynolds, Steven J., Mary E. Shepherd, Arun R. Risbud, Raman R. Gangakhedkar, Ronald S. Brookmeyer, Anand D. Divekar, Sanjay M. Mehendale, and Robert C. Bollinger. 2004. "Male circumcision and risk of HIV-1 and other sexually transmitted infections in India." *Lancet* 363:1039-1040.

Rhodes, Tim. 1997. "Risk theory in epidemic times: Sex, drugs and the social organisation of 'risk behaviour.'" *Sociology of Health and Illness* 19 (2):208-227.

Richards, Audrey I. 1982. *Chisungu: A girl's initiation ceremony among the Bemba of Zambia*. London, UK: Tavistock Publications Ltd, Faber & Faber.

Richens, John, John Imrie, and Andrew Copas. 2000. "Condoms and seat belts: The parallels and the lessons." *Lancet* 355 (9201):400-403.

Rimal, Rajiv, D. Johnson, and June Flora. 1997. *International HIV/AIDS public service announcements: An assessment of behavior and social content.* Unpublished manuscript.

Robins, Steven. 2009. *Mobilising and mediating global medicine and health citizenship: The politics of AIDS knowledge production in rural South Africa.* IDS Working Paper 324. Brighton, UK: Institute of Development Studies.

Robins, Steven. 2010. *From revolution to rights in South Africa: Social movements, NGOs, and popular politics after apartheid.* Durban, South Africa: University of Kwa-Zulu Natal Press.

Rödlach, Alexander. 2006. *Witches, westerners, and HIV: AIDS & cultures of blame in Africa.* Walnut Creek, CA: Left Coast Press, Inc.

Rödlach, Alexander. 2011. "'AIDS is in the food': Zimbabweans' association between nutrition and HIV/AIDS and their potential for addressing food insecurity and HIV/AIDS." *Annals of Anthropological Practice* 35 (1):219-237.

Rodriguez, Monica R., Rebecca Young, Stacie Renfro, Marysol Asencio, and Debra W. Haffner. 1995. Teaching our teachers to teach: A SIECUS study on training and preparation for HIV/AIDS prevention and sexuality education. *SIECUS Report 28, no. 2.* http://www.ascd.org/publications/educational-leadership/oct00/vol58/num02/Working-Together-for-a-Sexually-Healthy-America.aspx

Rogers, Everett M., James W. Dearing, and Soonbum Chang. 1991. "AIDS in the 1980s: The agenda-setting process for a public issue." *Journalism Monographs* 126.

Rogge, Mary Madeline, Marti Greenwald, and Amelia Golden. 2004. "Obesity, stigma, and civilized oppression." *Advances in Nursing Science* 27 (4):301-315.

Romero-Daza, Nancy. 1994a. "Migrant labor, multiple sexual partners, and sexually transmitted diseases: The makings for an AIDS epidemic in rural Lesotho." Doctoral dissertation, State University of New York at Buffalo.

Romero-Daza, Nancy. 1994b. "Multiple sexual partners, migrant labor, and the makings for an epidemic: Knowledge and beliefs about AIDS among women in highland Lesotho." *Human Organization* 53 (2):192-205.

Romney, A. Kimball, Tom Smith, Howard E. Freeman, Jerome Kagan, and Robert E. Klein. 1979. "Concepts of success and failure." *Social Science Research* 8:302-326.

Rompel, Matthias. 2001. "Media reception and public discourse on the AIDS epidemic in Namibia." *Afrika Spectrum* 36 (1):91-96.

Rose, Nickolas. 1999. *Powers of freedom: Reframing political thought.* Cambridge: Cambridge University Press.

Rose, Nikolas. 2007. *The politics of life itself: Biomedicine, power, and subjectivity in the twenty-first century.* Princeton, NJ: Princeton University Press.

Ross, Michael W., E. James Essien, and Isabel Torres. 2006. "Conspiracy beliefs about the origin of HIV/AIDS in four racial/ethnic groups." *Journal of Acquired Immune Deficiency Syndromes* 41 (3):342-344.

Ryan, Gery W., and H. Russell Bernard. 2000. "Data management and analysis methods." In *Handbook of qualitative research*, edited by Norma K. Denzin and Yvonna S. Lincoln, 769-800. Thousand Oaks, CA: Sage.

Sabatier, Renee. 1988. *Blaming others: Prejudice, race and worldwide AIDS.* Philadelphia, PA: New Society Publishers.

Sachs, Jeffrey. 2005. *The end of poverty: Economic possibilities for our time.* New York, NY: Penguin.

Saethre, Eirik, and Jonathan Stadler. 2009. "A tale of two 'cultures': HIV risk narratives in South Africa." *Medical Anthropology* 28 (3):268-284.

SAMP. 2010. Lesotho migration to South Africa: Facts and figures. Pretoria, South Africa: Southern African Migration Programme

Sampson, Robert J., Stephen W. Raudenbush, and Felton Earls. 1997. "Neighborhoods and violent crime: A multilevel study of collective efficacy." *Science* 277 (5328):918-924.

Sangaramoorthy, Thurka. 2012. "Treating the numbers: HIV/AIDS surveillance, subjectivity, and risk." *Medical Anthropology* 31 (4):292-309.

Sangaramoorthy, Thurka. 2014. *Treating AIDS: Politics of difference, paradox of prevention.* New Brunswick, NJ: Rutgers University Press.

Sangaramoorthy, Thurka, and Adia Benton. 2012. "Enumeration, identity, and health." *Medical Anthropology* 31 (4):287-291.

Sanson-Fisher, Robert William, Billie Bonevski, Lawrence W. Green, and Cate D'Este. 2007. "Limitations of the randomized control trial in evaluating population-based health interventions." *American Journal of Preventive Medicine* 33 (2):155-161.

Sapa. 2000. "I froze blood that had HIV." *Sowetan*, 25 May.

Sartre, Jean Paul. 1947. *Situations 1*. Paris, France: Librairie Gallimard.

Scalway, Thomas. 2003. *Missing the message? 20 years of learning from HIV/AIDS*. London, UK: Panos Institute.

Schneider, Helen. 2002. "On the fault line: The politics of AIDS policy in contemporary South Africa." *African Studies* 61 (1):145-169.

Schoepf, Brooke G. 1996. "Health, gender relations and poverty in the AIDS era." In *Courtyards, markets and city streets: Urban women in Africa*, edited by Kathleen Sheldon, 153-168. Boulder, CO: Westview.

Schoepf, Brooke G. 1997. "AIDS, gender and sexuality during Africa's economic crisis." In *African feminism: The politics of survival in sub-Saharan Africa*, edited by Gwendolyn Mikell, 310-332. Philadelphia, PA: University of Pennsylvania Press.

Schoepf, Brooke G. 1993. "Anthropologists, AIDS prevention and research ethics in Africa." Annual meeting of the American Anthropological Association, Washington, DC, November.

Schutz, Alfred. 1964. "'The well-informed citizen': An essay on the social distribution of knowledge." In *Alfred Schutz, collected papers, volume 2, studies in social theory*, edited by Arvid Brodersen, 120-134. The Hague, The Netherlands: Martinus Nijhoff.

Scorgie, Fiona. 2002. "Virginity testing and the politics of sexual responsibility: Implications for AIDS intervention." *African Studies* 61 (1):55-77.

Scott-Sheldon, Lori A., Tania B. Huedo-Medina, Michelle R. Warren, Blair T. Johnson, and Michael P. Carey. 2011. "Efficacy of behavioral interventions to increase condom use and reduce sexually transmitted infections: A meta-analysis, 1991 to 2010." *Journal of Acquired Immune Deficiency Syndromes* 58 (5):489-498.

Seidel, Gill. 1993. "The competing discourses of HIV/AIDS in sub-Saharan Africa: Discourses of rights and empowerment vs. discourses of control and exclusion." *Social Science & Medicine* 36 (3):175-194.

Seiter, John S., Harry Jr. Weger, Mandy L. Merrill, Mark R. McKenna, and Matthew L. Sanders. 2010. "Nonsmokers' perceptions of cigarette smokers' credibility, likeability, attractiveness, considerateness, cleanliness, and healthiness." *Communication Research Reports* 27 (2):143-158.

Semetko, H., and E. Goldberg. 1993. "Reporting AIDS in the US and Britain." In *Media and public policy*, edited by Robert Spitzer, 171-186. Westport, CT: Praeger.

Sepulveda, Jaime, Harvey Fineberg, and Jonathan Mann, eds. 1992. *AIDS prevention through education: A world view*. New York, NY: Oxford University Press.

Setel, Philip. 1999. *A plague of paradoxes. AIDS, culture, and demography in northern Tanzania*. Chicago, IL: University of Chicago Press.

Shapin, Steven. 1994. *A social history of truth: Civility and science in seventeenth-century England*. Chicago, IL: University of Chicago Press.

Shelton, James D., Daniel T. Halperin, Vinand Nantulya, Malcolm Potts, Helene D. Gayle, and King K. Holmes. 2004. "Partner reduction is crucial for balanced 'ABC' approach to HIV prevention." *British Medical Journal* 328 (7444):891-894.

Sherman, Judith B., and Mary T. Bassett. 1999. "Adolescents and AIDS prevention: A school-based approach in Zimbabwe." *Applied Psychology: An International Review* 48 (2):109-124.

Shilts, Randy. 1987. *And the band played on: Politics, people, and the AIDS epidemic*. New York, NY: St. Martin's Press.

Shoemaker, Pamela J., and Stephen D. Reese. 1996. *Mediating the message: Theories of influences of mass media content*. 2nd ed. White Plains, NY: Longman Publishing.

Shorter, Aylward. 1991. *The church in the African city*. London, UK: Geoffrey Chapman.

Shripak, Danielle, and Liane Summerfield. 1996. HIV/AIDS education in teacher preparation programs. In *ERIC digest*. Washington, DC: ERIC Clearinghouse on Teaching and Teacher Education.

Sidibé, Michel. 2009. Mobilizing prevention as a movement for universal access. Geneva: UNAIDS, Programme Coordinating Board.

Siegfried, N., M. Muller, J. Deeks, J. Volmink, M. Egger, N. Low, S. Walker, and P. Williamson. 2005. "HIV and male circumcision: A systematic review with assessment of the quality of studies." *Lancet Infectious Diseases* 5:165-173.

Silin, Jonathan G. 1995. *Sex, death, and the education of young children*. New York, NY: Teachers College Press.

Singer, Merrill. 1994. "The Politics of AIDS: Introduction." *Social Science and Medicine* 38 (10):1321-1324.

Singer, Merrill, Scott Clair, Monica Malta, Francisco I. Bastos, Neilane Bertoni, and Claudia Santelices. 2011. "Doubts remain, risks persist: HIV prevention knowledge and HIV testing among drug users in Rio de Janeiro, Brazil." *Substance Use & Misuse* 46 (4):511-522.

Singh, Jerome A., and Edward J. Mills. 2005. "The abandoned trials of pre-exposure prophylaxis for HIV: What went wrong?" *PLoS Medicine* 2 (9):e234.

Singhal, Arvind, and Everett Rogers. 1999. *Entertainment-education: A communication strategy for social change*. Mahwah, NJ: Lawrence Erlbaum Associates.

Singhal, Arvind, and Everett Rogers. 2001. "The entertainment-education strategy in communication campaigns." In *Public communication campaigns*, edited by Ronald E. Rice and Charles K. Atkin, 343-356. Thousand Oaks, CA: Sage.

Singhal, Arvind, and Everett Rogers. 2002. "A theoretical agenda for entertainment-education." *Communication Theory* 12:117-135.

Singhal, Arvind, and Everett Rogers. 2003. *Combating AIDS: Communication strategies in action*. London, UK: Sage.

Singhal, Arvind, Michael Cody, Everett Rogers, and Miguel Sabido, eds. 2004. *Entertainment-education and social change: History, research, and practice*. Mahwah, NJ: Lawrence Erlbaum Associates.

Singizi, Tsitsi. 2011. Peer leaders take the initiative on HIV prevention among young people in Lesotho. Accessed 5 May, 2011. www.unicef.org/aids/lesotho_59656.html

Sitholi, J. 2001. Cultural approaches to AIDS in Africa. *African online services*. Accessed 1 December, 2009. www.aegis.com/news/afrol/2001/AO010306.html

Skerritt, Andrew J. 2011. *Ashamed to die: Silence, denial, and the AIDS epidemic in the South*. Chicago, IL: Lawrence Hill Books.

Smith, Daniel J. 2003. "Imagining HIV/AIDS: Morality and perceptions of personal risk in Nigeria." *Medical Anthropology* 22 (4):343-372.

Smith, Linda Tuhiwai. 1999. *Decolonizing methodologies: Research and indigenous peoples*. London, UK: Zed Books.

Soloski, John. 1989. "News and professionalism: Some constraints on the reporting of news." *Media, Culture and Society* 11:207-228.

Sontag, Susan. 1979. *Illness as metaphor*. New York, NY: Vintage.

Sontag, Susan. 1988. *AIDS and its metaphors*. New York, NY: Farrar, Straus & Giroux.

South African Truth and Reconciliation Commission. 1998. Chemical and Biological Warfare Hearings, 8 June to 31 July. Accessed 9 March, 2010. www.doj.gov.za/trc

Spradley, James P. 1979. *The ethnographic interview*. New York, NY: Holt, Rinehart & Winston.

Stadler, Johnathan. 2003a. "Rumour, gossip and blame: Implications for HIV/AIDS prevention in the South African lowveld." *AIDS Education and Prevention* 15 (4):357-368.

Stadler, Johnathan. 2003b. "The young, the rich, and the beautiful: Secrecy, suspicion and discourses of AIDS in the South African lowveld." *African Journal of AIDS Research* 2:127-139.

Staff reporter. 2003. "Culture undermines prevention efforts in Lesotho." *Public Eye*, 26 September, 10.

Staff reporter. 2011. "Lesotho's HIV prevalence rate falls." *Lesotho Times*, 24 February. www.lestimes.com/?p=5496

Steinberg, Jonny. 2011. *Three-letter plague*. New York, NY: Random House.

Stephens, Christine, and Mary Breheny. 2008. "Menopause and the virtuous woman: The importance of the moral order in accounting for medical decision making." *Health (London)* 12 (1):7-24.

Stephenson, Joan. 2001. "20 years after AIDS emerges, HIV's complexities still loom large." *Journal of the American Medical Association* 285:1279-1282.

Storey, Douglas, Yagya Karki, Karen Heckert, and Marsha McCoskrie. 1996. Nepal Family Planning Communication Survey, 1994: Key Findings Report. Kathmandu, Nepal: National Health Education, Information, and Communication Center, Department of Health Services, Ministry of Nepal.

Storey, Douglas, Marc Boulay, Yagya Karchi, Karen Heckert, and Dibya Man Karmacharya. 1999. "Impact of the integrated radio communication project in Nepal: 1994-1997." *Journal of Health Communication* 4:271-294.

Strathern, Marilyn, ed. 2000. *Audit cultures: Anthropological studies in accountability, ethics, and the academy.* London, UK: Routledge.

Sue, Derald W., and David Sue. 1999. *Counseling the culturally different: Theory and practice.* 3rd ed. New York, NY: Wiley.

Swidler, Ann, and Susan Cotts Watkins. 2007. "Ties of dependence: AIDS and transactional sex in rural Malawi." *Studies in Family Planning* 38 (3):147-162.

Sznitman, Sharon R., Jennifer Horner, Laura F Salazar, Daniel Romer, Peter A.Vanable, Michael P. Carey, Ralph J. Diclemente, Robert F. Valois, and Bonita F. Stanton. 2009. "Condom failure: Examining the objective and cultural meanings expressed in interviews with African American adolescents." *Journal of Sex Research* 46 (4):309-318.

Tallis, Vicci. 2000. "Gendering the response to HIV/AIDS: Challenging gender inequality." *Agenda* 44:58-66.

Tamale, Sylvia. 2005. "Eroticism, sensuality and 'women's secrets' among the Baganda: A critical analysis." *Feminist Africa* 5:9-35.

Tanser, Frank, Till Bärnighausen, Lauren Hund, Geoffrey P. Garnett, Nuala McGrath, and Marie-Louise Newell. 2011. "Effect of concurrent sexual partnerships on rate of new HIV infections in a high-prevalence, rural South African population: A cohort study." *Lancet* 378 (9787):247-255.

Tarnoff, Curt, and Marian Leonardo Lawson. 2011. Foreign Aid: An introductory overview of US programs and policy. Washington, DC: Congressional Research Service, Library of Congress.

Tarnoff, Curt, and Larry Nowels. 2005. Foreign Aid: An introductory overview of US programs and policy. Washington, DC: Congressional Research Service, Library of Congress.

Tashakkori, Abbas, and Charles B. Teddlie. 2003. *Handbook of mixed methods in social and behavioral research.* Thousand Oaks, CA: Sage.

Tawfik, Linda, and Susan Cotts Watkins. 2007. "Sex in Geneva, sex in Lilongwe, and sex in Balaka." *Social Science & Medicine* 64 (5):1090-1101.

Taylor, Bridget M. 1995. "Gender-power relations and safer sex negotiation." *Journal of Advanced Nursing* 22 (4):687-693.

The Global Fund. 2008. Training traditional healers to refer suspected TB patients to the nearest clinic in Lesotho. Accessed 8 May, 2012. www.theglobalfund.org/en/savinglives/lesotho/tb1/

The Global Fund. 2009. Global Fund Round 2 Grant: Strengthening prevention and control of HIV/AIDS and TB in Lesotho, Final Report. Maseru, Lesotho: The Global Fund.

The Global Fund. 2010. Report of the Finance and Audit Committee regarding Office of the Inspector General matters. Twenty-First Board Meeting. Geneva, Switzerland: The Global Fund.

The Global Fund. 2011. Board Chair cover note: Audit and investigation reports issued by the Global Fund's Office of the Inspector General on 1 November 2011. Geneva, Switzerland: The Global Fund.

Thege, Britta. 2009. "Rural black women's agency within intimate partnerships amid the South African HIV epidemic." *African Journal of AIDS Research* 8 (4):455-464.

Thetela, Puleng Hanong. 2002. "Sex discourses and gender constructions in Southern Sotho: A case study of police interview of rape/sexual assault victims." *Southern African Linguistics and Applied Language Studies* 20:177-189.

Thomas, Anne G., Bonnie R. Tran, Marcus Cranston, Maleratro C. Brown, Rajiv Kumar, and Matsotetsi Tlelai. 2011. "Voluntary medical male circumcision: A cross-sectional study comparing circumcision self-report and physical examination findings in Lesotho." *PLoS One* 6 (11):e27561.

Thomas, Felicity. 2008. "Indigenous narratives of HIV/AIDS: Morality and blame in a time of change." *Medical Anthropology* 27 (3):227-256.

Thompson, Sandra C., Clem R. Boughton, and Gregory J. Dore. 2003. "Blood-borne viruses and their survival in the environment: Is public concern about community needlestick exposures justified?" *Australian and New Zealand Journal of Public Health* 27 (6):602-607.

Thornton, Robert. 2008. *Unimagined community: Sex, networks and AIDS in Uganda and South Africa*. Public Anthropology series. Berkeley, CA: University of California Press.

Tichenor, Phillip J., George A. Donohue, and Clarice N. Olien. 1970. "Mass media flow and differential growth in knowledge." *Public Opinion Quarterly* 34 (Summer):159-170.

Timberg, Craig, and Daniel Halperin. 2012. *Tinderbox: How the West sparked the AIDS epidemic and how the world can finally overcome it*. London, UK: Penguin Press.

Tomaselli, Keyan, Lauren Dyll, and Michael Francis. 2008. "'Self' and 'other': Auto-reflexive and indigenous ethnography." In *Handbook of critical and indigenous methodologies*, edited by Norma K Denzin, Yvonna S Lincoln and Linda Tuhiwai Smith, 347-372. Thousand Oaks, CA: Sage.

Traquina, Nelson. 1996. *Portuguese journalism and HIV/AIDS: A case study in news*. Association for Education in Journalism and Mass Communication, Anaheim, August.

Treichler, Paula A. 1991. "AIDS, Africa, and cultural theory." *Transitions* 51:86-103.

Treichler, Paula A. 1988. "AIDS, homophobia and biomedical discourse: An epidemic of signification." In *AIDS: Cultural analysis/cultural activism*, edited by Douglas Crimp, 31-70. Cambridge, UK: MIT Press.

Treichler, Paula A. 1999. *How to have theory in an epidemic: Cultural chronicles of AIDS*. Durham, NC: Duke University Press.

Trotter, Robert T., and James M. Potter. 1993. "Pile sorts, a cognitive anthropological model of drug and AIDS risk for Navajo teenagers: Assessment of a new evaluation tool." *Drugs & Society* 7 (3-4):23-39.

Tsing, Anna. 2005. *Friction: An ethnography of global connection*. Princeton, NJ: Princeton University Press.

Tun, Waimer, Scott Kellerman, Senkhu Maime, Zukiswa Fipaza, Meredith Sheehy, Lung Vu, and Dawie Nel. 2010. "Conspiracy beliefs about HIV, attitudes towards condoms and treatment and HIV-related preventive behaviors among men who have sex with men in Tshwane (Pretoria), South Africa." XVIII International AIDS Conference, Vienna.

Turner, Victor W. 1957. *Schism and continuity in an African society: A study of Ndembu village life*. Manchester, UK: Manchester University Press.

Turner, Victor W. 1969. *The ritual process*. New York, NY: Cornell University Press.

Ukpong, Morenike, and Kris Peterson. 2009. *Voices from the field: A series of reports on the oral Tenofovir trials from the perspectives of active community voices in Cambodia, Cameroon, Nigeria, Thailand and Malawi*. www.nhvmas-ng.org/publication/TDF2.pdf

Ulrey, Kelsy Lin, and Patricia Amason. 2001. "Intercultural communication between patients and health care providers: An exploration of intercultural communication effectiveness, cultural sensitivity, stress, and anxiety." *Health Communication* 13:449-463.

UNAIDS. 1999a. Communications framework for HIV/AIDS: A new direction. Geneva, Switzerland: Joint United Nations Programme on HIV/AIDS, A Penn State Project.

UNAIDS. 1999b. "Sexual behavior change for HIV: Where has theory taken us?" In *Best Practice Collection*. Geneva, Switzerland: Joint United Nations Programme on HIV/AIDS.

UNAIDS. 2000. "Collaboration with traditional healers in HIV/AIDS prevention and care in sub-Saharan Africa: A literature review." In *Best Practice Collection*. Geneva, Switzerland: Joint United Nations Programme on HIV/AIDS.

UNAIDS. 2005a. Intensifying HIV prevention: UNAIDS policy position paper. Geneva, Switzerland: Joint United Nations Programme on HIV/AIDS.

UNAIDS. 2005b. The 'Three Ones' in action: Where we are and where we go from here. Geneva, Switzerland: Joint United Nations Programme on HIV/AIDS.

UNAIDS. 2007. International experts review male circumcision. Accessed 8 January, 2014. www.unaids.org/en/resources/presscentre/featurestories/2007/march/20070307mcpt4/

UNAIDS. 2009a. Michel Sidibé calls for prevention revolution in opening address at UNAIDS' governing body meeting. Accessed 27 December, 2011.   www.unaids.org/en/resources/presscentre/featurestories/2009/december/20091208pcb/

UNAIDS. 2009b. Total Contributions 2009 [Donor contributions]. Geneva, Switzerland: Joint United Nations Programme on HIV/AIDS.

UNAIDS. 2010a. Getting to Zero, 2011-2015 Strategy. Geneva, Switzerland: Joint United Nations Programme on HIV/AIDS.

UNAIDS. 2010b. Global report: UNAIDS report on the global AIDS epidemic 2010. Geneva, Switzerland: WHO Library Cataloguing-in-Publication Data.

UNAIDS. 2010c. "Joint United Nations Programme on HIV/AIDS." Accessed 12 March, 2010. www.unaids.org/en/KnowledgeCentre/HIVData/default.asp

UNAIDS. 2012. Global report: UNAIDS report on the global AIDS epidemic 2012. Geneva, Switzerland: Joint United Nations Programme on HIV/AIDS.

UNAIDS. 2013. Global report: UNAIDS report on the global AIDS epidemic 2013. Geneva, Switzerland: Joint United Nations Programme on HIV/AIDS.

UNDP. 2011. Human Development Report 2011, Sustainability and Equity: A better future for all. Geneva, Switzerland: United Nations Development Program.

UNESC. 1995. Paper E/1995/71, May 19. Geneva, Switzerland: United Nations Economic and Social Council.

UNICEF. 2002. Young people and HIV/AIDS: Opportunity in Crisis. Geneva, Switzerland: The United Nations Children's Fund.

Upchurch, Dawn, Carol S. Aneshensel, Clea A. Sucoff, and Lene Levy-Storms. 1999. "Neighborhood and family contexts of adolescent sexual activity." *Journal of Marriage and the Family* 61:920-933.

USAID. 2007. Costing male circumcision in Lesotho and implications for the cost-effectiveness of circumcision as an HIV intervention. Washington, DC: United States Agency for International Development.

Valente, Thomas W. 1997. "On evaluating mass media's impact." *Studies in Family Planning* 28 (2):170-171.

Valente, Thomas W., and Walter P. Saba. 1998. "Mass media and interpersonal influences in a reproductive health communication campaign in Bolivia." *Communication Research* 25 (1):96-124.

Van Damme, Lut, Amy Corneli, Khatija Ahmed, Kawango Agot, Johan Lombaard, Saidi Kapiga, Mookho Malahleha, Fredrick Owino, Rachel. Manongi, Jacob Onyango, Lucky Temu, Modie Constance Monedi, Paul Mak'Oketch, Mankalimeng Makanda, Ilse Reblin, Shumani E. Makatu, Lisa Saylor, Haddie Kiernan, Stella Kirkendale, Christina Wong, Robert

Grant, Angela Kashuba, Kavita Nanda, Justin Mandala, Katrien Fransen, Jennifer Deese, Tania Crucitti, Timothy D. Mastro, and Douglas Taylor for the FEM-PrEP Study Group. 2012. "Preexposure prophylaxis for HIV infection among African women." *New England Journal of Medicine* 367 (5):411-422.

Van Damme, Lut, and Michael Szpir. 2012. "Current status of topical antiretroviral chemoprophylaxis." *Current Opinion in HIV and AIDS* 7 (6):520-525.

Van der Vliet, Virginia. 2001. "AIDS: Losing the "new struggle"?" *Daedalus* 130 (1):151-184.

Van Lettow, Monique, Wafaie Fawzi, and Richard Semba. 2003. "Triple trouble: The role of malnutrition in tuberculosis and human immunodeficiency virus co-infection." *Nutrition Reviews* 61 (3):81-90.

Vance, Carole S. 1991. "Anthropology rediscovers sexuality: A theoretical comment." *Social Science & Medicine* 33 (8):875-884.

Vandemoortele, Jan, and Enrique Delamonica. 2002. "The 'education vaccine' against HIV." *Current Issues in Comparative Education* 3 (1):6-13.

Vaughan, Peter W., Everett M. Rogers, Arvind Singhal, and Ramadhan M. Swalehe. 2000. "Entertainment-education and HIV/AIDS prevention: A field experiment in Tanzania." *Journal of Health Communication* 5 (Suppl):81-100.

Vaz, Rui Gama, Stephen Gloyd, and Ricardo Trindale. 1996. "The effects of peer education on STD and AIDS knowledge among prisoners in Mozambique." *International Journal of STD & AIDS* 7 (1):51-54.

Vincent, Louise. 2008a. "'Boys will be boys': Traditional Xhosa male circumcision, HIV and sexual socialisation in contemporary South Africa." *Culture, Health & Sexuality* 10 (5):431-446.

Vincent, Louise. 2008b. "Cutting tradition: The political regulation of traditional circumcision rites in South Africa's liberal democratic order." *Journal of Southern African Studies* 34 (1):77-91.

Visser, Maretha J., Johan B. Shoeman, and Jan J. Perold. 2004. "Evaluation of HIV/AIDS prevention in South African schools." *Journal of Health Psychology* 9 (2):263-280.

VOICE [MTN-003]. 2011. "Microbicide Trials Network." Accessed 28 November, 2011. www.mtnstopshiv.org/news/studies/mtn003

Wagner, Gunter. 1949. *The Bantu of North Kavirondo*. London, UK: International African Institute.

Wakefield, Melanie, Barbara Loken, and Robert Hornik. 2010. "Use of mass media campaigns to change health behaviour." *Lancet* 376 (9748):1261-71.

Walters, Lynne, and Timothy N. Walters. 1996. "Life on the edge of the precipice: Information subsidy and the rise of AIDS as a public issue, 1983-1989." Association for Education in Journalism and Mass Communication, Anaheim, August.

Wamai, Richard G., Brian J. Morris, Jake H. Waskett, Edward C. Green, Jyotirmoy Banerjee, Robert C. Bailey, Justin D. Klausner, David C. Sokal, and Catherine A. Hankins. 2012. "Criticisms of African trials fail to withstand scrutiny: Male circumcision does prevent HIV infection." *Journal of Law and Medicine* 20 (1):93-123.

Ward, Charles D., and Elliott McGinnies. 1974. "Persuasive effects of early and late mention of credible and noncredible sources." *Journal of Psychology* 86 (1):17-23.

Wardlow, Holly. 2008. "'You have to understand: Some of us are glad AIDS has arrived': Christianity and condoms among the Huli, Papua New Guinea." In *Making sense of AIDS: Culture, sexuality, and power in Melanesia*, edited by Leslie Butt and Richard Eves, 187-205. Honolulu, HI: University of Hawai'i Press.

Warwick, Donald P. 1983a. "The KAP survey: Dictates of mission versus demands of science." In *Social research in developing countries: Surveys and censuses in the third world*, edited by Martin Bulmer and Donald P. Warwick, 349-364. Chichester, UK: John Wiley & Sons.

Warwick, Donald P. 1983b. "On methodological integration in social research." In *Social research in developing countries: Surveys and censuses in the third world*, edited by Martin Blumer and Donald P. Warwick, 275-298. Chichester, UK: Wiley.

Watkins, Susan C. 2004. "Navigating the AIDS epidemic in rural Malawi." *Population and Development Review* 30:673-705.

Watney, Simon. 1991. "Discourses around HIV/AIDS." In *AIDS: Responses, interventions and care*, edited by Peter Aggleton, Peter Davies and, Graham Hart, 54-72. London, UK: Falmer Press.

Watts, L. 1993. "Coverage of polio and AIDS." *Ohio Journalism Monographs* 4.

Weed, Stan E. 1995. FACTS project year-end evaluation report, 1993-1994. Prepared for the US Office of Adolescent Pregnancy Programs. Kearns, UT: The Institute for Research and Evaluation.

Weed, Stan E. 2001. Title V education programs: Phase I interim evaluation report to Arkansas Department of Health. Salt Lake City, UT: The Institute for Research and Evaluation.

Weed, Stan E., Jerry Prigmore, and Raja Tanas. 2002. The Teen Aid Family Life education project: Fifth year evaluation report. Salt Lake City, UT: The Institute for Research and Evaluation.

Weed, Stan E., Joseph A. Olsen, Jacqueline DeGaston, and Jerry Prigmore. 1992. Predicting and changing teen sexual activity rates: A comparison of three Title XX programs. Prepared for Office of Adolescent Pregnancy Programs. Salt Lake City, UT: The Institute for Research and Evaluation.

Weeks, Jeffrey. 1999. "Myths and fictions in modern sexualities." In *A dangerous knowing: Sexuality, pedagogy and popular culture*, edited by Debbie Epstein and James T. Sears, 11-24. London, UK: Cassell.

Weiss, Helen A., Daniel Halperin, Robert C. Bailey, Richard J. Hayes, George Schmid, and Catherine A. Hankins. 2008. "Male circumcision for HIV prevention: From evidence to action?" *AIDS* 22 (5):567-574.

Weiss, Helen A,. Maria A. Quigley, and Richard J. Hayes. 2000. "Male circumcision and risk of HIV infection in sub-Saharan Africa: A systematic review and meta-analysis." *AIDS* 14 (15):2361-2370.

Weiss, Helen A., S. L. Thomas, S. K. Munabi, and Richard J. Hayes. 2006. "Male circumcision and risk of syphilis, chancroid, and genital herpes: A systematic review and meta-analysis." *Sexually Transmitted Infections* 82 (2):101-110.

Weller, Susan C., and A. Kimball Romney. 1988. *Systematic data collection*. Vol. 10, *Qualitative research methods*. Newbury Park, CA: Sage.

WHO. 1986. The Ottawa Charter for Health Promotion. Geneva, Switzerland: World Health Organization.

WHO. 2005. Summary Country Profile for HIV Treatment Scale-up: Lesotho. Geneva, Switzerland: World Health Organization.

WHO. 2006. Preventing HIV/AIDS in young people—A systematic review of evidence from developing countries, edited by David A. Ross, Bruce Dick and Jane Ferguson. Geneva, Switzerland: World Health Organization.

WHO. 2009a. Country Cooperative Strategy at a glance: Lesotho. Geneva, Switzerland: World Health Organization.

WHO. 2009b. Rapid advice: Antiretroviral therapy for HIV infection in adults and adolescents. Geneva, Switzerland: World Health Organization.

WHO/UNAIDS. 2004. "The 3 by 5 initiative." Geneva: World Health Organization and UNAIDS. Accessed 4 June, 2012. www.who.int/3by5/en/

Wierzbicki, Anthony S., Scott D. Purdon, Timothy C. Hardman, Ranjababu Kulasegaram, and Barry S. Peters. 2008. "HIV lipodystrophy and its metabolic consequences: Implications for clinical practice." *Current Medical Research and Opinion* 24 (3):609-624.

Williams, Brian G., James O. Lloyd-Smith, Eleanor Gouws, Catherine A. Hankins, Wayne M. Getz, John Hargrove, Isabelle de Zoysa, Christoper Dye, and Bertran Auvert. 2006. "The potential impact of male circumcision on HIV in sub-Saharan Africa." *PLoS Medicine* 3 (7):e262.

Wilson, Amanda, Billie Bonevski, Alison Jones, and David Henry. 2009. "Media reporting of health interventions: Signs of improvement, but major problems persist." *PLoS One* 4 (3):e4831.

Wilson, David. 2000. Peer group education guidelines, Volume 1. Harare, Zimbabwe: Department of Psychology, University of Zimbabwe.

Wingood, Gina M., and Ralph J. DiClemente. 1996. "HIV sexual risk reduction interventions for women: A review." *American Journal of Preventive Medicine* 12 (3):209-217.

Wolf, Angelika. 2007. Medical dialogue between traditional experts and biomedical health workers in Kasungu, Malawi. In *Medical Dialogue, HIV Practice Collection*. Eschborn, Germany: Deutsche Gesellschaft für Internationale Zusammenarbeit (GIZ).

Wolf, R. Cameron, Linda A. Tawfik, and Katherine C. Bond. 2000. "Peer promotion programs and social networks in Ghana: Methods for monitoring and evaluating AIDS prevention and reproductive health programs among adolescents and young adults." *Journal of Health Communication* 5 (Suppl):61-80.

Wood, Katherine, and Rachel Jewkes. 1997. "Violence, rape and sexual coercion: Everyday love in a South African township." *Gender & Development* 5 (2):41-46.

World Bank. 2000. Lesotho: The development impact of HIV/AIDS-selected issues and options. Unpublished report. Geneva, Switzerland: World Bank Macroeconomic Technical Group.

World Bank. 2010. Information and Communication Techonology (ICT) at a Glance Table: Lesotho. Geneva, Switzerland: World Bank.

Wreford, Jo Thobeka. 2008. *Working with spirit: Experiencing Izangoma healing in contemporary South Africa*. New York, NY: Berghan Books.

Youde, Jeremy R. 2007. *AIDS, South Africa, and the politics of knowledge*. Burlington, VT: Ashgate.

Young, James C., and Linda Y. Garro. 1982. "Variation in the choice of treatment in two Mexican communities." *Social Science & Medicine* 16 (16):1453-1465.

Zimmerman, Rick S., Seth M. Noar, Sonja Feist-Price, Olga Dekthar, Pamela K. Cupp, Eric Anderman, and Sharon Lock. 2007. "Longitudinal test of a multiple domain model of adolescent condom use." *Journal of Sex Research* 44 (4):380-394.

Note: Page numbers in Boldface type indicate illustrations; those followed by *n* indicate notes.

Nicola Bulled has a Ph.D. degree in anthropology from the University of Connecticut and a MPH degree from the Boston University School of Public Health. She has a growing track record in health-related publications and in health research among several populations in the United States, Lesotho, and South Africa. Prior to pursuing her doctoral degree, she worked in public health with state and city HIV prevention programs, including the Boston Needle Exchange. Originally from South Africa, Dr. Bulled has a keen interest in the region. She became acutely aware of the effects of global health communication when she worked in Lesotho in 2004 establishing an U.S.-funded HIV-testing clinic on a college campus. Her research was funded by the Fulbright Foundation.